The **Mystery Patient's**

GUIDE TO

Gaining & Retaining Patients

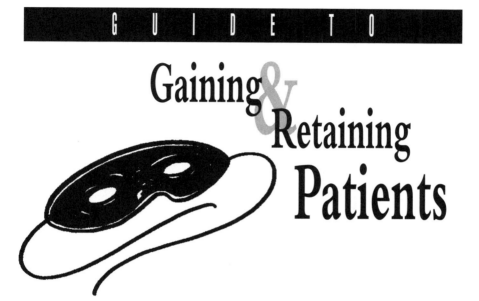

The Mystery Patient's

GUIDE TO

Gaining & Retaining Patients

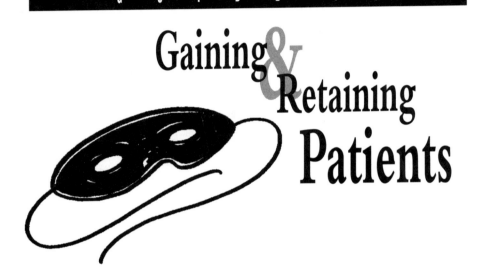

SUZANNE BOSWELL

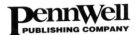
PennWell
PUBLISHING COMPANY

DENTAL ECONOMICS

PennWell Publishing Company
Tulsa, Oklahoma

Previously published by Suzanne Boswell:
Menswear: Suiting The Customer, Regents/Prentice Hall,
Englewood Cliffs, NJ, 1993

The author gratefully acknowledges the following for permission to use portions of
her articles which they previously published: *Dental Practice & Finance, Dental
TeamWork, Journal of the Massachusetts Dental Society, Journal of the California
Dental Society*

Oh, The Places You'll Go! by Dr. Seuss, copyright 1990 by Dr. Seuss Enterprises,
L.P., reprinted by permission of Random House, Inc.

References to the Social Style Model, Social Style Profile, and Social Style Concepts
are used with the permission of the TRACOM Corporation. Any use of the
copyrighted material without the expressed written permission of The TRACOM
Corporation is strictly prohibited.
Illustrations by Wanda Bedford

Copyright 1997 by
PennWell Publishing Company
1421 South Sheridan Road/P.O. Box 1260
Tulsa, OK 74101-1260

Boswell, Suzanne, 1947-
    The mystery patients guide to gaining & retaining patients / by Suzanne Boswell.
        p.   cm.
    Includes index.
    ISBN 0-87814-654-7
    1. Dental care–Marketing. 2. Dentist and patient. I. Title.
RK58.B557 1997
617′ .0068′8—dc21
DNLM/DLC
                                                                                        96-50954
                                                                                        CIP

Printed in the United States of America
1 2 3 4 5 01 00 99 98 97

DEDICATION

This book is dedicated to the patients who offered their opinions and preferences so openly in focus groups and to the exceptional dental teams who care and listen!

Contents

ACKNOWLEDGMENTS

It is not without a great deal of input and assistance that a book like this is created. I have many, many people to thank for their support, energy, ideas, and encouragement! There are two major groups from which the roots of the book sprouted: patient focus groups and audiences consisting of dental professionals. Without the hundreds of patients who so openly shared their perspectives, the book would not exist. The audiences of organized dentistry provided a key sounding board to understanding the issues and concerns of greatest import to them.

Once the outline of the book was established, there were numerous friends and colleagues who were very kind in providing invaluable insights, feedback, and ideas for implementation. Each person listed here contributed to this book and I express sincere words of appreciation to you all:

Fred Aurbach, DDS
Jan Balsiger, DDS, FAGD
Amy Baxter
Wanda Bedford
Norton Bicoll, DDS, MAGD
Alton Bishop, DDS
R.W. Buchert, DDS, Foundation of the Greater St. Louis
    Dental Society

Linda Byrd, T.H.E. Design
Steve Carstensen, DDS
Terry Daugherty, DDS
Harry Demaree, DDS
Terry Dickinson, DDS, FAGD
Hugh Doherty, DDS, CFP
Joey Fischer, Art Research Institute, Ltd.
Bob Frazer, DDS
Mark Friedman, DDS
Nathan Friedman, DDS, USC School of Dentistry
Ron Goldstein, DDS
Susan Hollar, DDS, FAGD
Gerry Kress, PhD, Baylor School of Dentistry
Joe Lancellotti, Camelot Professional Services
Paul Landman, DDS
Roger Levin, DDS
Tom McDougal, DDS
Sally McKenzie, CMC
Mitch Moore, DDS
Linda C. Niessen, DMD, Baylor School of Dentistry
Jim Pride, DDS
Risa Pollack-Simon, CDA
Charles Pugh, DDS
Jim Reisman, DDS, FAGD
Naomi Rhode, RDH, CPAE
Karen Cortell Reisman
Dave Roberts, DDS
Steve Schwartz, DDS
Alan Selbst, DMD
Debbie Seznik, DDS
Jeff Shapiro, DDS
Cherilyn G. Sheets, DDS
Jerry Stigall, The TRACOM Corporation
Jack A. Weichman, DDS, JD
Betsy Wheat
Robin Wright
Bob Zampieri, DDS
Edwin Zinman, DDS, JD

Colleen Gleason and Jim Bramson, DDS of the American Dental Association, for their support, interest, assistance, and friendship. My friends and contacts at the Dallas County Dental Society, Greater Houston Dental Society, and the Texas Dental Association.

There are other key individuals who significantly aided in bringing this book to fruition: Kirk Bjornsgaard of PennWell Books who was *always* there with prompt answers and support; I sincerely appreciate your guidance, patience, your wit and your way with words. Hands down, you've got the record for fastest e-mail responses in the Internet! A special thank you goes to "Dr. Review", who provided incisive commentary, support, and suggestions that helped to make this a better book. My assistant, Lou Jimmerson, for her unending support ; her enthusiasm and interest in what we do; her ability to tackle, overcome, and survive constant technology challenges; her skill with and love of the written word; and her unflagging good humor. Mary Rae Hoskins for her fortitude in transcribing the many muffled audiotapes dictated while I was in flight from one seminar to another. My husband, Herb, for understanding my strengths and my weaknesses and loving me anyway and for his support and belief in what I do, no matter how offbeat it may initially appear! Thank you all.

Foreword

BY TOM McDOUGAL, DDS

Within these pages, Suzanne Boswell offers the dental profession a vitally important perspective on how to ensure practice success. Her insight into dentistry stems from many sources. Her creative "Mystery Patient" visits to offices throughout the United States provide important feedback to help dental teams improve their practices. She gained further perspective on dental patients by conducting focus groups to uncover prevailing attitudes and preferences. Through hundreds of patient interviews, Suzanne has sought the "real" message from patients about their satisfaction vs. dissatisfaction in order to disseminate it to aware dental teams. In her informative and highly innovative seminars at major dental meetings from coast to coast she offers a revealing perspective on patient issues and attitudes.

She has gathered all of this valuable research and wisdom into a truly unique book. The reader will learn the "inside story" on patient views of the dental office and dental team. Our profession has not been privy to such insights before and the wise practitioner will recognize the opportunities offered by a thorough study of them.

For those who delight in reading the end of a novel first, take a look at the final chapter, "Top Tips from

Patient Focus Groups". Aside from providing a valuable checklist, this section will give you a hint of the topic breadth covered in this book. You'll see that understanding what this book teaches you can move your dental team in the direction of true caring, ultra service, and exceptional quality for your practice.

Suzanne's work is extremely timely in today's dental marketplace, in which practices are continually challenged by health care consumerism. As never before, the quality-oriented practitioner must use every strategy possible to insulate the practice from outside control, and by reading this book you'll learn patient-friendly ways to do so. The more a practice can fine-tune service to meet and exceed patient needs and desires, the more likely the practice will survive and prosper in these challenging times.

Staff attitudes, communication skills, office ambiance, trends affecting dentistry, staff and patient stability, importance of patient retention, patient perception of quality and service—all of these formidable challenges are addressed in this excellent text. Gaining an understanding and control of these factors is critical to differentiate a practice in the patient's mind.

I believe *The Mystery Patient's Guide to Gaining & Retaining Patients* also provides an excellent resource for the dentist to use in staff meetings. Each section and chapter can be used as the jumping-off point for team discussion and brainstorming. The principles presented in this book will provide dental teams an incentive to delight, not just please, each patient who enters their doors. *The Mystery Patient's Guide to Gaining & Retaining Patients* is required reading for all dentists and team members who aspire to be the "best of the best".

Introduction

The writing of this book has been a labor of love. The book has been writing itself in my mind for several years, although words had not been put on paper. I've always stopped myself with the thought, "I can't do it yet. There are still more questions to ask, more issues to talk about with patients, more offices to visit, and more surveys to conduct." But I finally realized that the journey will never be finished! Just as society changes so do the issues, so do the patients, and so do the practices! Better to send the message to dental teams now, to communicate the perspective of patients now. Future seminars, books and articles will update the ever-changing market.

THE PURPOSE

My goal is to remove the mask from your patients, to enable you to hear their comments and concerns. I hope that with this knowledge, you'll be better able to manage the challenges and related opportunities that present themselves daily. It is very easy in any profession to become so entrenched in one's own responsibilities and formidable tasks, that one may lose perspective—the "can't see the forest for the trees" syndrome.

It's a tough marketplace right now for the profession of dentistry. You're forced to manage issues unimagined 10 years ago, and these same issues may test your fortitude. The more you understand your patients, the more you investigate what your alternatives are, then the more manageable the situation can be. I do not mean to oversimplify today's conditions, just to offer another perspective, one which I believe will enable you to see new opportunities in your practice.

THE PERSPECTIVE

The viewpoint in this book is probably quite different from that of the typical reader. You probably come from the dental profession; however, your patients do not. They are not concerned about behind-the-scenes management of the dental practice unless it has a direct impact on them. They only are concerned about their relationships with the practice. How you develop and manage those relationships are the keys to gaining and retaining your patients. Patients do not see the practice from the inside looking out in the same way that a dental professional might. Through this book you will see your practice from the outside looking in... through objective eyes that are unbiased in the same way that your patients' eyes are.

Some readers might ask, "Well, you don't come from dentistry, you don't have a dental background. How can you possibly understand our problems?" I don't come from dentistry, and that's my strong point in bringing this information to you. I don't carry the baggage of thinking about the dental practice as an "insider." I see your offices in the same manner as your patients do. I recall a comment from an audience member on a seminar evaluation. It said, "How can you relate to our problems—

you've got to understand how difficult and challenging our jobs really are." That's exactly my point: your patients don't know this, and frankly they don't care! For the most part they're concerned about their own problems and are looking to you for solutions! Like it or not, it's a "buyer's market." The patient doesn't need to understand you, but it's vital to the life of your practice that you understand the patient.

If I were the reader of this book, I would want to know what qualifies the writer to present this information and this perspective to you. Before you read the book, I believe it is important to understand where I come from and how my background benefits you.

THE PAST

Since 1970 I have been involved in customer relations, communications, self-presentation, and impression management. When I say customer relations, I mean the front lines—managing all consumer relations phone calls and communications for an international menswear firm for over 13 years. At the same time I was a designer for this company and responsible for the design, construction, quality, and manufacturing specifications for garments made in the United States and Mexico. For 11 years I taught art history, consumer relations, self-presentation, and retailing concepts on a post-secondary level while starting my own seminar and consulting business. As a consultant and a professional speaker, I helped a wide range of business clients present themselves and their companies in the most positive manner possible.

I was presenting seminars on self-presentation, customer relations, and marketing topics nationally when the Dallas County Dental Society contacted me to present a program on self-presentation at the Dallas MidWinter Meeting. In doing research for my first dental seminar I visited several dental practices as a patient to gain a better understanding of current issues. The program was very well received; one presentation led to another and over the years I have made contact with some exceptional practitioners whom I consider to be key mentors. I feel fortunate indeed to have gained important insights from these mentor-friends. Throughout this period I visited dental offices undercover to understand patient-practitioner issues. I had very high dental bills; however, the state of my oral health and my smile were dramatically improved!

The "mystery patient" as a concept had not developed yet, not until I was invited to present at the California Dental Association's San Francisco Symposium. While at a luncheon there, a clinician asked me what I did. I was struggling to describe this process, and I mumbled, "Well, I guess I'm sort of *a mystery patient.*" When every fork stopped in mid-air and every eye looked at me, I realized that maybe I had something here!

Throughout this period I was still speaking to many other non-dental groups. One of the niches I developed was in the hospitality industry. I assisted image-aware organizations like Marriott to fine-tune services and self-presentation of staff members, and I became an undercover guest at hotel properties, reporting to management on guest relations and impression management. I also worked closely with marketing groups, especially those in advertising. These groups were interested in marketing themselves as salespeople as well as their products and services in a customer-friendly manner. All of this background would ultimately come together in the development of the seminars and consulting for dentistry. You will recognize the influence and the value of this varied background throughout the book.

I started focusing on dentistry and I realized that my own personal experiences as a patient, while extremely helpful and pertinent, were not complete. It would be necessary to gain a wider perspective of how patients view their dental experiences, how others make decisions, and what they look for in a dental practice. It was at this point I initiated a process of quantitative and qualitative analysis of dental patients with a focus on comparing their attitudes and preferences with those of the practitioner. As the workload increased and the needs dentists have for this information became more pronounced, I assembled a team to assist in both research and focus group development.

In 1994 we completed two written surveys to compare patient and practitioner perspectives. The patient survey had 236 questionnaires returned with 70% national and 30% Texas respondents. The survey of dentists had 197 respondents from throughout the state of Texas (See Appendix A for demographic information). These two surveys were structured in a parallel format with similar questions asked of both groups. However, the practitioners were queried on how they thought the patients would respond to the questions. Interestingly, we found that often the practitioners' grasp of patient preference was quite different from the patients' reality. This meant it was crucial to gain more insight into the unspoken attitudes of patients and bring those viewpoints to the practitioners. It was at this point that we initiated the focus groups series. Through this venue we were able to gain a very clear view of what patients like and don't like, what they want and don't want. Also it afforded the opportunity to take the results of the quantitative analysis and refine it through qualitative input. It has been through the focus groups that we gained the greatest insight into patient attitudes.

THE PRESENT

It is in the focus groups where patients really open up and tell us how they feel. It's clear that patients do not frequently talk this openly with members of the dental team (though they *are* more open with staff members than with the dentists!). But if they are about to leave a practice, it's unlikely that the practice will learn the real reason. If they stay with a practitioner, it's unlikely that the practitioner knows exactly why. Also it's unlikely that the practitioner recognizes those patients who may depart the practice due to managed care issues, or what it might take to regain their loyalty. The focus groups are the foundation for learning more about changing patient attitudes. Now when I am hired to visit an office undercover, I see the practice not only through my own eyes, but through the eyes of the hundreds of patients we've interviewed!

THE PATIENTS

You might ask, "Where do the patients in the focus groups come from?" It is an important question; after all, you will read throughout the book about different demographics that we included in our survey groups. We contact nonprofit groups like schools, charitable organizations, and professional groups that seek non-dues revenue. Our meetings are fund-raisers for the contracted groups.

The groups we work with are known to represent the demographics sought. For example, if we want to interview clients of pediatric or family dental offices, we contact the PTA's of elementary schools. We then provide the PTA with a very specific list of participant criteria we seek, including age, gender, dental appointment frequency, socioeconomic background and more detailed specifics if the group topic is highly specialized. With the example above, we would specify age of children in the household, and the type of dental practice visited. Focus group participants are formed from volunteers to the organization.

Groups include 8-15 participants and are held for two-hour sessions which are audio taped. The nonprofit group is paid for each qualifying participant who attends the session. Participants volunteer their time and the nonprofit group benefits by bringing in non-dues revenue. We believe this is a win-win proposition as funds are given to a worthwhile group in the community where the meeting is held and we gain valuable insights for the dental profession.

THE PROFESSIONALS

Though this process is initiated through dialogue with patients, it continues with the professional dental community. The information and insights gained in our focus groups and through my own mystery visits are then fed back to dental teams in seminars from coast to coast. When we first started the focus group concept, I envisioned the information flowing from the patients to the practitioners. However, we've experienced an interesting evolution: Once the data is provided to the dental teams in seminars, new questions and issues are generated from the audiences. These questions are ones which often provide fodder for future focus groups. When we know *your* questions and concerns, we're able to be more productive and effective in this on-going dialogue. In essence, as a speaker, I've become a conduit between the two groups.

THE PROMISE

Although my speaking and consulting started in other fields, I find that dentistry offers the greatest personal satisfaction. It is with no other group that I'm able to use all aspects of my background so fully. But putting that aside, I feel a very strong connection with the exceptional people in the dental profession. My admiration for the profession and the dental teams I meet continues to grow. I feel privileged to be a part of the continuing education programs and to be able to consult and assist practices nationwide.

Dentistry is now the major center of interest for me. However, I will never eliminate the work I do with hospitality and marketing groups. For I find that maintaining these relationships provides valuable insights into how other businesses with similar challenges manage those challenges. Many of their solutions can be translated successfully into the dental arena. Having an open mind to different ways of solving similar problems results in some valuable Ah-ha's!

Therefore, my promise to you is to continue to open a window on the ever-changing attitudes of patients. Whether it is in the form of seminars, audiotapes, videotapes, articles or books, be assured that we will continue to seek out and disseminate the trust-builders and trust-breakers from the patient's perspective. Once the insights are gained, my goal will be to present the information in the most effective manner possible and hopefully one which is entertaining as well!

In many ways, I feel like a patient advocate. I want you to know and understand how patients think, what they want, and how you can provide the most effective service from the patient's point of view. I also feel like an advocate for the professional dental team. I hope to help you retain your patients in these challenging times, and gain new patients as well. Also I hope to provide information that will result in patients obtaining the treatment they want and need from a team that communicates genuine interest and care.

And Finally . . . Putting it into Practice

At this point the educator kicks in. When you put down this book, I hope it is with a plan to implement, not just for yourself, but for the entire team. Within the team reside the heart and the mind of the practice; only minor change occurs in isolation. Significant change can occur within a cohesive and focused group.

Below, I've listed some ways to use this book for the benefit of the entire team and for the benefit of the patient. These suggestions can form the foundation for numerous staff meetings. Your progress is my progress and I want that for us both! Also, I'm interested in knowing what questions *you* want asked of the patients!

Putting This Book to Work in Your World: Suggestions for the Team

• Address each chapter on societal trends and how these trends might be affecting your community and your practice. How do you see these trends reflected in the faces of your clients, prospects, or in other businesses. Brainstorm and make a list of the opportunities that may exist and investigate avenues to reach new patients and gain greater loyalty with patients of record.

• Evaluate your self-presentation on an individual and group basis. Determine your behavioral styles (chapter 15) and how these styles influence team dynamics. Discuss the strengths of each style and recognize the strengths each style brings to the group. Structure a procedure to determine the style of each patient of the practice and communicate in an appropriate manner with each patient.

- Discuss the apparel of each of the three office categories and determine if they are congruent with the image of the office. What changes, if any, would be necessary to increase patient confidence based on appearance of the team.
- Thoroughly evaluate your collateral materials and how congruent they are with the image of the practice. What steps would you need to take to bring them into tighter focus for patients? Lay out a long-range plan with a deadline date by which your image on paper will be congruent and consistent.
- What is the first impression of your office for new patients? Have each team member become a patient at some time during the busy part of the day. Start with entering the front door as if you'd never been there before. Note what you first see, what you like, what you don't like. Sit in the reception area and hear what patients hear. Take notes. When all members have gone through this process compare notes and make changes as needed.
- Take a tour of the office as a group. Have different team members introduce each area and explain the patient benefits of that area. Ensure that all team members know and understand how to present these marketing elements to patients.
- Have a "show and tell" team meeting wherein each team member gives a "bio-background" on himself/herself so that the entire team knows more about each other and can send a cohesive, knowledgeable message to patients. The understanding of each other's strengths can go a long way toward building the confidence of the team as a unit. It is especially powerful in building patient confidence and credibility when patients view this mutual team respect and team pride in the practice.
- Have 10 different contacts call the office at various times to offer feedback on telephone image and protocol.
- Discuss "Immersion" (see chapter 18) and its impact on the patient. Address how team cohesiveness can influence patient comfort and confidence in the practice.

Brainstorm on how the team can most effectively and genuinely immerse new patients into your practice.

- Make a list of the 10 most common questions callers pose and discuss the most patient-friendly way to market the practice through professional answers to the questions.
- Formulate and conduct your own in-office survey to gain patient feedback. Make sure that patient anonymity is maintained.
- Consider having your own patient focus group or advisory group wherein you discuss major patient-centered issues in the practice.
- Evaluate where and how treatment plans and patient finances are discussed. These are often the reasons that patients leave a practice.
- Role play the case presentation and discussion of fees in a group. Give feedback as to both verbal and nonverbal cues and responses. Also observe the *patient* and discuss what the patient nonverbal cues could mean.
- Make a list of the top 10 marketing concepts of the practice. Discuss these at length and ensure that every team member deeply understands the significance of each item and could confidently discuss these with patients.
- Discuss and list the ways that the practice can continue to build strong relationships with patients after appointments. In morning huddles discuss the building of relationships with daily patients. Determine what you can learn about the patient that can aid in developing patient relationships.
- Review each of the Top Tip boxes at the close of each chapter. Rate yourself on a 1-10 basis as to how well you address these issues. Give yourself a nice pat on the back for those areas in which you score high, and draft a *to do* list for those areas that are weaker.
- Review chapter 22 as a group. Discuss each listed item and determine how the team can maximize the issue in reinforcing the relationship with patients.

IT'S ON PURPOSE

An aside about "the mask". Is it a marketing technique? It might be by default, but not by design. I've had so many people ask me about this, that I'll answer the question here. The mask had, and still has a very real purpose: unless you knew me or had seen me speak, you probably wouldn't recognize me! It helps to maintain some degree of anonymity for me. It also represents the fact that *all* your patients are mystery patients. Getting behind their masks and into their heads is vital to the life of your practice.

I've found a very nice side benefit though: I don't have to "live up" to a picture. How many times have you heard people say about another person, "Hey, he/she doesn't look *anything* like that picture!" Well, I don't either and . . . it's on purpose!

We welcome your feedback and inquiries! Information on The Mystery Patient Process, seminars, team retreats, consulting, custom focus groups, surveys, and additional continuing education products may be obtained by contacting:

Suzanne Boswell Presentations
3767 Forest Lane, Suite 116-470
Dallas, TX 75244-7100   USA

Phone: (972) 243-2086
Fax: (972) 406-8738
E-mail: DentalPt@aol.com

Our mission is to aid the dental team increase patient retention and treatment acceptance through finely tuned patient relations and through understanding the attitudes of today's patients.

PART 1
Societal Topics and Trends

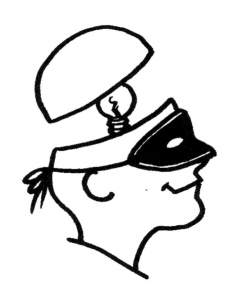

"The only unchangeable certainty is that nothing is unchangeable or certain."
—JOHN F. KENNEDY

"Change is the only thing that offers new opportunity."
—ROSS SHAFER

Change. It's inescapable. To deny its existence is to deny reality. To embrace it as opportunity is a mind-set that can lead to an exciting and productive future. Tom Peters, business guru, perhaps put it best, "Excellent firms don't believe in excellence, only in constant improvement and constant change."

As the community, the profession, and the world change around you, your practice must change also. That means it's crucial to keep your fingers on the pulse of the public. It is vital to understand what's happening to your patients in terms of the issues that are affecting their lives as they also will affect your practice. It is important for the entire dental team to be aware of societal issues in addition to being up-to-date on clinical treatments and techniques. The degree to which patients are affected by the news, by the media, and by society is the same degree to which these issues will affect your practice. Patients carry this assorted *baggage* into the dental practice with them. The entire team then must manage any issue-laden patient. That is not to say that all patients are so encumbered, or that those who are, carry all issues with them.

The following topics are just a few of the factors that are affecting dentistry and business in general today. There are many more and, just like the world around us, they will change as well. The following chapters offer methods to constructively approach challenging issues and, in the process, meet the needs of your patients more effectively. The challenges that face your patients as they enter your practice are probably quite different than the challenges which faced them 10 years ago. Likewise, the societal issues that will be influencing all of us in 10 years will differ from those we experience today. The future just isn't what it used to be! Be prepared.

There are three important concepts at work in relation to dealing with changing societal issues and how they affect the dental practice. With these three steps deeply ingrained, a practice can weather the majority of challenges presented:

Goals for Part One:
1. Recognize the changes that occur in society and the evolution in consumer attitudes.
2. Recognize the opportunities that can exist as a result of those changes.
3. Develop creative solutions to the challenges that meet the needs/wants of your patients and that also help your practice move in a positive direction.

CARPE DIEM!

1

An Aging Society

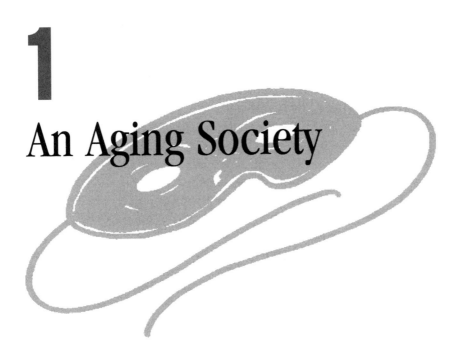

""It takes about 10 years to get used to how old you are."—Author Unknown

Of all the societal trends that affect the practice, none will have such a significant impact as the aging of society. This is an indisputable issue: we will get older. As life expectancy increases, you can expect that the average age of your patient base will age and you'll be presented with new challenges. Our perspectives change as do our bodies. Our attitudes change as do our clinical needs and wants. Expectations of an older client base differ appreciably from that of the younger groups. Moving into the year 2000 and beyond, the "Baby Boomers" and the upcoming "Generation X" will have enormous impact on the bottom line of your practice.

The Older Patient. Who is this "aging" patient base made up of? There are three general groupings all of which would fall under the category of the "older" patient. The first age group is 65 to 74. "These individuals are new to retirement and the designation of *senior citizen,* among other things."[1] The second group falls in the age range of 75 to 84 where health may vary widely from being quite active to being infirm. The third group is individuals over 85 years old. "This group, after years of managing chronic diseases, is usually more frail physically."[2] Of the three groups, this third oldest group is the fastest growing segment of the older population.

The American Association of Retired Persons (AARP), is one of the most powerful lobbying groups in the United States. Their political clout is being felt more and more strongly as Baby Boomers march toward their retirement years. How does this affect the dental practice?

You may have already experienced the fact that older patients today are far more vocal than patients of the same age 10 to 15 years ago.[3] If they're unhappy with your service, or with treatment by the doctor or any member of the team, they are more likely to voice it than they were in the past. Also they are more likely to make changes and to move to another practice than they would have 10 to 20 years ago. Understanding their mind set and responding in an appropriate manner to this powerful group is important to gaining and retaining these patients.

In a focus group we conducted of older patients, several commented on the patronizing attitude that is sometimes displayed towards older individuals. Because they value their independence so much, many older patients will resent or may respond negatively to assistance if it's given but not asked for. It is important to recognize that many feel that much is being taken away from them like their cars, homes, spouses, and kids. Allowing them to maintain their self respect and a feeling that they have *some* control is a critical matter for them. With the advent of managed care programs, offices may need to help their elderly in understanding their options. For example, the elderly patient who was going to leave her dentist because "my plan says I'm supposed to". The confusion surrounding these issues can be particularly disconcerting for this group of patients.

Baby Boomers. Though we presently have a significant and growing older population, the power of this Baby Boomer group has not yet truly shown its numbers. It is with the Baby Boomers that we will see significant changes in our society. Marketing your practice, helping your patients feel comfortable in the office, communicating effectively with your patients, and certainly the clinical issues that you'll be presented with will change. In addition, you'll be dealing with a group of patients who have a unique perspective.

The Baby Boomers have a totally different mind set than preceding generations at the same age. The dental team must recognize these differences and meet the changing needs of this demographic group. In his book, *Age Wave*, Ken Dychtwald, Ph.D., puts it this way,

> *Once a sleeping giant, older America is now awakening to its social and political power. In doing so it is throwing off the biggest myth, the sum of all the others, which states that the old American is unimportant, invisible, politically weak, socially discountable, and economically insignificant.*

The Baby Boomers are more health conscious and active longer than preceding generations. As result, they tend to be more independent and are becoming even more so. A most important element of their mind-set is the importance they place on value of the services they use and the products they buy.

No longer does the consumer look just for price, and that is particularly true of the aging segment of society. They're now interested in the value they get for their dollars, and for today's consumer that "value" is based on the quality that is received for the price paid. While our society is moving away from conspicuous consumption, the aging segment of the society feels most strongly about this. It is important to avoid a message of "glitz for glitz' sake" in your practice. The Boomers movement is in a very serious "back-to-basics" mode. They will be judging your practice on the value they receive.

In conjunction with the back-to-basics values that are so appreciated by this group, there is also a greater understanding and sensitivity towards people in general and the challenges presented to society on the whole. One might liken this to the *earth children* of the sixties who have now come of age and have been tested by reality. They appreciate honesty, straight forwardness, and a willingness to be of help to one another.

That is not to say they have lost an interest in issues of image and appearance. A sizable segment of the aging group will have a very serious interest in oral health, cosmetic dentistry, and maintaining a youthful appearance. They know they are living longer lives and they want to continue to look good. In the focus groups that we conduct with patients, we found that the Baby Boomer group is divided almost in half in this area. That is, nearly 50% of Baby Boomer patients will have some degree of interest in cosmetic dentistry.

However, some do not want the practitioners to raise the subject matter. When questioned about this, interested focus group participants voiced varying opinions as to the appropriateness of a practitioner bringing up cosmetic procedures as suggestions. Many individuals felt it should be up to the patient to raise the subject matter because this could be a sensitive area and the practitioner could be perceived as being judgmental or worse, as "pushing treatments" on the patient.

In addition, though some patients may have an interest in cosmetic dentistry, they may not be in a position to afford it or to spend the money on themselves. Before treading into unknown waters, be sure to seek out the attitudes of your patients. When I had an appointment as a "mystery patient" in one dental office, the doctor handed me a mirror and said, "If you had a magic wand, is there anything you'd like to change in relation to your smile?" This is a non-judgmental way of approaching this subject matter. You'll find out how patients view their appearances and how receptive they are toward suggestions.

Recognize also that this group will be more skeptical than their predecessors at the same age. They've seen it all, "They're sick of the hype and are seeking the simple truth ..."[4] This group will try out more products, more services, they'll do more research and they'll be skeptical until they believe all the information is in.

Research has shown that this group is more likely to spend money on their children than on themselves.[5] If the patients you're dealing with have children who are still in school or for whom they still have financial responsibilities, then these same patients, though interested in cosmetics, may not invest in themselves. They may however, invest in their children's dental work.

Influentials. A significant element of the Aging Society has been identified by research marketers. These are the "Influentials", the group of individuals who have typically self-actualized; they are past the difficult decisions of starting a career and family. They are well educated, often involved in their communities, are more than twice as likely as the average person to be "top talent" or professionals, and twice as likely to own their own businesses. They are interested in technology, travel frequently, and often are asked their opinions by others.

This is a significant group for dentistry as this demographic group includes those at the upper end of the socioeconomic scale, who are interested in their health, appearance, and have the money to invest in their own dental care and that of their children.[6] This group is financially able and willing to take risks, though they are typically calculated risks. They've done their research and they'll try and compare products and/or services until they're sure that the correct decision has been made.

This is a key group to understand. They are willing to pay fee-for-service rates, but want to be sure that there is value. With this demographic group, it's crucial that there be very solid value offered. If there are any doubts, they are perfectly willing to move on to another provider to determine if the value offered is better there. Ross Goldstein, a San Francisco-based psychologist who specializes in tracking generational trends says, "The old advertising adage is that you sell the sizzle, not the steak. With this group you can still maybe sell the sizzle, but there had better be a good steak underneath."[7]

Respect and the Aging. Feedback in focus groups as well as in seminars we conduct nationwide have validated this group's demand for respect. This is seen very clearly in the older segment of the aging society in relation to use of their names. Many patients in focus groups have commented on a younger practitioner or team member referring to them by their first name when, in fact, the team member was never given permission to do so. One patient in a focus group who was about 65-years-old commented, "It was my first time to visit this dentist, he entered the room and I was surprised at his age, he looked young enough to be my grandson. But he introduced himself like this, 'John, my name is Dr. Smith, how are you doing today?' I told him that I'd be happy to call him Dr. Smith so long as he referred to me as Mr. Jones!"

You will not go wrong if you use a more formal term in introducing yourself but you could well go wrong by assuming it's appropriate to use the patient's first name with this group. Anything that smacks of lack of respect for the aging patient may be cause for them to move to another practice. Also, the issue of respect and civility really goes beyond age. A Roper poll indicated that there is "a growing focus on manners and politeness" in conjunction with the realization that "codes and customs are part of what enables society to function."[8]

The dignity of the patient must always be considered. This is crucial in respect to elderly patients. In a seminar I conducted, an audience member related an incident that involved one of her associates who was assisting an elderly female patient. The patient became clearly distraught before treatment began. The staff member, sensing the patient's mounting tension, drew the patient out. She learned that the patient had grown upset when seated because she noticed that her white shoes were scuffed and she was embarrassed. The assistant offered to help. She quietly took the shoes to the break area and cleaned them so the patient would feel more at ease.

This is an example of a staff member's awareness of the patient's anxiety and also sensitivity to maintaining the patient's dignity. Handling this in the quiet and caring way she did, enabled the assistant to help the patient become more comfortable and effectively receive clinical treatment. You can be sure that this small act went a long way in building patient confidence in the team and in the practice. Though the staff member did not perform this act for "marketing purposes", the outcome was a patient who felt a stronger alliance with the practice and was more likely to refer the practice to friends and family.

Because our society is being educated by the media, patients are highly aware of what is considered appropriate communication between practitioner and patient. Today's patients realize that the practitioner has obligations to educate and to inform the patient on conditions and treatments. The more educated the patient is, the more aware and sensitive he/she is to how you communicate with him/her. Respecting the intelligence of these patients will be crucial to your retaining them.

Beyond the formal relationship of patient to practitioner, this group values practitioners who verbalize an interest in the patient as a person not just as a "case". They value being recognized as an individual and appreciate the interest that is communicated to them about their personal activities, their personal interests, and their work. It is important to realize that although your patients may be 65-years-old, this group is remaining employed longer than previous generations. The team should not assume they are retired. They may still be actively employed and proud of it. Therefore, acknowledging their involvement as an active, significant part of our society is important to retention of this group.

There is a tendency for society to look at the elderly as fragile. Perhaps society may say, "This person is no longer cuddly—she's beyond touch." It's up to caring people and caring practitioners to tear down the "don't touch" signs.[9] The great anthropologist, Ashley Montagu, wrote of the increased need of touch as we age, a need that applies to men as much as to women. It is in old age that we again become dependent on others for human support, yet society seems unwilling to accept the fact of aging. It is with the aged, that a conventional handshake cannot replace a caressing hand, "the only touch of love".[10] Practitioners must regain the ability to communicate and reach patients in this most caring of ways especially as the client base of the practice ages.[11]   Patients have commented in focus groups about the positive impact of touch. When offered in a sincere, caring manner and combined with verbal reassurance, a comforting touch can greatly reduce patient anxiety.

Changing Values. Once adults reach middle age their values start to shift. It is this changing value system that is crucial to understand in marketing to this patient. Five key values which form the basis for motivating older individuals are: autonomy and self sufficiency, social and spiritual connectedness, altruism, personal growth, and revitalization.[12] Of these five, revitalization may be the most significant in relation to dentistry. You must communicate with this group in a manner that recognizes them as vital, and at the same time, indicate the benefits of treatment as contributing to their quality of life. The majority will respond to a more subjective approach than they might have in their earlier years.

There are many ways that you can address the special needs of your elderly patients. For your patients who are in the oldest age group, consider offering a pick-up service. Make sure that the typeface is large and readable on any documents given to these older patients. Ensure that your reception area chairs have arm rests and are firm, yet comfortable. Avoid rugs that could cause a fall. Rest rooms should be equipped with hand rails next to the toilet. Use fixtures that are patient-friendly for those who may have arthritis or impaired dexterity.[13]

Those dentists who recognize and respect the magnitude and power of the aging segment of society will find a highly receptive and agreeable group of patients. Dentists may consider contacting AARP chapters or high-end retirement centers to offer slide and informational presentations for these groups. Some doctors offer a courtesy fee reduction to the seniors because these patients are able to schedule appointments with some degree of flexibility.

STRAIGHT FROM THE PATIENT'S MOUTH: PATIENT SURVEY AND FOCUS GROUP COMMENTS

"They talked to my daughter about my treatment instead of to me ... like they thought I was beyond the ability to understand what they were talking about. I was very offended." (75-year- old male patient whose daughter had driven him to the dental office)

"My doctor is just about my age and I like that.....he understands me." (62-year-old female)

"I've finally come to a point were I feel totally comfortable with my appearance. I'd be offended if a dentist brought up the space between my teeth. If I wanted it fixed I'd tell him!" (47-year-old female)

"I was forty-five when I had braces put on my teeth. I was always embarrassed of my crowded teeth as a child and I'm so glad I did this. My dentist brought up the idea and I'm glad that he did. Without his encouragement I would probably have not done it." (49-year-old female).

"Every time I go to my dentist's office, the staff shouts at me. They think I can't hear them, so they talk really loudly to me. They are all in their 20's. I've watched them with younger patients and they don't shout at them. It actually makes me feel older!" (70-year-old male who appeared much older than his age.)

"I was interested in implants. The dentist wanted to do a bridge and was trying to discourage me from having implants. He made it sound like the bridge might be better because I'm so old that, considering the costs involved, I might not be around long enough to get the full benefit of the investment! I can easily afford them, but I'd never go back to that dentist because of his attitude." (72-year-old male)

TOP TIPS:

1. Know and talk "value" of the practice and of the treatment. This is particularly important to Baby Boomers.
2. Address patients by the honorific, Mr., Mrs., Ms., Miss, until invited to use the patient's first name.
3. Avoid references to age or terms that may offend the ageless-minded patient like, "elderly", "older". If necessary, "senior" and "mature" are less offensive.
4. Avoid a patronizing tone, it will be perceived as demeaning by many, particularly if there is a wide age difference.
5. Ensure that the office is patient-friendly: easily accessible with convenient parking, good lighting, door handles and washroom faucet handles that are easy to turn, chairs that are easy to get out of, reading matter of interest to this age group, and staff members that reflect a range of ages.
6. Being comfortable is a major need of the older customer; convenience and access may be as important as the service provided.
7. Listen closely to complaints offered and respond in an appropriate service manner.
8. Security and safety are key factors in the older patient's choice of a dental practice location.

9. Do not pre-judge what the patient wants because of his/her age. Recognize the patient's perspective in relation to quality of life.

10. Older patients will respond well to seeing a range of ages represented in the team, particularly mature team members.

REFERENCES

[1] Niessen, Linda, D.M.D., M.P.H.; Mash, L. Kay, D.D.S.; Gibson, Gretchen, D.D.S. "Practice Management Considerations for an Aging Population", *Journal of the American Dental Association*, Volume 124, 1993.

[2] Niessen, Linda, D.M.D., M.P.H.; Mash, L. Kay, D.D.S.; Gibson, Gretchen, D.D.S. "Practice Management Considerations for an Aging Population", *Journal of the American Dental Association*, Volume 124, 1993.

[3] Speer, Tibbett L. "They Complain Because They Care," *American Demographics*, May, 1996.

[4] Murray, Kathleen. "Getting Older, Getting Better," *American Way*, American Airlines publication.

[5] Research of Yankelovich Partners, Yonkers, NY, 1992.

[6] "Influential Americans: Trendsetters of the New Millenium," A report based on 5000 interviews by Roper Starch Worldwide, and co-sponsored by *The Atlantic Monthly*, September, 1995.

[7] Murray, Kathleen. "Getting Older, Getting Better," *American Way*, American Airlines publication.

[8] "Sixteen Numbers to Know for 1996," *The Public Pulse*, Roper Starch Worldwide, Inc., 1996.

[9] Boswell, Suzanne. "Back to Basics: Staying in Touch with the Patient," *Journal of Esthetic Dentistry*, Volume 7/Number 1, 1995.

[10] Montagu, Ashley, "The Human Significance of the Skin," Harper and Row, New York, NY, 1978.

[11] Boswell, Suzanne. "Back to Basics: Staying in Touch with the Patien" *Journal of Esthetic Dentistry*, Volume 7/Number 1, 1995.

[12] Wolfe, David. "Targeting the Mature Mind," *American Demographics*, March, 1994.

[13] Niessen, Linda, D.M.D., M.P.H.; Mash, L. Kay, D.D.S.; Gibson, Gretchen, D.D.S. "Practice Management Considerations for an Aging Population," *Journal of the American Dental Association*, Volume 124, 1993.

2
Becoming Culturally Competent

"Who is a wise man? He who learns of all men."
— THE TALMUD

It was the morning break at the seminar and I had just completed discussing the impact of cultural diversity on the dental practice. When the audience left the room for coffee, Dr. Tom Orent, of Framingham, MA, came up to talk. He related a most fascinating journey on which he'd taken his practice and it related directly to the subject I'd just addressed.

He showed me two versions of his business card, one was written in English and one in Portuguese. He explained that he recognized that he had a high proportion of Brazilian patients in his practice and that for a significant number of the recently immigrated Brazilians, language was a major barrier to treatment. Dr. Orent decided to actively pursue this market—what might have been a problem to some became a challenge to him. The path he took to connect with this group was remarkable. Over a span of seven years he hired Brazilian staff and had a brochure translated into Brazil's Portuguese language. He purchased books and tapes to teach himself Portuguese well enough to explain dental conditions and treatments, and to understand the patients. He and his wife even hosted three International Exchange students from Brazil.[1]

If you were newly from Brazil and lived in this community, which dental office would you select? You'd choose the office that appeared welcoming and the one where you felt the most at ease. Dr. Orent recognized the changing face of his client base and he rose to the occasion to meet the changing needs. It is this kind of visionary thinking that recognizes an opportunity where others might see an insurmountable problem.

Adjusting to the Changing Face of Your Community

Because the face of our society is changing so rapidly, it is imperative to recognize how the face of your patient base also may be changing. How can you increase patient comfort in your office? Conventional wisdom says that people like and respond to people who are like them. Social psychologists confirm that this is a reality. Initial attraction and "likeability" include a recognition of similarity in backgrounds, similarity in interests, and a perception of shared experiences.[2] To help your patients feel comfortable and at ease in your office, having a staff which reflects the face of your community is important. If you have a high percentage of African American patients, then staff members who share this commonality will increase patient comfort level. The common thinking is, "We come from the same place, therefore it is more likely that you will understand me." Likewise, having a variety of ages represented on your staff is a good idea if you treat patients from different age groups.

In the landmark book, *Megatrends 2000*, Naisbitt and Aburdene note that as the world becomes smaller, there is a greater need for each culture to own and value its heritage.[3] That is coming to fruition. Today there is a resistance to the concept of a "melting pot" wherein all cultures blend. Instead there is a great desire for each culture to maintain its roots while fitting into the overall multi-cultural picture. Therefore, recognizing and valuing the differences among ethnic groups and cultures is an important mind-set in communicating effectively with all. If your office is located in an ethnically diverse area, you might consider investing in team attendance at a diversity or sensitivity training seminar to increase awareness and understanding. Otherwise, the communication challenge may be one of "asking the service people to adopt behaviors that are incongruent with their cultural programming.[4]

ETHNICITY VERSUS DIVERSITY

When the term cultural diversity is used, more often than not people think in terms of ethnicity. However, cultural diversity encompasses far more than just ethnic origins. The concept also includes various nationalities, lifestyles, gender, religious preferences, physical abilities, and so on. Any of your patients may fall into more than one cultural group. For example, you might have an Hispanic patient who is a wheelchair-user. This patient brings to the office, pertinent issues surrounding those who are physically challenged as well as the traditions of his heritage.

A very powerful statement to patients is having a team member who is physically challenged. This a statement to all patients that the practice is a caring and sensitive one and recognizes the abilities of all people. A significant benefit of having staff members that reflect a wide range of cultural groups is that the entire team becomes sensitive and aware of the issues and the strengths of all people. The world is reflected more accurately through the faces of this diverse team.[5]

As an undercover patient in one office I visited, I noticed that the doctor's business cards were printed in English on one side and in Japanese on the other. As I waited at the front counter, I looked around the reception area. I noticed that there were also Japanese newspapers on a reception table. I asked the receptionist about this. She said, "Our [Anglo] dentist is married to a Japanese woman and we have many Japanese patients. They appreciate our having reading matter specifically for them." As in Dr. Orent's practice, this office was communicating value and respect for this group of patients. To other visiting patients, this made a statement about the sensitivity of the practitioner.

The Journal of the California Dental Association published an article, "A Multiple-Language Health History For Dental Practice."[6] Accompanying the article were patient history forms in numerous languages. (Fig. 2-1) The forms were published in such a way that they could be duplicated by readers and used in the dental practice. For a practice with a high percentage of a specific ethnic group, these forms would be welcomed by patients and certainly communicate an appreciation and value for those patients.

I mentioned this in a seminar and one of the audience members commented, "But we wouldn't be able

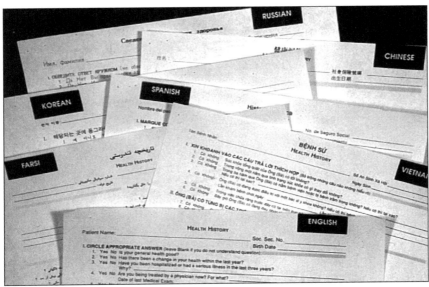

Fig. 2-1 Health history forms in the languages of your client base increase patient comfort. (Courtesy California Dental Association)

to read the forms ourselves." However, the questions on each form were numbered sequentially in the same order as the English Health History form. The columns of the "Yes" and "No" responses were identical as well. Anyone comparing a foreign language form with the English form would be able to understand the responses. The only area that would require interpretation would be those questions which called for a subjective, written answer by the patient. This corroborates the importance of having staff members who are able to communicate in the language being addressed.

How one approaches a patient of a particular ethnic group may be largely influenced by the age of the patient or how long the patient has lived in the community. In a focus group we conducted with Hispanic patients of various ages, we learned that the younger age ranges who were third generation Americans were less likely to be steadfast to long-term traditions than the older patients who might be first generation in the United States.

However, there is no hard, fast rule on this; every patient is a unique individual. Age is not necessarily a determining factor for attitude or for preferences. The important point is that an awareness of the uniqueness of the culture is very important.

MEETING THE NEEDS OF PATIENTS WHO ARE PHYSICALLY CHALLENGED

In relation to the physically challenged group, there are many issues to be addressed, some of them are verbal, some of them are nonverbal, and some relate to the actual design and layout of your office. Amy Baxter, Ms. Wheelchair America 1996, is a patient of orthodontist, Dr. Alton Bishop in Bedford, TX. I visited the office with Amy and experienced the practice from a totally new perspective. Amy spoke about the way the staff related to her, "The staff here asks me if I want or need help instead of pushing my chair or physically moving me. Most disabled patients are going to respond to an openness in communication. I mean, they'd much prefer you to *ask* if the patient wants help. Saying something like 'how can we help make your visits more comfortable for you?,' will be appreciated by them." (Fig. 2-2)

As time goes on, the issues of office design will become more important in relation to this group. Because the group is growing in size, it is likely that more patients who use wheelchairs will be visiting offices in the future. Ease of accessibility and comfort in the office will be crucial. A doctor in a seminar audience commented, "I've never had a patient in a wheelchair come to my office." His statement was countered by another dentist who said, "We had a couple of patients in our practice who used wheelchairs and made adjustments to accommodate them.

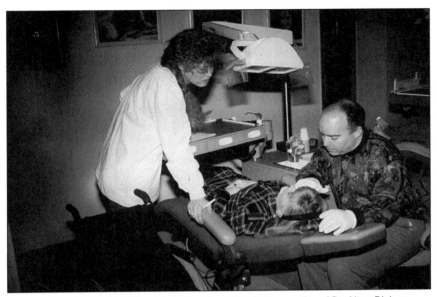

Fig. 2-2 Amy Baxter, Ms. Wheelchair America 1996, in the practice of Dr. Alton Bishop of Bedford, Texas.

As a matter of fact, we put a ramp that led directly into the treatment hallway at the back door of our office. Patients in wheelchairs can enter the practice readily from the parking area via this ramp. As a result, we've had many more referrals from patients who use wheelchairs and this segment of our practice has grown significantly. These are very responsive and loyal patients."

Amy Baxter has commented on the height of the counters. In her orthodontist's office there is a lower counter area where she feels more comfortable, as does the staff.

GENDER ISSUES

Gender is another issue which is a vital factor in your office. Not only because a significant percentage of your patient base is female and they tend to make many of the decisions on healthcare providers for the family, but in addition, the majority of dental practice staff members are female.

How the male or female practitioner communicates with the female patients is an issue of interest and concern to both the patients and the media today. Doctors have been targeted in the media as to their manner of discounting verbalized concerns of women. Television and newspapers have reported on not only the poor communication skills and poor listening skills used by physicians with women, but also have addressed the resultant physical complications that can occur due to poor communications.

It is not uncommon for female patients to feel "not heard" in relation to their practitioners. Because of the sensitivity and patient awareness toward this matter, it will be crucial that the members of the dental team not only communicate openly with female patients, but most importantly, that they *listen* to them. The female patient who feels discounted by the dentist is a possible candidate for "grazing" to another practitioner who has better communication skills.

The male patient may not be as likely to communicate openly about sensitive subjects as female patients do. The team may need to recognize and learn how to encourage patient communication from such patients. One male focus group patient noted, "I always felt very uneasy in the dental office, but the assistant has helped me to talk about my concerns a little more. Just talking about my anxiety has helped and I know that they understand and care." Of course this holds true for all people, though female patients may be more likely to verbalize it than male patients.

LEARNING MORE ABOUT YOUR PATIENTS

Learning more about the communication styles of your patients will be key to gaining and retaining them. One of the ideal ways to get your fingers on the pulse of your patients is to develop your own patient focus groups, or establish an advisory group that represents the predominant cultures in your patient base. Getting feedback from patients of different cultural groups will help you understand the ways to modify your own behavior in relating to that group, whether it is your body language, your speech pattern, and/or the ways in which you can increase patient comfort in the office.

Changing the face of your practice and changing the way you communicate with your patients will be crucial to your continued success with a constantly evolving marketplace. The subject of cultural diversity is an enormous one and there are so many facets of it that it is impossible to address all of them in this chapter. Most importantly, in order to truly understand the impact of cultural diversity on your practice, it is strongly suggested that some type of sensitivity training be considered for the team. This is particularly important when your office is located in a city or area where there are numerous cultural groups. Remember, the term "cultural" should be observed in the broadest perspective. That is, it encompasses issues of ethnicity, gender, physical abilities, religions, and lifestyles.[7]

STRAIGHT FROM THE PATIENT'S MOUTH: PATIENT SURVEY AND FOCUS GROUP COMMENTS

"I don't have a problem about going to a white doctor, so long as I'm treated just like all the other patients in the office ... and I mean from the staff too." (28-year-old African-American female patient)

"This [Anglo] dentist has a lot of Chinese patients ... I like to have my teeth cleaned by the Chinese hygienist, we live in the same area and know a lot of the same people." (35-year-old Chinese female)

"My family has gone to this doctor [Hispanic] for ages ... he's worked on my parents and we all keep going to him ... he speaks Spanish to my parents .. and English to the rest of us." (32-year-old Hispanic male)

"I can tell as soon as I walk in the door what to expect ... if I get an attitude at the front desk, it's probably going to be that way all through the office." (31-year-old African-American male patient of visiting a non-African-American dentist's office)

"It's really not an issue for me ... I just want the best treatment I can get ... I'm not worried about being best friends with my dentist." (Hispanic male)

"I felt like he really didn't want to touch me ... I could tell he was tense and uncomfortable ... I never went back." (38-year-old African-American female patient relating emergency visit to a white, male dentist)

"If I'm considering going to a dentist who may be from another country, then I'm going to want to know more about the doctor's education and experience. I'll probably ask more questions about his background." (50-year-old white male)

"Gender is really not an issue for me ... I'm more concerned about the quality of care, not the gender." (45-year-old male)

TOP TIPS:

1. Recognize the changing face of your clientele via staff members that reflect this changing community.
2. Acknowledge clientele diversity through reception area magazines and amenities that reflect the interest and languages of the group.
3. Have signage and printed matter in multiple languages if a significant percentage of the clientele warrants this.
4. If you have a sizable client base of another ethnic group, acknowledge their holidays and/or celebration days with tasteful decorations. Ask patients for suggestions.
5. Make available to staff members professionally-conducted cultural awareness or sensitivity training.
6. Actively listen to all patients and especially ensure that female patients have expressed verbally their concerns and been given feedback indicating your level of understanding.

REFERENCES

[1] Orent, Tom. *1000 Gems, The Book*, Gems Publishing, Framingham, MA, 1996.

[2] Kleinke, Chris L. *Meeting and Understanding People*, W.H. Freeman and Company, New York, NY, 1986.

[3] Naisbitt, John; Aburdene, Patricia. *Megatrends 2000*, William Morrow and Company, New York, NY, 1990.

[4] Albrecht, Karl.. *At America's Service*, Dow-Jones Irwin, Homewood, IL, 1988.

[5] Morrison, Ann. *The New Leaders; Guidelines on Leadership Diversity in America*, Josey-Bass, Inc., San Francisco, CA, 1992.

[6] Jacobsen, DDS, Ph.D., Peter, L.; Fredekind, DMD, Richard. "A Multiple-Language Health History For Dental Practice", *The Journal of the California Dental Association*, Volume 21/No.5, 1993.

[7] O'Hare, William P.; Frey, William H.; Fost, Dan. "Asians in the Suburbs," *American Demographics*, May, 1994.

3

Visions of Value

"Quality in a service or product is not what you put
into it.
It is what the client or customer gets out of it."
— PETER DRUCKER

J ust as beauty is in the eyes of the beholder, so is
value. The vision that one patient has in relation to
value of a service or of the practice may be very
different than the vision that another patient has of the
very same service or practice. Getting an accurate read on
what "value" is, is as easy as hitting a moving target. Yet
the trend exists within all socio-economic groups. There is
an increased desire for, and awareness of the importance
of, greater value. With a tougher economy and with the

public tightening the purse strings the dental practice must take new steps to communicate *real value* to all levels of patients.

As discussed in chapter 1, the Baby Boomers are having an enormous influence on the concept of value in services and products. The boomers do point the way for society in a major backlash to the excesses and the vulgarities sometimes seen in the "glitzy eighties." This trend can be expected to continue into the second millennium.[1] Society today has recognized that status and prestige are not surrogates for quality and value.

The conventional wisdom in earlier years was "the more it costs, the better it must be." Not so today—it's much more complex. Today's consumers are far more knowledgeable and savvy than those of the past; they are also skeptical in general. The media has heightened their awareness and concerns about costs and value in health care.

WHAT DO YOUR PATIENTS VIEW AS VALUE?

Today's dental patient wants quality for a reasonable price on an everyday basis. This is not nearly as simple as it might sound. The issue is greatly complicated by the concept of "usual, customary, and reasonable." Today's patient looks at price, quality, value, and questions if they are receiving their dollar's worth.

The challenge here is not just for the patient, it's also for the practice, the dental team. In patient focus groups that we conduct, there are frequent discussions of fees and concerns about the possibility of being overcharged. Because patients don't know how to judge the quality of dental care, they are more confused by fees. So here we have a fairly sophisticated consumer who is placed in what he/she perceives as an alien environment, trying to evaluate clinical expertise and skill that he/she knows little about. This is frustrating for the patient to say the least. If we match what they value with the dental treatment they need, then the patient and the practice both win.

The patients who communicate perceptions of high value of the practice and the greatest trust in dental team are those patients who are most likely to accept treatment and have been well educated by the team. One patient in a focus group put it this way, "My dentist does a wonderful job explaining what she's going to do and how it's going to help me. She explains in a way that I can understand. Once I know how the procedure is going to help me and what the *long-term* benefit is going to be, then I feel better about what is being proposed." An important note here is this patient had been with her dentist for many, many years. The doctor had established a high degree of trust with the patient, had an excellent track record with the patient, and had proven her clinical skills through excellent work. So this patient's perception of value was built on a trusting relationship.

THE TREATMENT COORDINATOR AND COMMUNICATING VALUE

One effective way to communicate the value of the practice and value of treatment is through a treatment coordinator. There is a higher perception of value, a clearer understanding of the recommended treatment, and the patient is educated when both new and recall patients experience a skilled, professionally trained treatment coordinator. This individual can help educate the patient as to the benefits of the practice, the clinical skills of the practitioners, and the quality level of treatments provided. In addition, patients often perceive the treatment coordinator to be a valuable ally, one they can contact with questions, concerns, and requests for information. From the doctor's point-of-view, this individual can also be a valuable ally in handling patient telephone calls and questions as a communication liaison.

Practice management consultants can assist in the training of coordinators. McKenzie Management in Dublin, OH, for example, is one of the consulting firms that offers such services.

In one office where they had trained a treatment coordinator, a patient commented about the benefits of working with this staff member,

> *Before working with Jane, I always felt as though the dentist was explaining to me in words that I couldn't understand. I felt like I was getting a lecture on the condition and the treatment, and so I couldn't come to a decision on treatment. Now Jane explains the treatment in language I can relate to; I feel more confident in making decisions and getting the treatment that's right for me.*

Many patients comment that they feel more at ease asking questions of the treatment coordinator than of the dentist. But most importantly, they understand the benefits of the treatment and the perceived value rises as well.

As an undercover dental patient, I've experienced the benefits of being introduced to the practice as a new patient by a treatment coordinator. A knowledgeable treatment coordinator who has strong interpersonal skills and an in-depth knowledge of the practice can go a long way toward instilling credibility and trust within the patient.

In one office I visited, the treatment coordinator was particularly adept. I had been seated in the reception area just moments when a well-dressed and well-groomed woman crossed the reception room and introduced herself. She shook hands warmly and welcomed me to the practice. She explained that she was my treatment coordinator and she would like to introduce me to the practice. She led me to a consultation room where she first took a patient history, gave me the opportunity to discuss my concerns and interests in relation to dentistry, and then she addressed each question that I had. She gave me detailed information about the practitioners, about the practice, and about what I would experience in this first visit.

After this introduction, she took me on a tour of the practice, introducing me to other team members when they were available. She gave me her business card and invited me to contact her any time I had any questions relating to the practice or the treatments that I was having done. In the 25 minutes that I spent with this woman, she elevated my perception of the entire practice and the value that I would receive as a patient in this office. Most importantly, she came across as warm, kind, and knowledgeable. She predisposed me to feeling good about the team before the clinical exam ever began. Whether you use a treatment coordinator or not, it is the responsibility of the entire team to communicate value to the patient early in the process.

VALUE VERSUS FEES

For the dental team working with a new patient, or for a younger practice, the challenge is greater in establishing a "vision of value". More responsibility is placed on the team for effectively educating the patient.

This is an extremely important point. If the patient does not understand the value of your office, your service, your treatment, your clinical skills, you must ask yourself, "Have we really given all the necessary information to the patient? Are we communicating in the most effective manner for this patient? Are we exhibiting a deeply-felt service attitude?" Take the responsibility yourself first, then if you've done all you can, consider the following:

- You have a patient who is looking solely for price.
- You may not be educating the patient properly.
- There is a communication breakdown with the patient.
- Your services are overpriced for the value provided.

It is the last item that is of the greatest concern to the patient. But fees typically will not be a problem if you are dealing with a patient who is looking for quality, if you educate the patient properly, and if you communicate effectively.

Though fees are inextricably tied to the concept of value, it is fees that practitioners talk about most in relation to patient's perceptions of value. For example, one doctor put it this way, "I think patients are deciding about treatment based solely on how much it costs." In fact, patients often counter this concept with statements like, "Well, if that's the kind of service the practice is going to offer, why not go to an office that will be less expensive; I can be treated the same way and pay less for it!"

Frequently patients include non-clinical services and the quality of patient-practitioner relationship in evaluating value. It is critical that the practitioner recognize that the patient is not judging value by fee alone. So much of value is also placed on the non-clinical, the service that is provided. This includes attendance to interpersonal skills. Since patients do not know how to judge the clinical, they use other means to determine the quality of the treatment. The verbal and non-verbal elements that are discussed at length in Part 2 of this book will influence the patients' perceptions of service and consequently, influence their perceptions of value in what you provide. It's what occurs over the long haul that produces the reality in the consumer's mind today. In other words, if your service is excellent but your clinical treatment is not perceived to be on the same level, then the patient feels short-changed. This can result in disillusionment and the possibility of moving on to another practice. The two concepts must work hand-in-hand effectively to reach the patient; service and clinical quality must both be perceived as high value for the fees charged.

Patients in focus groups have discussed their feelings about fee increases, particularly when they've been patients of a practice for a long time. One patient put it this way, "I've gone to my dentist for over 11 years. In that time, it seems like the cost of a regular cleaning goes up every other visit. The only difference I've seen is that the office has been redecorated! There's been no difference in service." Patients must see, hear, and understand the value for their dollars. Perception plays an important part. If the patient perceives no differences, then he may see this as an arbitrary fee hike. If the practice educates the patient to benefits of the treatment and of the practice, then the perception of value rises.

This concept becomes even more important if you increase your fees. Remember this, if there is a fee increase, the patient must feel confident that the new fee is justified. It's the responsibility of the team to make that justification a reality for the patient.

THE SAVVY HEALTH CARE CONSUMER

You are dealing with a far more savvy patient base than in the past. Since the 1950's consumers have moved from:

- buying what they were told to buy and could afford to buy, to
- proving they would buy whatever they felt like buying, to
- becoming the world's most competent buyers.

Deep at the heart of the vigilante consumer trend is a wish that companies could somehow be more *human*. Consumers are willing, even eager to say, "anyone can make a mistake ... after all, you're only human." If the organization responds in a "human" way, it's not so much "what happened", but whether or not you fixed it— quickly, responsibly, and honestly.[2] To put it mildly, today's healthier consumers are "mad, and they won't take it anymore." They'll either voice their complaints vehemently, or they'll walk away without giving you a hint of what was wrong, but they'll tell everyone they know. The little things make an enormous difference today. Perceptions of value vary with every patient. Listening closely, understanding what they really want and responding appropriately will be the key to gaining and retaining patients.

VALUE AND DEMOGRAPHICS

To add one more element to this challenge of communicating value, the entire team must have a basic understanding of the mind-set, motivations, needs, and preferences of the different demographic groups represented in the client base. An entire book could be written on this topic alone, for it includes issues of regional trends and preferences, cultural groups, psychographics, preferences by age, socioeconomic segmentation etc. Some of these issues have been addressed in chapters 1 and 2.

In the *American Demographics* article, "Dentists Are Forever," attitudes and preferences of different demographic groups were mentioned in relation to accepting dental treatment.[3] Though socioeconomic levels and statistics can give clues to patient attitudes, they will not speak for the specific attitudes of the patients in your own practice. Patients are different, their decision-making processes will differ, and their decisions are based on the team as well as many other factors. Transplanting your entire patient base to the office of another practitioner might result in a quite different decision-making process. Much depends on how well you are able to communicate.

Consumer Reports published the book, *The Complete Guide To Dental Health; How To Avoid Being Overcharged And Over Treated.*[4] This book title indicates the concerns and attitudes of many of our "super consumers" today. To get your message of value across to your patients, the entire dental team must focus on communicating with your patients as never before.

Straight From the Patient's Mouth: Patient Survey and Focus Group Comments

"I've been to my doctor for 27 years. I trust him and so I don't need a lot of "proof" [of condition] ... If he told me I needed two crowns, I'd get them. It's that simple."

"When I saw that picture [monitor view on intraoral cam-era] I could see what he was talking about and I realized the seriousness of the problem."

"After my last cleaning I saw that there was a separate charge added to my bill for an infection control fee. They had never done this before and I really feel it was just a way of increasing their fees and trying to justify it. I mean, weren't they sterilizing everything before they started charging this fee?"

"The doctor kept pushing for a gold crown. I didn't want that gold color in my mouth and I told her so. I think she just wanted the gold because it was a higher fee."

"The doctor was interrupted during my appointment by a phone call. When he came back, he said that it was a con-tractor who was putting in his Jacuzzi. I thought to myself, 'I'm paying for that.' The next time I went to his office for a cleaning, the fee had gone up."

TOP TIPS:

1. Recognize the patient as consumer and respect the intelligence of today's consumer.
2. Tell the truth in a straight-forward, up front manner.
3. Verbalize value in the context that will be most meaningful to the specific patient. This will vary from

patient to patient depending on demographic group, lifestyle, etc.

4. Increase patient education, particularly in relation to increased fees.
5. Ensure patient comprehension of education and value by encouraging patient feedback.
6. Ensure that every team member recognizes the value of the practice and of treatments. Patient trust is shaken if staff can't credibly reinforce the value of accepting treatment.

REFERENCES

[1] Research of Yankelovich Partners, Yonkers, NY, 1992.

[2] Popcorn, Faith. *The Popcorn Report*, Doubleday, New York, NY, 1991.

[3] Mogelonsky, Marcia. "Dentists Are Forever," *American Demographics*, August, 1990.

[4] Friedman, Jay W. *Complete Guide to Dental Health: How to Avoid Being Overcharged and Over Treated*, Consumer Reports Books, Yonkers, NY, 1991.

4
Comfort and Safety as a Patient

"I like this office because it's attractive, comfortable, and soothing. I go early to get away from the kids and read magazines in peace!"

—FOCUS GROUP PARTICIPANT

O n entering the office I was caught completely off guard. A feeling of anxiety crept over me as the waiting room began to look like "discomfort"! The only seating available was high-backed wooden benches which, while they were visually attractive, were decidedly uncomfortable. The floor was wood and there were no rugs to soften the sounds. Walls were tan and moldings were stained dark brown; the area seemed dark, even somewhat depressing.

The front office area was walled-in and patient communication was via a translucent, sliding glass window. Decor was stark Early American and seemed to be designed for the benefits of the practice, not for the patients. This appeared to be a reception area requiring little maintenance, and offering a high degree of privacy for the staff with little regard for patient needs or comfort. Indeed, it seemed more like a w-a-i-t-i-n-g room than a reception area. Patients would certainly be aware of the length of time spent in this area.

The term cocoon is used to describe any of various protective coverings usually found in nature. The term is also used to identify the societal trend whereby the public feels a need to build a warm, safe, comfortable cocoon around itself. Relating this to the dental practice, cocooning means establishing an environment in which the patient feels comfortable and is surrounded by warm, nurturing people within a patient-friendly physical setting. In this sense, comfortable is safe.

"Crime has surfaced on public opinion polls as American's number one concern, whether or not the high level of anxiety is statistically warranted. Forty percent of those responding to a 1993 *Time/CNN* poll think that crime is as serious in the suburbs as it is in the cities."[1] Though the perception may not be accurate, the issue is that society has become safety-obsessed. Safe is comfortable. Each time we interview a focus group, a key gainer/retainer is that the patient should feel "cocooned"; the patient is safe, comfortable and can trust the doctor and staff. People are making business decisions every day based on where they feel safe. It is for this same reason that we see an increase in gated communities and secured retirement centers.

Because of the anxieties frequently associated with a visit to the dentist, patients have always appreciated an office that has a comfortable and serene atmosphere. But the desire for this has increased and today it is near requisite. Not only do your patients want comfort, nurturing, and a pleasant office, but they also want their safety ensured. To meet the challenge, we must first take a proper inventory and to accomplish this, we'll investigate the issue by breaking it into cocooning for comfort and cocooning for safety.

COCOONING FOR COMFORT

The patient-friendly office must present itself as a place of comfort as well as clinical care. The patient is going to be influenced by both the physical environment of the office and the communications skills of the entire dental team.

When a patient enters your office, how "welcoming" is your reception area? This is a topic frequently brought up by patients in focus groups. When we ask patients, "What is important to you in the appearance of the reception area?," the patient often talks about, and describes an environment very similar to a living room. They like and appreciate chairs that are comfortable rather than the hard-backed, plastic variety reminiscent of hospital emergency rooms. They prefer individual chairs over couches, and lighting which is conducive to reading, but is not harsh or intense. Individual room lamps along with soft overhead lighting tend to create a friendly, warm, home-like environment. "'Comfortable', 'casual', and 'cozy' are the three descriptions that Americans find most appealing in a room."[2] Making your reception area a warm cozy cocoon will be very appealing to your patients (See chapter 12 on decor and amenities.)

ATMOSPHERICS

The atmosphere you create influences patients' emotions, moods, and perception of you, the practitioner. "*Atmospherics* describes the conscious designing of space to create or reinforce specific effects on buyers, such as feelings of well-being, safety, or comfort."[3]   Based on your choice of designed atmosphere, the patient has learned just a little bit more about you. In addition to influencing the patients' emotions, you are telling them how much you care about them and their comfort in your office.

Patients are highly aware of the sounds and the smells of the office. One patient in a focus group commented, "I walked into a general dentist's office for the first appointment and I was hit in the face by a very strong, medicinal odor. It was overwhelming and it reminded me of the office that I used to go to as a child, where I was terrified! I had to wait 20 minutes to see the doctor. By the time I sat down in the chair, my tension level was sky-high just from the smell. I never went back to that doctor again." This is a dramatic illustration of the power of odor in influencing patients.

Aromatherapy has long been used in the retail environment and is moving into service businesses as well. "At the Sloan-Kettering Cancer Center in New York City, technicians are so convinced that scent has an effect on mood that they use sweet-smelling vanilla fragrance during some medical tests."[4]   This same concept is being responded to very positively by dental patients as it not only aids in covering any medicinal odor, but in the process it can aid in the reduction of anxiety. Aromatherapy units are now available with a wide variety of subtle scents that can aid in creating a soothing and positive environment for your patients.

One office I visited communicated a high attentiveness to odor. In a tour of the office, I saw a bread making machine in the staff area. I was told that they frequently baked bread just for the wonderful "homey" odor that it produced in the office. Another office commented that during the holidays, they kept a pot of spiced cider simmering, and that wonderful smell infiltrated the whole office. I've also heard about offices that periodically make popcorn because of the mouth-watering aroma it produces. There are pros and cons about this one, but there's no denying that it is a wonderful smell!

As an undercover patient, and a researcher of dental patients, I have experienced many of these same smell and sound factors firsthand. In one office I visited, as I sat in the reception area I could hear the sounds coming from the treatment room down the hall. Not only did I hear the sounds of the instruments, but I heard the muffled responses of a patient in some discomfort. This is the kiss of death for patients sitting in your reception area. Ensure that the area is free of sounds and discussion from the treatment rooms. A pleasant tape or CD playing subtly in the background can diminish the perception of time spent waiting, in addition to covering background noise.

In the office of my dentist, Dr. James Reisman, there is an alcove built into a part of a treatment room. (Fig. 4-1) In the alcove is a reclining chair with a lap blanket draped over it. On a side table are beautiful coffee table books with lovely photographs in them. In addition, there is a telephone on the table and a window facing a pleasant, green expanse. This alcove area is used for patients who are in the office for longer treatments and can be used during interim rests. Not only are the creature comforts of the patient attended to here, but the area literally looks like a cocoon.

Patients frequently comment in focus groups about their appreciation for the creature comforts that are offered in the dental office. These creature comforts might be in the reception area or in the treatment rooms, but in either

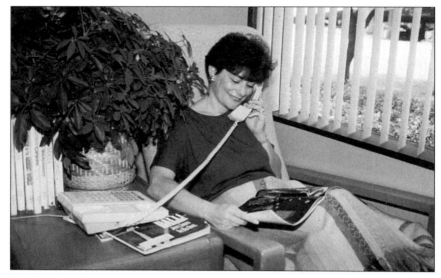

Fig. 4-1 A patient receiving a long treatment relaxes between procedures.

case, it shows an interest in, a value for, and a caring of, the patient. Some of the amenities most valued are:

- Telephone in reception for patient use
- Beverages (healthy ones only, please) available for patients
- Lap blanket for patients in the treatment room
- Small desk with straight-back chair for writing
- Head sets or distractions during treatments
- A good selection of up-to-date periodicals
- Pleasant, soothing music

Inherent in insuring that your office is OSHA-compliant, there are barriers built in between the patient and the dental team. Although these barriers offer safety-measures, they may present to the patient a rather cold and sometimes forbidding environment. So from the patient's perspective, the dental office and the dental team must work a little bit harder in building a "connect" to compensate for this environment.

An extremely important part of creating a "cocoon-like" office for your patient involves the people skills of your staff. No matter how warm and welcoming you make the office physically and visually, that appearance will be superficial at best if the staff comes across in a cold or uncaring manner. Congruence is key here. Staff must come across with a genuine caring attitude toward patients. The chapters on communications skills in Part 2 of this book delve into that area in great depth. However, as it relates to "cocooning", it is important to look at the individuals who represent the office and are in direct contact with the patients.

It is very difficult, if not impossible at times, to teach interpersonal skills. We can teach the steps to take, but how those steps are taken by the staff member is another story entirely. People have to *want* to fine-tune their interpersonal skills; it doesn't happen by accident or by dictate. Those people who have innate people skills, a genuine warmth and caring for other human beings, are the ones you need in your front-line positions. They help to reinforce an environment of comfort for the patient. You may have a staff member who has the ability to communicate well with patients but just needs a little bit fine-tuning, or polishing. The individual who would prefer to work with data and details instead of people, will serve you best *not* being on your front lines. In many cases, these same employees would rather not be in the spotlight, juggling interpersonal issues.

COCOONING FOR SAFETY

Matters of patient safety at your practice vary greatly depending upon where your office is located, whether you are in a metropolitan or rural area, or whether you are in the north or south. In any case, maintaining patient safety in your locale is crucial to your patients and to your practice from a litigation point of view.

Your choice of location and the ease of reaching your office is important. From a safety point of view there should be adequate parking, as well as easy ingress and egress to ensure patients feel comfortable in reaching your office and their safety is maintained as well.[5]

If you are located in a metropolitan area or any area where there may be a possibility of crime, and that could be anywhere today, it is important to take steps to ensure patients feel at ease in visiting your office. This includes offering parking that is easily and quickly accessible to the entrance of the building, having adequate outside lighting during evening hours or during the winter when it gets dark earlier. If you're in an area where there are icing conditions during colder months, it will be key to your patients that parking and sidewalks be sanded adequately. Although you may not be responsible for these things yourself, your patients will *perceive* that you are responsible, at least in part.

In some metropolitan cities, you may be located in office buildings where there is a great deal of foot traffic. Fear of crime may be particularly high among the city-dwellers and this is readily evidenced by the number of key chains that sport mace or pepper sprays. Recognize the significance of this and as much as possible, take steps to ensure your patients feel at ease in coming to your office. If you hear frequently voiced concerns from your patients, take heed, this is an important message and the issues revolving around this can be serious enough to send your patients to other practitioners. The more you hear patients communicate about this subject in relation to your office, the more important it is that you communicate back with them about what you do, or the steps that you take to ensure their safety. It is verbalizing that you are attending to their safety, and bringing it to the awareness of your patients that can help to instill a sense of caring from you and a sense of value of your practice.

STRAIGHT FROM THE PATIENT'S MOUTH: PATIENT SURVEY AND FOCUS GROUP COMMENTS

"I really like the headset ... it helps me to separate my mind from what's being done."

"It's the sounds and the smells that unnerve me in the dental office."

"My doctor is a very compassionate person ... he touches me on the shoulder and checks how I'm doing during treatment."

"I won't go back 'cause the waiting room was uncomfortable, the staff was unfriendly, and the doctor acted rushed."

"My kids like to go to our dentist because she's fun, painless, and there's a great play area for them."

"I drive by my dentist's office every morning on the way to work. They always have fresh coffee and muffins for morning patients ... I drop in sometimes and get a coffee "to go". I love my dentist!"

"The reception area is lovely. It's very clean and I like the unusual selection of magazines they have."

"... the fish tank is soothing for me, and my kids are fascinated ... keeps them quiet!"

"I appreciate the phone ... I can check in with the office and feel like I'm still in touch with them even though I'm not there."

TOP TIPS:

1. Ensure that the office is void of medicinal smell.
2. Be aware of sounds in reception and between treatment areas that may negatively influence patients.
3. Create a reception area that communicates the warmth and comfort of a living room.
4. Offer "creature comforts" and amenities for patients.
5. Back up the warm physical environment with a staff that helps the patient feel welcome and a part of the dental family.
6. Ensure that your office locale is as safe as possible.

REFERENCES

[1] Nichols, Paula. "If Sex Won't Sell, Try Safety," *American Demographics*, Ithica, NY, June, 1994.

[2] Nichols, Paula. "The Public Pulse," Roper Starch Worldwide, Inc., January, 1996.

[3] Kotler, Philip; Clarke, Roberta. *Marketing for Healthcare Organizations*, Prentice-Hall, Englewood Cliffs, NJ, 1987.

[4] Wilkie, Maxine. "Scent of a Market," *American Demographics*, Ithaca, NY, August, 1995.

[5] Edwards, Frank. "Marketing Professional Services," Louis Allen Associates, Inc., Mountain View, CA, 1991.

5

Lack of Loyalty

"If I can't tell a difference between two dentists, I'm going to the less expensive one."

— FOCUS GROUP PARTICIPANT

As a professional patient and consultant, I find it interesting that sometimes practitioners opt for the costly "fix" instead of the one that is the most meaningful to patients and the most patient-friendly. Sometimes an expensive "Band-Aid" won't cure the condition. If you are presented with a high percentage of your patient base "grazing," look at the practice from a patient's perspective. Take the following incident, as an example.

I had been hired as an undercover patient by a practice. It was clear throughout the entire process, that there was a serious lack of "people-connect" with the patient. The feeling was true throughout the office from the moment of the first phone call to the moment I walked out the door after my appointment. I'd had contact with five people in the practice, including the dentist. None of them exhibited any desire to build a relationship with this new patient. There was no sense of cohesion among the team; they were coldly robotic in their interpersonal transactions with each other.

Following the appointment, the doctor confided in me that he was very concerned about patient retention. This came as no surprise! If I'd been a "real world" patient I wouldn't have wanted to return either. Ninety-five percent of the problems experienced in the phone calls and visit to this office were people-related. In discussion of the solutions, the doctor said, "I'm willing to throw some money at it, but I want to get it 'fixed' soon." However, the core problem in this office could not be solved by a quick money fix. These were people problems; they take more effort, time, and hard work to resolve. The idea of the "easy solution" is appealing, but does not often offer the most solid solution. Sometimes it doesn't take money at all to resolve the areas of concern— it may take heart and time. "You don't have time", you say? If you don't *make* time, all you may *have* is time!

The solution for the doctor in question? A reevaluation of the staff that he had hired and a refocusing on how he had come to the decisions he'd made. "She's really knowledgeable about financial matters, but she told me in the first interview she's not a 'people-person'." This was a mistake the doctor made and it was affecting the bottom line of his business. In addition, he needed to conduct staff meetings periodically as well as invest in team-building activities or programs. Perhaps most importantly, the team did not have a common purpose. They needed to jointly script a mission statement that would define their purpose and give them direction. All of these issues were having an impact on patient retention in the office.

Dental Professionals' View of the Challenge

Dr. Tom McDougal who presents seminars nationwide on the topic of "Ultra Quality Service" is recognized for his ability to develop long-term relationships with patients. Dr. McDougal comments that "dentistry must move from *commodity* delivery to relationship establishment with each patient." It is the value, confidence, and trust that comes from a people-based relationship that will help to keep patients coming back.

Dr. Steve Carstensen of Bellevue, WA, put the same concept this way, "The office must stress the practice's commitment to the long-term goals for the patient's health." This statement goes beyond addressing transitory treatments of a filling or a crown, to caring about the quality of life of the patient. The patient who understands this commitment by a team will be far more likely to want to remain in the care of that practice.

The real irony in dealing with the present lack of loyalty by patients, is that it will take the very same trait, loyalty, in order to retain patients. It will be perseverance and loyalty to patients that will enable practitioners to keep patients today. On one hand patients are confused by healthcare challenges; they are being forced to make decisions that they are not fully equipped to make. Society encourages consumers to change, to try new products, concepts, and services. On the other hand, practitioners are being challenged by these same factors and are being forced to make difficult decisions as well. The entire team daily juggles the many challenges that occur from the first appointment until the time the office closes.

Risa Pollack-Simon, CDA, a dental practice consultant and editor for the ADA's *Dental Teamwork* magazine, states that it's easy for the team to get "so caught up in the every day grind of accomplishing required tasks that they tend to forget about the patients for whom they are performing those tasks."[1] Maintaining equilibrium, meeting the needs of patients, and staying on schedule, indeed require that the entire team understand this delicate balance.

WHO MAKES UP YOUR CLIENT BASE, GRAZERS OR LOYALISTS?

Researchers have found that the health of a healthcare organization can be measured by the loyalty of its patient base.[2] Kotler and Clarke have identified four groups of patients in regard to healthcare organization loyalty:

(1) *hard core loyals* who are devoted to the organization;

(2) *soft core loyals*, who are devoted to two or three organizations;

(3) *shifting loyals*, who are moving from favoring one organization to favoring another; and

(4) *switchers*, who show no loyalty to any organization.[3]

Taking these concepts into the dental practice, the patients who feel the greatest bond with the practice probably fall in the hard core loyals and the soft core loyals groups. The switchers are not likely to desire a bond with the team; they may not have a high dental IQ or put value on dentistry as much as the first two groups. Then the shifting loyals are those who are "at risk" in the practice today. They are the ones who infrequently reveal their real feelings or motives to the practitioners.

PATIENTS' ANSWER TO THE "BIG QUESTION"

At the close of every patient focus group we pose the following scenario to participants:

> *You are happy with your dentist. You've been a loyal patient of this dentist and have had no complaints. The team has been caring and treatments you've received all have been successful. You've had no reason to change practitioners until ... your spouse announces that a managed dental plan is available through the company. Here's your quandary, your doctor is not on the list. Do you leave the office of the practitioner where you have been happy?*

And so, dear reader, what do *you* think the majority of patients say? I pose this same question to audiences at some of the practice management presentations I make. Granted, it's a tough question, and it's a tougher answer. In an ideal world, the majority of patients would say, "No, I won't leave a place where I feel secure and have been well cared for. I opt to stay with the practitioner in whom I've placed my trust." However, we don't live in an ideal world. Dental team audiences are tentative and somewhat mixed in relation to guessing how patients would answer this question. It's an unsettling issue for a team that has worked hard to win the trust of patients. However, the objective dental team members recognize the challenging reality.

So here it is: In focus groups the majority of patients respond that they *would* opt to accept the managed plan. Please don't shoot me, I am just the messenger! It may be an unpleasant message, but I want to make the patient perspective perfectly clear:

- No, not *all* patients say they would change practitioners, but a significant majority would do so.
- The patients who said they would *not* accept a plan were those that had the strongest relationships with their dental teams. The teams had built strong bonds of trust.

What was the primary reason that satisfied patients would leave their dental offices? Money. I'm confident that you knew the answer! It's a harsh reality. It's a reality that must be faced and managed by the entire team. Knowing the reasons that patients might accept this alternative are important to recognize.

Here are some comments we hear repeatedly on this subject:

I've only been a patient in the practice for a short time and I don't really have a history with this doctor, so it's not a big deal to change.

To stave off this type of thinking, you've got to "immerse" the patient into the practice family as early in the patient-practice relationship as possible. Infusing a sense of value and the uniqueness of your office is crucial so that the patient recognizes this is a special place. This requires an investment of time and energy in the patient early in the process. (See chapter 18 for more on "Immersion.")

I've been a patient in the practice for a long time, but it seems that the service has

*deteriorated. I feel like a number. If that's
the way it's going to continue, there's no
reason for me to stay! I'll opt to save the
money!*

A long-term patient of record may be at risk of
being "taken for granted." The thinking of the team may
be, "Mr. Jones has been with us so long. He must be happy
here and so we don't need to worry about him." So the
team focuses on gaining new patients, putting out fires,
and oiling the "squeaky wheels." IBM has a philosophy
that could be transferred effectively to dentistry, "Treat
each customer as if it's the customer you're about to lose."
With today's healthcare consumer mentality, this is a
healthy philosophy for every practice to adopt.

*When my wife came home with the man-
aged care materials, it made me think
about a problem I had at my last appointment. They never apologized or even recognized that they had made a mistake
and were at fault.*

When patients are presented with a managed care
option, they typically reflect on how they have felt about
past clinical treatment and patient service. They think
about inconsistencies of service, how they were treated in
emergencies, how problems are handled, how "fair" the
practice is with them. What is crucial is how the team
manages patient problems. When the practice comes
through tough times for the patient, the patient feels
greater allegiance toward the practice. It's here where
patients pause to think about your past performance.

All of the above situations are manageable. But
they can't be managed with a "Band Aid" mentality. Trying
a quick fix on a relationship that has been floundering for
a while won't typically save you when a patient is
presented with the managed care scenario. Managing
these situations means having in place a practice

philosophy and mission that is understood and lived by every member of the team every day. It means that the entire team must understand deeply the goals of the practice. When patients see and feel staff believe in the practice, when they experience the power of a loyal team, it builds patient confidence and patient loyalty.

TEAM LOYALTY AND PATIENT LOYALTY

Patient loyalty is a concept that is frequently addressed in continuing education sessions. But there is another side of the loyalty issue that will have an impact on your patient retention, and that is staff loyalty to the practice. When we ask patients to "tell us what you really like about your dental office", they frequently counter with discussion of the office staff. The long-term patients of a practice will often comment that some degree of comfort comes by way of "seeing the same familiar staff faces" at each of their office visits. This brings us back to the issue of relationships. There is a perception of security and stability that comes by way of staff continuity. Patients often feel a greater intimacy with staff than with the dentist(s) and that comfortable bond can be a very strong one. As with a cohesive blood-line family, this bond can weather challenging times more readily than the practice that has not effectively developed relationships with its patients.

The inclination for patients to graze is one of the biggest concerns I hear from the practitioners I work with today. But the steps that I hear being taken often indicate greater concern for getting new patients in the front door instead of retaining present patients of record. Sales organizations are highly aware of the costs involved in getting new customers, and this concept is drummed into salespeople. It is smarter and far less expensive to work on retaining the patients you already have.

Robert Frazer, Jr., DDS, of Austin, TX, conducts seminars for dental teams on practice management issues and strategic planning. He agrees with the applicability of this concept in the dental practice. He cites that, "20-25% of your patients account for 75-80% of your fee revenue directly or through referral." In addition, he indicates the absolute need for the office to build long-term relationships with patients. This is verified by our focus group research. Patients repeatedly indicate that those who are the happiest with their dental offices are those who think of the entire team as "friends and family." If you've done a good job of educating your patients and building a sense of value for your practice, you've made a significant investment in that patient and one that needs to be nurtured and maintained.

WHY PATIENTS "GRAZE"

Besides the more obvious issue of a patient moving from the physical area of your office, what are some of the reasons that patients give for moving away from a practice? Responses gathered from our surveys and focus groups spotlight the following as top offenders;

- Doctors who do not listen to the patients (requires better communication skills)
- Dental work that does not last as long as the patient *perceives* it should last (assuming excellent clinical treatment has been provided, this requires education and explanation on the part of the practitioner to the patient)
- Fees that do not seem to be in line with the patient's perception of the value received

(requires an understanding of the patient's value system, finely tuned patient education, and excellent communication skills on the part of the entire team)

• Practitioners who do not thoroughly explain what is going to happen before proceeding with the clinical procedure (requires better communication skills)

• Offices that consistently seat the patient more than fifteen minutes past appointment time (may require a review of scheduling procedures or refining of interpersonal techniques that result in running late)

• Offices where the patient is treated as a tooth and not a person (requires better interpersonal skills)

• Offices that do not assist or educate in relation to insurance benefits (requires policy or procedural decision-making, then requires good communication skills)

• Offices that do not look clean (requires objective view of the office and appropriate actions taken)

• Dental team member(s) who are not neat and/or organized (requires objective view of the team as well as strong interpersonal, management, and communication skills)

• Practitioners who are perceived as dogmatic about treatment (requires an objective view of priorities in the practice as well as better interpersonal and communication skills).

• Offices where there is tension or the dental team does not seem cohesive (requires objective view of the team as well as interpersonal, management, and communication skills)

- Offices that do not apologize for an error or injustice when appropriate to do so (requires greater awareness and sensitivity to the patient's viewpoint as well as excellent communication and interpersonal skills)
- Offices that appear more concerned about the schedule than about their patients (requires an objective look at priorities in the practice and better impression management techniques)

Patients in focus groups have talked about all of these issues. Take another look at this list and you'll find that almost all of them relate to non-clinical matters. The entire list is manageable. In other words, these issues should not be left to fate. They can be managed by members of the dental team to ensure that patients are satisfied with treatment, clinical and non-clinical, in the office.

THE IMPORTANCE OF RELATIONSHIP MANAGEMENT

Betsy Wheat, a practice management consultant from Plano, TX, says that relationships with patients should be managed on a continuing basis. She suggests that this issue be addressed at each morning briefing. The entire team must work on building the relationship with each patient including noting personal information in the patient's record. Patient loyalty is earned ... and re-earned at each appointment.

Some of the ways to manage these challenging issues are:

- Conduct patient surveys to solicit information on patient attitudes.

- Communicate the changes that your office makes in order to meet your patients' needs.
- Communicate on-going appreciation to new patients, patients of record, and to prospective patients.
- Verbalize your interest in the patient as a person, as well as a client of your practice.
- Ensure that the team communicates as a cohesive whole.
- Take all steps possible towards ensuring that the patient's visit to your office is painless including learning how to give a painless injection and offering distractions that help the patient feel more at ease in your office.
- Establish your own focus group(s) or advisory group.

Dr. Frazer has implemented the practice focus group concept with great success, and refers to this as his "Select Client Group". His group meets every 18 to 24 months and discusses what the practice is doing and how to improve. In addition, they discuss ways for the practice to locate other prospective patients like themselves. Besides the obvious sense of family or community that occurs in this group of patients, they also feel a commitment to, and investment in, the practice. This results in a strong allegiance by this key group and a desire to see the practice succeed.

When patients feel they are listened to, heard, and their opinions seriously evaluated, they feel a bond with the practice. In one patient focus group we conducted, a patient said, "The doctor was taking a poll on how patients felt about changes in the reception area ... what our preferences were. He was going to make changes based on the poll consensus. I was impressed that he cared enough to ask us about our feelings and I'm interested in seeing the outcomes!" This was a doctor who was communicating patient importance and a responsiveness to patient opinions.

You might also consider utilizing a consultant to help you find and fine-tune weak areas. The time you spend with an objective consultant who is experienced with practices and situations similar to yours can be highly cost-effective in the long run. In the dental profession, there are consultants who specialize in highly focused areas such as financial issues, new patient process, ergonomics, marketing, and developing a practice identity. Other consultants may have a more "holistic" view of the practice and be able to offer valuable assistance in numerous areas.

You may rate yourself positively in all the areas listed above, and you still may have patients move away from your practice. The issue of managed care also comes largely into play here. If your patients communicate to you that their reason for leaving is to go to a managed care provider or to move to another managed care provider on their list, it is important that you handle this issue adroitly. It is possible that after leaving your practice and moving to another office, your patient may regret this decision. Comparisons between the two offices may result in a desire to move back to your care.

MAKING THE DIFFERENCE FOR THE PATIENT

It's a challenge, yes. But there is something you can and must do now to prepare for this possibility. You must fine tune your service and your patient communication in order to increase patient-perceived differences between you and the other guys! Managed care practitioners are not insulated from the challenge of patient grazing. After all, patients have those lists from which they choose providers. If they are unhappy with one dental office, they can easily refer to the list for another option.

Your goal needs to be: build the greatest void between you and others so that if/when patients leave the practice they consciously recognize the differences between your office and the new office. If patients experience no difference between you and others, then they have no specific reason to return to your care. To encourage the return of patients, you must ensure that patients will experience a significant contrast. That is when patients encounter the mind-expanding "Aha!" That is the purpose of this entire book—to give you tools with which to build the exceptional experience for your patients.

The likelihood of that patient coming back to you can occur only if the patient feels at ease with you and if you leave the door open to him. This means that in the initial announcement of departure, you must verbalize an appreciation for this individual as a patient and as a person.

> *Ms. Smith, I understand that you will be moving to another dental practice. I just want you to know that our door is always open to you. We value you as a patient in our practice and we will always welcome you back. If, for any reason, you find that the practice where you're going does not meet your specific needs, or if you want to return for a specific treatment please call us. We will always consider you a part of our dental family.*

Your communication skills to this departing patient can make the difference between whether he or she feels comfortable in returning to your practice or not.

Trust and Value. It all boils down to these two concepts. No matter the amount of external marketing a practice does, nothing can be as powerful to gain referrals and retain patients as value offered within a trusting relationship between patient and the entire dental team. With trust and value in place, a patient who grazes away will recognize what is missed and will want to return to this special place and to the exceptional experience of feeling truly cared for.

STRAIGHT FROM THE PATIENT'S MOUTH: PATIENT SURVEY AND FOCUS GROUP COMMENTS

I was sitting in the hygiene room and I overheard a couple of the staff members talking about another patient. They were trying to figure out if the other patient was on a managed care program or not. Since I pay full fee, I really didn't like thinking that other patients were paying less for the same treatment. It made me wonder about the ethics in this office and I'm not sure I want to stay there. My confidence has been shaken.

I really like the doctor in this practice but he's got one person at the front desk who is very snippy. She's the one I have to deal with on my payments and my appointments. I'm about ready to leave that office just because of her.

The last two times I went to have my teeth cleaned I never even saw the doctor. If that's the way it's going to be, maybe I'll find a less expensive office.

We just moved and there are a number of dental offices closer to our home now. Since I never had a really strong relationship with my present dentist, I'll probably change to one who's closer.

Whenever I go in, the doctor seems so rushed. He's running from room to room and I just end up feeling like a number.

My wife, my children and I all went to the same dentist. But his fees got really high and I don't think his service or quality got any better. I moved our whole family to another office where the doctor really explains what he's doing.

The doctor got really dogmatic. He insisted that I needed a crown and that there were no other "smart" options. I don't like being told the way it has to be, I think that there were alternatives but he just talked about what he wanted to.

TOP TIPS:

1. Recognize each patient as an individual and communicate in ways that are comfortable for them. (See chapter 15.)
2. Communicate with each patient as a person, not as a case.
3. Act promptly in relation to any patient concerns; maintain open lines of communication with patients.
4. Explain a treatment thoroughly prior to proceeding clinically.
5. Be in the moment; focus on the patient during the appointment.
6. Call patients following an involved or difficult procedure.
7. Ensure that all team members understand and reflect a patient-centered practice philosophy.

REFERENCES

[1] Pollack-Simon, CDA, Risa. "Positive Impressions Breed Loyalty," *Dental Teamwork*, American Dental Association, February, 1996.

[2] Kotler, Philip; Clarke, Roberta. *Marketing for Health Care Organizations*, Prentice Hall, Englewood Cliffs, NJ, 1987.

[3] Kotler, Philip; Clarke, Roberta. *Marketing for Health Care Organizations*, Prentice Hall, Englewood Cliffs, NJ, 1987.

6

Eco-Awareness in the Dental Office

"We shape our buildings: thereafter they shape us."
— WINSTON CHURCHILL

The public has become far more aware of the importance of "saving the planet." In the United States, it is the Baby Boomer generation that truly fuels this trend towards environmental awareness. As discussed in chapter 1, it's clear that as the Boomers have started to move into middle age, they are shifting their focus away from consumerism as an end in itself and are expressing greater concern about the quality of life and personal fulfillment. Because they may feel guilty about earlier acquisitiveness contributing to environmental ills, their social values are increasingly driving their decision making.[1]

How Does this Affect the Dental Practice?

By 1990, nearly one-half of Americans had taken some kind of environmental consumer action. The public has had its awareness raised by the media in relation to this topic and there's a growing sensitivity nationwide to the environmental issues. So what does this mean in relation to the dental practice? It doesn't mean that all patients have an eye on saving natural resources or that they practice recycling, but the likelihood is great that they know about and for the most part, respect, efforts being made to do so.

Roper Starch Worldwide, Inc. found that public response to improvements in national environmental performance varied among government, consumers, and business. In his book, *A Deeper Shade of Green*, Peter Stisser notes, "Business still receives the greatest level of complaints about environmental performance." It appears clear that both consumer and governmental groups will continue to monitor the attentiveness of business to environmental issues with increased interest.[2] Your patients may inquire about these issues and you must be prepared to answer those questions.

Our focus groups show that some people may be attracted to your office if you show environmental awareness in your operations and communications. One easy way to accomplish this is through the use of recycled paper. The environmentally aware patient will appreciate the conservation and other patients will not feel they are being "preached at".

How "greening" affects dentistry is far more subtle than other trend-issues. It's easier to relate this to products and packaging. For example, in the grocery store there is an obvious movement to downsize packages, to make them recyclable and to communicate the benefits to the consumer. The movement is still new in the area of services. Also there are significant regional differences in responsiveness and interest in conservation. For example, in the Pacific Northwest there is a very high awareness of conservation and recycling. In many cases, sensitivity to this issue is not just respected, but expected!

However, increased awareness and sensitivity is growing nationwide. The public will, no doubt, also value the businesses that attend to ethical use of our natural resources. Societal trend researcher, Faith Popcorn, sites this by giving the "good guy" a pat on the back. She notes that the public appreciates the "Ethical Man who makes it his business—both literally and figuratively—to make the world a better place. Timely heroes!"[3]

REGIONAL AWARENESS AND SENSITIVITY TO ENVIRONMENTAL ISSUES

Public concerns about these issues do seem to be highly regional. Responsiveness and attentiveness to environmental matters vary greatly from community to community and from state to state. In her book, *Green Marketing*, Jacquelyn Ottman recognizes the fact that appreciation and attendance to environmental issues varies from coast to coast.[4] She notes that the typical "green consumer" is:

- An educated, affluent, politically liberal woman
- Lives in the northeast, west, or a midwest suburb
- Is between the ages of thirty and forty-nine and has children age six and over and
- Is likely to be influential in the community and is possibly an activist for environmental or social causes.[5]

Regardless of the locale of the consumer, or patient, it's important to recognize that the individual with these interests has buying power and is frequently in a position to influence other "green consumers."

PERSPECTIVES OF FOCUS GROUP PATIENTS

In the focus groups that we've conducted, this subject matter has been brought up several times by patients. The topic has related to the use of plastic and all of the disposable items that effect barriers between people or between patient and equipment. One patient commented, "If they change all that plastic and throw it away after every patient, what is that doing to the landfills?" This subject matter had not been raised by patients in our focus groups prior to 1995. But in our group discussions about infection control and sterilization, this issue is mentioned approximately 20% of the time. It is typically raised by a female who is well educated.

An interesting story was related by one patient in a focus group. She talked about her thirteen-year-old daughter who had just returned from a dental appointment. The daughter and an assistant had gotten into a conversation regarding all of the plastic that was used in the treatment room. The staff member explained that this was for the protection of the patient and that the materials were changed after each patient was treated in this room.

The daughter remarked to her mother that she was concerned about the waste and about the possibility of slowly decomposing plastic. Parents of school age children are frequently gaining insights from their children today regarding this topic! The environment and the issue of precious natural resources is being discussed more and more in schools. It is not unusual for the children of a family to be the ones who encourage recycling within the home. This certainly points to upcoming generations who will be more aware of how a business runs in relation to saving natural resources.

You are presented with a challenge here—maintaining the barriers that are important and required by OSHA, while ensuring that your practice and the profession maintain an awareness and sensitivity to the issue of conservation. As you take the steps, small though they might be, your patients also will be learning from you. At the same time, you will be reinforcing the message you are indeed a caring practitioner.

COMMUNICATING WELL WITH YOUR PATIENTS AND YOUR COMMUNITY

The following are areas to consider in relation to your usage of products and natural resources in your office. Ask yourself, how can your office:
- Conserve natural resources
- Minimize waste and prevent pollution
- Minimize use of materials unnecessarily
- Use renewable resources
- Use recycled materials
- Use energy efficiently and
- Consider biodegradability in supplies purchased.

Some of the things you can do to aid in this movement and also communicate positively about your practice to your patients include:
- Use recycled paper in your letterhead, business cards and all printed items,
- Make purchasing decisions of supplies based on the ability to recycle,

- Maintain separate trash receptacles for those items which are not being placed in the biohazard receptacles,
- Use energy efficient electrical appliances wherever possible,
- Encourage staff and patients to be judicious in use of water,
- Encourage staff in turning off lights, for example, in the break area, if that area is not going to be used for a while.

STRAIGHT FROM THE PATIENT'S MOUTH: PATIENT SURVEY AND FOCUS GROUP COMMENTS

I only do a little recycling, but since I travel a lot, I've become more aware of recycling in other parts of the country ... they seem more advanced than near my home.

I believe in all the environmental efforts, but I don't like it if I think a business is promoting "green" in a token manner. Don't play on my emotions and then charge me twice as much for the product or service!

Honestly, I'm not really good about this myself [recycling etc.] ... but I resent what I see business doing in an arbitrary manner. It's business that pollutes the air, water and creates landfill problems.

TOP TIPS:

1. Use recycled paper and make your patients aware of this by incorporating the appropriate recycling symbol if you produce newsletters or promotional pieces.
2. Have unobtrusive signage for patients regarding your environmentally (energy) aware office.
3. Purchase disposable supplies.
4. Use recycling receptacles for non-biohazard items.
5. Ensure that staff knows and can converse with patients who are interested/concerned about what you do in these areas.

REFERENCES

[1] Ottman, Jacquelyn A. *Green Marketing*, NTC, Business Books, Lincolnwood, IL, 1993.

[2] Stisser, Peter. "A Deeper Shade of Green," *American Demographics*, March, 1994.

[3] Popcorn,Faith, *The Popcorn Report*, Doubleday, New York, NY, 1991.

[4] Ottman, Jacquelyn A. *Green Marketing*, NTC, Business Books, Lincolnwood, IL, 1993.

[5] Ottman, Jacquelyn A. *Green Marketing*, NTC, Business Books, Lincolnwood, IL, 1993.

7

Mind-Body Connect: An Evolving Patient Attitude

"The secret of the care of the patient is in the caring for the patient." — FRANCIS W. PEABODY, MD

"Ｎew age stuff ... bah, humbug!" you might say. Whether you personally like it or not, patient awareness of the mind-body connect is something you may have to address in one way or another. There is a significant movement that is changing the way the public looks at healthcare. It may be influencing patients in your area, it may not, but we are hearing its impact in focus groups. In one group, one middle-aged business executive expressed his changing attitudes this way,

> Well, I'm much more open to alternative
> means of prevention and treatment than I
> was 10 years ago. I think maybe our fore-

*fathers did have some answers in natural
treatments. And I've been impressed with
some of the eastern philosophies about
prevention and treatment. Besides, with
the skyrocketing costs of healthcare today,
I think it's pretty pragmatic to explore all
avenues possible.*

THE MIND AND WHOLE BODY HEALTH

You are treating a patient base that is experiencing
a mind-changing evolution in relation to healthcare.
Receptivity to this wave of change depends on your
demographic group. Attitudes vary greatly based on your
locale, but the reality exists. There *is* a significant
movement at work, and one with high public acceptance
to the relation between mind and body.

The cover of *First Magazine* announced, "Beat
your fear of the dentist!" with an article, "An Amazingly
Easy Cure for Dental Phobia."[1] In this mainstream
magazine, the reader would gain insights into the use of
hypnosis in the dental office. The reader could be your
patient ... the same patient who avoids treatment because
of fear of possible pain. Are you prepared to deal with the
patient who enters your office with questions after reading
such an article or after hearing about it on TV? Be
prepared. If you haven't been approached with questions
or conversation related directly or indirectly to the mind-
body connect, you or another member of the team will be!

The subject of the mind-body connect is one that
can be taken in many directions, especially in the dental
practice. This concept of the mind as it relates to the body
reaches into areas including verbal and nonverbal

communication, self presentation, impression management, patient anxiety, and pain management.

Increasing your awareness of how this concept can affect your practice is key to understanding and meeting the needs of your patients. Here are some of the ways that this movement may affect you:

- Patients want to be in the care of a dental practice where importance of the patient's overall health is recognized. Take a full health history of the new patient and update it on a set schedule via a face-to-face interview. The taking of patient blood pressure positively influences patient perceptions of the practice. The office is likely to be viewed as one that truly cares about the patient. This is a significant way to increase patient perception of value as he or she thinks, "This office is professional and concerned enough to monitor and track my vital signs as they relate to oral health."

- When you conduct an oral cancer exam, explain what you are doing and why it is important to the patient. Ensure that the patient knows you are a physician of the mouth; you will increase patient perceptions of your value as a practitioner when you educate the patient while you conduct an oral exam. One doctor explained to me that he did not tell patients he was conducting a cancer exam for fear of scaring the patient. On the contrary, patients will feel *more* cared for. If the last dentist discussed this part of the exam with the patient, and you don't, the patient may think it's being overlooked.

- If you are attending a fearful patient, initiate a dialogue to encourage the patient's expression of concerns. Meaningful open dialogue indicates your desire to address the needs of this patient.

You see the individual as a whole person, not just as a tooth or a case.

• Include information in your reception area that indicates an interest in overall health. Magazines like *American Health* or *Prevention* provide a clue to patients that this is an office of an aware healthcare provider.

• If you provide refreshments, ensure that you're sending a positive message to patients. Offer healthful options like decaffeinated coffee, bottled waters, fruit. You are a role model and what you choose to offer is making a statement to your highly aware patients.

• If a patient asks questions or indicates interest in alternative treatments or what you might think of as "fringe philosophies" be careful how you address this. Avoid being dogmatic. Realize that although you may not agree with this patient's point of view, it is important to the patient. Minimizing the patient's perspective can be perceived as condescending and can work against you in the long run. If you don't agree, at least listen and let the patient air his/her views. You'll benefit by gaining insight into an attitude that may be shared by other patients. The more you know about your patients' changing attitudes the more quickly you can adjust to meet their changing needs.

MAINSTREAM SOCIETY'S VIEW OF THE MIND-BODY CONNECT

Good Housekeeping magazine, a long-standing bastion of logic and sense, acknowledged the public interest in alternative treatments in its extensive article, "Living Well—Alternative Medicine." In it, the pros and cons of numerous therapies were defined and addressed. One of the subset articles was on "Hypnosis and Biofeedback." In this segment authors cited the relevance of these therapies, "If you still think of hypnosis as some hocus-pocus, mumbo-jumbo technique, think again. The American Psychiatric Association, The American Psychological Association and the American Dental Association all have endorsed the technique. Thousands of U.S. doctors now use hypnosis to overcome the pain of chronic headaches, backaches, childbirth, cancer, severe burns, as well as neutralizing dental phobias, and more."[2]

A significant percentage of the public has accepted and embraced the ideas of the psychology of mind-body connect. "An estimated one in three adult Americans used an unconventional therapy at least once in 1990,"[3] and we can expect to see this number increase. Public interest can be seen by perusing mainstream magazine stands, the windows of bookstores, and scanning best seller lists. You probably have magazines in your reception area right now that include articles on the subject! The interest in this and related topics is regarded in some circles as "new age quackery". However, researchers, scientists, doctors, and philosophers have studied the concept for years. Hippocrates, the father of medicine, noted that, "The natural healing force within each one of us is the greatest force in getting well."

The cover of another mainstream publication, *Ladies Home Journal* was strongly supportive with an article, "Mind Over Pain."[4] In it, authors Domar and Dreher report on research into pain and pain management. Domar who researched and practiced mind-body medicine at Harvard Medical School's Division of Behavioral Medicine, suggests that "pain signals can become programmed into our central nervous systems and that people who change their mind-sets about pain can change the actual experience of pain."

THE PRACTITIONER AND THE HEALTHCARE PROFESSIONS

Relating the mind-body connect to medicine and dentistry can require a grand leap for the practitioner. It has been long associated with traditional western therapies that the practitioner *fix* or *do something* to alleviate patient pain and disease. There may be a "subtle but real bias against approaches that lessen the patient's dependence upon the doctor and his procedures."[5]

In interviewing some dentists on this topic, I found a wide range of responses. One dentist commented on the regional interest in the subject and the fact that some patients are more extreme than others.

> *Many dental professionals have trouble with some of the alternative views and acceptance by the public can vary depending on region of the country and whether one is in a metropolitan city or a rural area. I'm from a pretty open-minded area and there is wide acceptance locally, yet I know some of my peers who scoff at patients who come to the office with these ideas.*

Another dentist commented,

*Many of my colleagues have a lot of trou-
ble with the more alternative views. I deal
with it every day and I find that it doesn't
matter what patients think, when it comes
to clinical dentistry I can still provide
excellent clinical treatment. But in terms
of relationship, it is critical for the
patients to know they are being listened to
and taken seriously. Several doctors I've
told stories to express that they'd laugh at
the patient for a similar expression or
point of view. Tolerance is required.*

This tolerance needs to be understood and
practiced by all members of the dental team.

A third practitioner offered a unique way of
measuring the possible interest in his area. He said,

*We've noticed in the past five years a seri-
ous increase in health food stores and
courses offered in Yoga and Meditation.
Also, we've found that a lot of patients
who are into fitness are also aware of the
mind-body connect, because they experience it on a very personal level. So if there
are a lot of exercise clubs or gyms in the
area, there may also be a higher receptivity to mind-body philosophies.*

Professionally, care should be taken of spreading
oneself so thin that credibility is lost. If a patient enters a
practice and finds health food, vitamins, and various other
non-dental products for sale, the patient may start to view
the practice as one seeking alternative forms of income,
instead of offering alternative forms of treatment. If
patients view the practice as a "store" more than a place of
treatment, then the practitioner may have "crossed the
line" of credibility and patient trust. When patients have
been queried about this in our focus groups, the majority

found the idea unappealing. This was most offensive with patients of higher educational and socioeconomic levels. If the product did not relate directly to dentistry, patients found it confusing and questionable.

APPLICABILITY IN THE PRACTICE

View of the patient as a "whole person" can take many forms. As a "mystery patient", when I find a sign-in sheet at the front desk of the practice, there is frequently a check-off question in relation to health changes. When the public is dealing with voice mail and lack of human touch, we would prefer to be asked about health changes by a humanistic person who will show interest and communicate sincere care in any discussion that ensues. But a check off list that says, "I've had health/medication changes since my last visit: yes/no" is much like that voice mail system that doesn't allow the caller to ever talk with a human being, or the answering machine that will not take messages.

It may not be feasible or necessary to conduct such an interview on each patient appointment. However adding such a segment to an annual appointment when x-ray updates are made would increase patient perception of a "whole body" dental office, and one that takes a sincere interest in the health of its patients.

A patient in one of our focus groups addressed this issue as follows:

I'd been a patient of the practice for about two years and the office was okay ... I just went in for regular six-month cleanings. But the last visit there was a new hygien-ist—she was incredible, really warm and responsive. What I remember most was that before she did anything, she sat down

*and talked to me as a human being! She
went over my past history and asked specific questions about my medication and
a surgery I'd had. She was extremely professional and I felt like she cleaned my
teeth better too.*

It was interesting that after the positive
interpersonal transaction and the personalized updating of
the patient's history, there was a perception of excellent
clinical skills, as well. This same patient also made
negative comparisons of previous hygienist skills as
opposed to this new, more attentive, practitioner.

MIND-BODY AND FEAR

Nathan Friedman, DDS, Clinical Professor and
Founder of the Department of Behavioral Dentistry at
University of Southern California School of Dentistry in Los
Angeles, CA has developed the Iatrosedative Process
wherein the dental practitioner can relate to and treat the
patient's dental fear. This involves a specific pattern of
communication techniques that results in the patient's
sense of greater control and in a stronger relationship
between patient and practitioner. In this process the
patient participates in a structured interview with the
practitioner wherein a bond of trust develops.[6] This is
certainly another application of the mind-body connect
that aids in patient confidence and belief in the practitioner
and in the practice.

In dentistry, what is the most significant and
widely accepted application of mind-body connect relates
to verbal and nonverbal communication. It is a matter of
seeing the patient as a whole person, not just a tooth.

Patients in focus groups note the way they feel about their experiences in their dental offices with comments like,

- "I sat in that chair for three hours and I felt like a 'thing.' They didn't talk to me, or ask me how I was feeling. I felt like a car up on an auto rack!"
- "I could hear the dentist in the next room talking about a patient. He said . . . 'Beth Jones? Oh yeah, you mean the extraction!' She wasn't a person, she was a tooth!"
- "It was the first time any doctor had treated me that way; she was caring and gentle and asked me frequently during the treatment, 'How are you doing?'"

HYPNOSIS AND BIOFEEDBACK

The understanding and application of the mind-body connect has been long recognized in the study of anxiety and pain management as in the use of biofeedback and hypnosis. A cover story of *AGD Impact* addressed this topic. William W. Howard, DMD, MAGD suggested,

> *I feel strongly that every dentist should benefit by receiving at least some instruction in hypnosis ... a good course in hypnosis should deal with principles of patient management that should make any practice more enjoyable for both dentists and patients.*[7]

There even exists an association specifically for clinical practitioners who use hypnosis as a part of therapy. The American Society of Clinical Hypnosis (ASCH) has components across the United States and Canada. The ASCH offers workshops and accreditation for professionals.[8]

Biofeedback and other modalities can afford patients a measure of awareness and control in situations that might otherwise produce a high stress response. Research study of biofeedback by dental patients was conducted by Dr. Richard Hirschman. Dr. Hirschman used an electromymyographic (EMG) device with his patients and trained them on its use as well as in relaxation techniques. He found that those patients who were trained in this technique were less anxious than those who were not trained.[9,10]

Reasonably priced biofeedback devices are now available for purchase through retail outlets and mail order companies that offer high technology and health products. The Association for Applied Psychophyfiology and Biofeedback can offer additional information on the subject.[11]

FOCUS GROUP RESPONSE

The interest in alternative medicine and treatment has become so widespread, that we decided to introduce the subject into some of our dental focus groups. The majority of the participants indicated a basic understanding and belief in the concepts. When we talked about application via communication, the practitioner helping to alleviate fear and anxiety through non-pharmacological means, these same patients were highly enthusiastic, though somewhat questioning of how that could be effected. Some of them were aware of biofeedback and its use in clinical treatments.

Most interesting, however, were the responses in relation to hypnosis. Before using the word *hypnosis,* we talked about the process of controlling one's inner state to help to reduce anxiety and pain response. Focus group participants were responsive to the concept. As we progressed into applying the word *hypnosis* to this, there was a decided drop in positive responsiveness. The expressed concern related to perceptions of hypnosis as a process where one would "lose control" of the self. Some patients drew parallels to the images one might see in a Las Vegas stage show. A much smaller percentage of the group remained confident in this process once this word was used in relation to it. With increased understanding and awareness of how hypnosis can be used in a professional, clinical environment, I believe we will see greater acceptance of the word as well as the process.

A doctor spoke to me privately after I had addressed this issue in a state seminar. He noted that he used techniques of hypnosis with *all* his patients, but that he no longer used the word in applying the methods. He said that 20 years earlier he had studied application of hypnotic techniques in reducing patient anxiety. He tried to convince patients of the benefits of hypnosis, but through this disclosure of intent, he unwittingly drove some patients away from his practice. He still used the basic concepts without using the word. This affirmed what we learned in focus groups.

STRAIGHT FROM THE PATIENT'S MOUTH: PATIENT SURVEY AND FOCUS GROUP COMMENTS

I mentioned to the hygienist that I was on a macrobiotic diet and that my internist wasn't able to help me manage my disease. The next time I went in for a cleaning, the hygienist said she'd talked with the dentist and that most of these "oddball" techniques [macrobiotics] didn't work and that the dentist had another internist for me to try. I was really offended. I didn't say anything, but I never went back. They had no idea how insensitive that was; they thought they were being helpful!

The dentist I went to when I was a kid was clueless when it came to anxiety ... or he just didn't care. My dentist now really knows how to help me feel more at ease; she talks to me about how I'm feeling emotionally; she knows my history of bad dental experiences. Even her voice is soothing! I don't feel embarrassed about my anxiety the way I used to because I know she understands.

They had a display of vitamins and it looked like multi-level marketing products. It really turned me off. It looked like a store, not like a dental office.

I'll try just about anything that will help me get a grip on my fear. It goes way back to childhood, but I've yet to find a dentist or medical doctor who has a reasonable solution that puts me in control of my emotions.

TOP TIPS:

1. You don't have to accept or "buy" alternative treatments or the idea of holistic therapies. However, it is critical to be knowledgeable about this trend so you can discuss the viewpoint with your patients with some understanding.
2. Monitor the attitudes in your area by watching for indicators like, health food stores, biofeedback, yoga and meditation classes, local/regional best-selling books, etc.
3. Listen to patient discussion topics and make notes in patient records as to attitudes and interests in this area.
4. Ensure that staff understands the significance of this movement and its possible impact on the practice. Make sure that no one on the team attempts to "correct" patient viewpoints which may not be in agreement with their own. Intolerance in the dental team won't be tolerated by patients!
5. Ask employees to bring into staff meetings any articles on alternative treatments that may influence patient attitudes, interests, or concerns. Also ask them to make note of any news reports on TV or radio. Discuss these at meetings so that the team is aware of trends.
6. Verbally check with patients on health and medication updates; reassure patients that you are sensitive to their overall health changes that may influence treatments.
7. Communicate with the patient as a "whole person" rather than as a "tooth" or a "case" by listening to their concerns and responding with care and sensitivity.

REFERENCES

[1] _____, "An Amazingly Easy Cure for Dental Phobia," *First Magazine*, Englewood Cliffs, NJ, September, 1994.

[2] _____, "Living Well: Alternative Medicine," *Good Housekeeping Magazine*, March, 1994.

[3] Squires, Sally. "The New Medicine," *Modern Maturity*, American Association for Retired Persons, October, 1996.

[4] Domar, Ph.D., Alice D.; Dreher, Henry. "Mind Over Pain," *Ladies Home Journal*, August, 1996.

[5] Ornish, M.D., Dean. *Stress, Diet and Your Heart*, Holt Rinehart and Winston, New York, NY, 1982.

[6] Friedman, D.D.S., Nathan. "Fear Reduction with the Iatrosedative Process," *Journal of the California Dental Association*, March, 1993.

[7] Howard, DMD, MAGD, William W. "All Dentists Should be Literate in Hypnosis," *AGD Impact*, Chicago, IL, July, 1994.

[8] The ASCH is based in Des Plaines, IL. Information may be obtained by calling (708) 297-3317.

[9] Ingersoll, Ph.D., Barbara D. *Behavioral Aspects in Dentistry*, Appleton-Century-Crofts, Norwalk, CT, 1982.

[10] Association for Applied Psychophyfiology and Biofeedback is located at 10200 West 44th Avenue, Suite 304, Wheat Ridge, CO, 80033, 1-800-477-8892.

8

Patient Rights and Informed Consent

"So what happens if I sign it and I'm one of those exceptions?
What if the worst case scenario happens to me?"
— Focus Group Participant

DISCLAIMER: Insights and opinions offered here are
not to be considered legal advice. An attorney should
be consulted in relation to any legal questions.

Patients are becoming more knowledgeable about
the issues of patients' rights. Also the public is more
litigious than they were in the past and perhaps
more so in the United States than in other countries. It is
wise for the dental practitioner to recognize these two
issues go hand in hand: patient rights and informed
consent. It is imperative that as patient knowledge evolves,

communication skills of the entire dental team must evolve also. It is key that practitioners become more knowledgeable in their responsibilities to deliver informed consent to patients in a patient-friendly manner.

PATIENT AWARENESS OF PRACTITIONER RESPONSIBILITY

I was conducting research on the Internet to investigate what information is available to dental patients. In one of the dental news groups I learned about a very interesting on-line site that was under construction. An individual who had experienced a catastrophic dental injury was in the process of establishing a "dental injury hot-line" to be set up as a computer bulletin board service. This patient was interested in providing data to other dental patients. The range of information he intended to cover was extensive, including case histories from other patients.

This was a patient who had a high level of involvement and personal interest in the issues of patient rights and informed consent. He was highly knowledgeable as well, including insights and viewpoints into the dental peer review process. He expressed his goal of developing an informational database to help advise patients on key issues. He also wanted to provide information to the dental profession about patient needs and concerns. No, this was not the average dental patient, but he had a voice that was being heard and responded to.

He represents a segment of the population who are seeking information of this type. The computer and the Internet are making the world smaller and the most vocal members of the community will find each other! The responses posted to this news group list indicated interest. His venue and his voice might be considered "fringe" now, but public interest indicates a stronger movement to come.

There is a strong patient movement toward using technology for health information and it could be misinformation. Needless to say, there will be more and more clinical information available to patients on the Internet. Doctors will be dealing with more educated consumers who will have the right questions to ask.

Patients are willing to ask more questions than in the past. Gone are the days when all patients thought that the doctor was always right. As one dentist put it, "In the past, practitioner-to-patient dialogue was like an adult-to-child communication, but today it's more of an adult-to-adult communication. Some patients are willing to challenge the practitioner and may feel comfortable in getting second opinions as well." Dr. Alan Selbst, lawyer and endodontist from Houston, TX, advised, "Every practitioner needs to be cognizant about patient activism, that it is critically important to engage patients into the decision-making process that affects their bodies."

Litigation has been a concern for all healthcare practitioners and organizations and for good reason; the public is quick to find fault and the court is frequently the meeting place for patients and practitioners who are both unhappy. Dentistry is not immune. "Dental malpractice litigation has increased significantly in the last few years." It is the area of "negligent non-disclosure" that may be cause of special concern. This occurs when a doctor "does everything right technically; however, he may be found negligent if he failed to inform the patient of the inherent risks of the procedure and one of those risks manifests itself."[1] Statutes and court decisions as to what constitutes informed consent can vary from state to state, and this makes the issue even more complex.[2, 3, 4]

PATIENT RIGHTS

The informed and empowered patient is apt to be a wise "consumer" of any healthcare service. Patients are learning what to question and what is appropriate and what is inappropriate in patient rights and practitioner communications. The National Health Council, a private, nonprofit group of health organizations produced a consumer information guide, "Putting Patients First: Patient Rights and Responsibilities". This booklet is a consumer aid in understanding rights in making healthcare decisions. The item listed first indicated that patients have the right to "Informed consent and treatment decisions, timely access to specialty care and confidentiality protections."[5] Other items include gaining information in relation to insurance coverage, cost of services, and information on providers. It is however, the first issue which is of primary concern to both patients and practitioners.

In the *Principles of Ethics and Code of Professional Conduct* published by the American Dental Association, item 1-L states that, "The dentist should inform the patient of the proposed treatment, and any reasonable alternatives, in a manner that allows the patient to become involved in treatment decisions."[6]

THE PATIENT'S PERSPECTIVE

As an undercover patient, I'm periodically presented with a very basic, very broad-based, generic consent-for-treatment form as a part of the new patient registration protocol. This form may indicate that "the doctor has advised me of the dental treatment that is needed . . . "—yet it is given to the patient *prior* to even meeting the doctor, and is verbalized in a generic manner to apply to any treatment. In some cases risks and complications are indicated—risks which are also broad-based and may relate to numerous types of treatments.

The first time I saw this I was quite surprised that a patient would be presented with such a form before any treatment plan is even discussed. I took the new patient form back to the front desk and gave it back to the receptionist. I'd completed the medical history portion, but left the generic consent portion blank and unsigned. The receptionist asked me about that segment of the form and I replied, "Well, I don't feel comfortable about signing this because I haven't seen the doctor yet." I've since seen this type of general consent on several occasions in relation to my new patient visits, and I've had reservations and concerns about this approach since.

In discussing this issue with dental patients in focus groups, there is a wide range of awareness related to this section of a new patient information form. Some patients remark that they arbitrarily sign it and may not even read what they are signing. Many patients are unaware of the differences between signing a broad informed consent that appears on a new patient form versus signing validation of the information they've just provided in the medical history.

In a number of my own undercover visits, I've refused to sign the consent form if it is a standard part of the new patient information form and I've not yet met the doctor. My interest has been to see how this might be handled by team members. I have never had any staff members balk at my refusal to sign, and I would be very concerned about the practice if any team member did.

Some practitioners have concerns about the amount of information to be provided to the patient. At what point does the type or amount of information create undue anxiety in the patient's mind? I polled a group of dentists nationwide to understand the practitioner's point of view. One dentist queried, "Does asking for the informed consent signature decrease patient trust? Could it inject an adversarial element to the relationship?" Another practitioner noted, "... information is power ... offer more information to patients and they'll feel more confident that they are armed to make the best decisions."

Then there is the perspective voiced by numerous practitioners polled: build relationships with patients, instill trust in the patient for the practice first, then dealing with the issue of informed consent will not be perceived as adversarial. The practitioners who offered this insight all had been in practice over 20 years and were known for their long-term relationships with patients and patient families. They were *not* suggesting that providing appropriate informed consent was not necessary, but that the process was easier and the likelihood of litigation decreased with development of positive patient relationships.

"Relationship, relationship, relationship", were the words of Dr. Fred Aurbach of Dallas, TX, who suggested that, " ... intent and ethics are questioned less in a relationship that has been built on trust." We have interviewed hundreds of patients nationwide on many, many topics, and I am a firm believer that this is an enormously important concept: the trusting relationship can weather difficult times far more readily than the weak affiliation. Dr. Edwin Zinman of San Francisco, CA, adds, "For the same reason, if trust is breached, the patient feels betrayed." For example, if the patient were not forewarned about the risks, or complications were minimized by the dentist, then patient trust is dissolved.

This perspective was also affirmed by dentist-attorney experts.[7] Dr. Jack Weichman, is an endodontist, attorney, and arbitrator for the Los Angeles Superior Court. In the seminars he conducts for dentists on the subject of informed consent, Dr. Weichman notes that, "Malpractice prevention can be broken down into two main categories:

Patient relations and Record keeping." He advises that when strong relationships are built with patients, there is less likelihood of a patient filing a lawsuit. "The dentist who calls the patient in the evening following a procedure, goes a long way toward communicating genuine care and enhancing that relationship." Although the record keeping may seem a nuisance at times, Weichman observes, " ... either you take the time now to put it in the records when the patient is there, or, you spend the time writing to your insurance carrier, answering interrogatories, having your deposition taken, and going to trial."

WHAT THIS MEANS TO THE PRACTITIONER

Dr. Norton Bicoll of Dallas, TX has been a member of the Dallas Peer Review Committee for several years. He notes that maintaining a trusting relationship is a key factor in avoiding legal complications with patients. The majority of cases that have come before the peer review relate to communications problems between practitioner and patient ... problems that might not have occurred had there been a warm, honest, and open relationship with the patient.

Of course you still must have records that indicate appropriate information given to the patient. Bicoll states, "I make sure I have three instances shown in our records of informing the patient. It could be a combination of written information provided to the patient, an office discussion, and a phone call to the patient, for example." He routinely calls the patient in the evening after a patient's appointment to ensure that there is patient comprehension of the information that was provided and to encourage questions from the patient. "If a practitioner has a strong track record of educating the patient and soliciting patient questions, there's less likelihood of running into problems." From the patient's point of view, the practitioner will be seen as a caring and very professional one as well.

Dr. Terry Dickinson of Houston, TX, is one of many practitioners who suggests that dentists ask patients questions that, "can't be answered with 'yes' or 'no', in other words, ask open-ended questions. Get answers to *how, why, what, when, where.*" These type of questions will give you greater insights into patient comprehension.

Although laws do vary from state to state, and it is crucial for the practitioner to know the law in the state where he/she practices, the following are typical common law elements of disclosure:

ELEMENTS OF DISCLOSURE[8]

The typical common law elements of disclosure are:

    1. nature of the procedure [in lay terms],

    2. inherent [foreseeable] risks of the proce dure, and

    3. anticipated benefits of the procedure.

It has been suggested that the following be disclosed:

    4. disclosure of the inherent risks of the alter native procedures, and

    5. a generalized opportunity to question the doctor about any of the above mentioned elements.

Dr. Zinman also suggests that patients be advised of the consequences of doing noth-ing.

THE POWER OF EFFECTIVE COMMUNICATION

Patients feel more cared for when there are open lines of communication and the doctor encourages the patient to voice thoughts, opinions, and questions. This process also "demonstrates that the treatment is being personalized to the patient's needs. By encouraging questions, informed consent allows patients to have an important part in controlling their own therapy."[9] There are certainly benefits for the practitioner, although disclosing data may be challenging for the doctor, patients feel that process of communication and mutual decision-making is valued [and represents] progress toward the dentist's professional ideal."[10] We took an informal poll of practitioners and experts in relation to the significance of effective communication in this matter.

Dr. Stephen Schwartz, an endodontist from Houston, TX, emphasizes the importance of the patient-practitioner relationship. He notes that if there is a depersonalization in the quality of care provided to the patient, "It's going to take away the patient's compassion that they might ordinarily have for an honest mistake. Honest mistakes are not going to be tolerated when you don't have any relationship at all with the caregiver."

A consultant and speaker on the subject of communications, Robin Wright of Evanston, IL has researched and written extensively on the topic of risk communications. Wright suggests,

> *Patients feel greater comfort and increased sense of power when they are involved in the treatment discussion. Lay people do not want a one-way communication of experts to the public. They seek two-way communication and full participation in making risk decisions. In addi-*

tion, two-sided messages, presenting both advantages and disadvantages are judged more trustworthy than when only advantages are presented.[11]

One respondent related a communication process he uses to provide total disclosure and build patient trust at the same time. He provides to the patient a detailed informed consent form that relates to the specific treatment. When he brings up a possible complication to the treatment, he immediately explains the steps he will take to avoid that complication. He has found this to be a highly successful method to help the patient through the decision-making process. Following this process, hopefully the patient thinks:

- the dentist told me why I need this treatment,
- there are possible complications with the treatment, and
- the dentist is aware of the complications and is going to do his best to confront and manage them. If they occur he will know what to do.
- If I don't have the treatment, my condition may worsen or I may have other related problems.

The practitioner has staved off unsettling patient concerns about complications by initiating discussion and then directly addressing the subject. Once a patient knows you are open to discussing an issue, you are more likely to gain the patient's respect. Also you are likely to gain access to what would normally be unspoken attitudes, enabling you to address patient fears or objections.

Some of the doctors who responded to our informal poll indicated a concern about scaring the patient. One posed, "Does the patient want to know, or need to know that the local anesthetic can cause death? I think the reasonable things the patient can expect should be considered ... not every extreme possibility, i.e., a brain abscess can result from the bacterium instigated by brushing and/or flossing their teeth!"

The dentist does need to "disclose all information that a reasonable person would find *material* or meaningful in making a decision whether to consent to a proposed treatment."[12] In most states there is no legal duty to inform the patient of remote risks. Experts in the combined fields of dentistry and law agree that disclosure is *not* an option, it is a given.[13] It is required that the practitioner give full disclosure to patients, and that includes addressing the topic of death in relation to the treatment, if that is a reasonable possibility. In some states the exception to this rule is if the patient requests, "don't tell me the risks." In the process of giving full disclosure it is crucial that the information be provided in language the patient understands. Many patients may be hesitant to ask a practitioner to explain technical terms and misunderstandings can result.

Dr. Selbst offered this insight,

How much and what you disclose varies from state to state, so it's important to know the requirements within one's own state. Adverse occurrences that are considered to be so rare and remote need not be disclosed to the reasonable patient. However, if one disclosed to the patient what a reasonable patient would expect to know: the risks, the benefits, and the options, and if those were somewhere memorialized in their records, I think that would constitute significant evidence of informed consent.

Key words here are: "reasonable patient" and "memorialized." Keep in mind that the standard of "reasonable" may vary from state to state. Nevertheless, a key factor in all of this is the memorializing in the record the instances of adequately and appropriately informing the patient.

MEMORIALIZING DISCLOSURE AND CONSENT

What are the ways that the disclosure and consent can be memorialized? There is far more involved in this process than can be, or should be, addressed in this book. To view the possibilities from the patient's point of view, however, the oral consent is arguably the easiest and quickest. The downside is that it may not stand up in court, and it lacks the message of patient value. That is, when you've taken the time to offer information on paper, you are educating the patient and also communicating the value and importance of the patient. You are memorializing in a manner which will have more meaning to a jury than an oral consent.

Numerous organizations offer preprinted consent forms that include information on the elements of disclosure.[14] Using customized forms specific to the treatment will aid in building credibility and patient trust.

Technology is coming into play in this area also. The consent form may be customized by computer to the specific treatment and to the specific patient, providing a highly credible document and one that communicates well to the patient. Videotape of treatment disclosure is starting to be used in this process as well. Videotapes are available that are specific to different procedures. A caveat here, however: if the patient leaves the office with the videotape, this does not prove that the tape was viewed by the patient, unless upon return of the tape the patient signs a form acknowledging having viewed the tape in its entirety. A tape that is viewed while the patient is in the office and so noted on the records would be perceived as more credible by a jury.

Video may be highly viable in the area of aesthetics as well. As with plastic surgeons, unrealistic patient expectations prior to treatment may result in dissatisfaction following a procedure. For this reason, the visual records are particularly valuable. Availability of video technology in the office provides another benefit. A microphone can be attached to the patient's chair in the treatment room. Conversation and actual treatment can be recorded on video. This can provide an excellent legal record.

Dr. Weichman adds an important point in relation to record keeping. "Keep full notes on everything that goes on, including phone calls from patients or relatives of patients. If you get an angry phone call stating, 'you ruined my mother's mouth', that should definitely be placed in the records. If profanity or foul language is used by patient or relative, that should be noted in the records also."

WHAT PART DOES THE TEAM PLAY?

Staff plays a very important role in communicating with patients, but the role of providing informed consent legally cannot be delegated to staff; the doctor must do this. Dr. Edwin Zinman tried a case wherein staff was entirely providing the disclosure. In the trial, the staff testified that if there were any patient questions, the dentist was available. The jury found that there was inadequate informed consent despite the fact that the consent form was signed and despite the fact the patient said he understood everything according to the consent form. Staff can supplement but not replace the dentist's duty. Dr. Jack Weichman suggests that staff members be in the treatment room when disclosure is given to the patient and that a staff member, and the doctor also sign the consent form.

Staff members are enormously important in influencing patient perceptions of the entire practice. Though the team members at the front desk are not involved in the clinical issues, they color patient viewpoints of the entire office. Attitude of staff can help to ease patient concerns about results of a treatment or can increase patient anxiety. All team members must recognize their responsibility to patients and to the practice.

STRAIGHT FROM THE PATIENT'S MOUTH: PATIENT SURVEY AND FOCUS GROUP COMMENTS

I get the 'consent' part, but I don't get the 'informed' part. When I sign the form, aren't I just giving permission to do the procedure?

I'm going to take my cues from my dentist. I really trust her and if she says there's little risk, then that's all I need to know.

If the doc is going to do a really serious surgery, then I've got to feel okay about him personally. I don't want to hear somebody I don't know or don't trust telling me that something could go wrong!

If they tell me all the bad things that can happen and I don't see that there are enough benefits for taking those chances, then I won't go through with the treatment.

I would never sue my dentist. Even if I signed the consent and something went wrong. I've been a patient there for over 22 years and they're like family to me.

TOP TIPS:

1. Develop genuinely caring and trusting relationships with patients.
2. Listen actively to patients and take notes when it seems appropriate to do so.
3. Ask open ended questions to increase understanding of patient's position.
4. Establish a pattern of consistently educating patients in all procedures.
5. Provide written information about treatments and potential likely risks specific to treatments.
6. Keep accurate notes in records about oral consent given.
7. Have a team member in the room when treatment information is given.
8. Ensure that the dentist is the primary source of information in relation to informed consent and that the dentist maintains the ultimate responsibility in such.
9. Ensure that the patient is given an accurate perspective with the benefits as well as the potential complications, alternatives, and consequences of non-treatment.

REFERENCES

[1] Selbst, DMD, MS, JD, Alan. "Understanding Informed Consent and Its Relationship to the Incidence of Adverse Treatment Events in Conventional Endodontic Therapy," *Journal of the American Association of Endodontists*, August, 1990.

[2] Selbst, DMD, MS, JD, Alan. "Understanding Informed Consent and Its Relationship to the Incidence of Adverse Treatment Events in Conventional Endodontic Therapy," *Journal of the American Association of Endodontists*, August, 1990.

[3] Bailey, JD, Beverly. "Informed Consent in Dentistry," *Journal of the American Dental Association*, May, 1985.

[4] Additional information specific to malpractice and how to avoid litigation may be found in *Malpractice: What They Didn't Teach You in Dental School* by Jeffrey J. Tonner, J.C., PennWell Books, Tulsa, OK, 1996.

[5] The brochure, "Putting Patients First: Patients' Rights & Responsibilities," is available from the National Health Council, Washington, DC, (202) 785-3910.

[6] Council on Ethics, ByLaws and Judicial Affairs, *ADA Principles of Ethics and Code of Professional Conduct*, American Dental Association, Chicago, IL, January, 1993.

[7] Interviews were conducted by Suzanne Boswell in the writing of this chapter, with Stephen Schwartz, DDS, MS; Norton Bicoll, DDS, Alan Selbst, DMD, MS, JD, Edwin Zinman, DDS, JD, and Jack Weichman, DDS, JD who is also an arbitrator-mediator and expert witness with the Los Angeles Superior Court.

[8] Selbst, DMD, MS, JD, Alan. "Understanding Informed Consent and Its Relationship to the Incidence of Adverse Treatment Events in Conventional Endodontic Therapy," *Journal of the American Association of Endodontists*, August, 1990.

[9] Council on Insurance, "Informed Consent: A Risk Management View," *Journal of the American Dental Association*, October, 1987.

[10] Ozar, Ph.D., David; Sokol, DDS, JD, F.A.G.D., David. *Dental Ethics at Chairside*, Mosby-Year Book, Inc., St. Louis, MO, 1994.

[11] Wright, MA, Robin. *Tough Questions, Great Answers: Responding to Patient Concerns about Today's Dentistry*, Quintessence Publishing Co., Inc., Carol Stream, IL, 1997.

[12] Rule, DDS, MS, James; Veatch, Ph.D., Robert. *Ethical Questions in Dentistry*, Quintessence Publishing Co., Inc., Carol Stream, IL, 1993.

[13] Interviews were conducted by Suzanne Boswell in the writing of this chapter, with Stephen Schwartz, DDS, MS; Norton Bicoll, DDS, Alan Selbst, DMD, MS, JD, Edwin Zinman, DDS, JD, and Jack Weichman, DDS, JD who is also an arbitrator-mediator and expert witness with the Los Angeles Superior Court.

[14] One organization that offers consent forms on a variety of treatments is, Stepping Stones to Success, located in Pueblo, CO. (719) 545-0511.

PART 2

Impression Management and Self Presentation

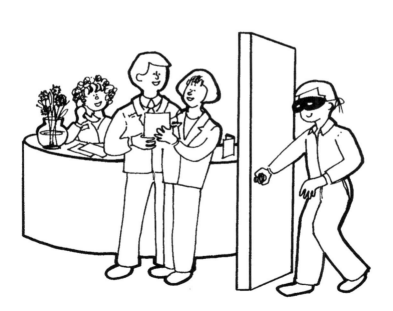

If I knew you and you knew me,
If both of us could clearly see,
And with an inner sight divine
The meaning of your heart and mine.

I'm sure that we would differ less,
and clasp our hands in friendliness
Our thoughts would pleasantly agree
If I knew you and you knew me.

— N I X O N   W A T E R M A N

How well do you really know and understand your patients? Understanding their issues, feelings, and concerns is vital to retaining your patients and gaining new ones. It means recognizing the outside world environment that your patients are dealing with, as addressed in Part 1. It also means understanding how the public might see your entire team and the office itself. It means looking at how you self-present and how well you and the entire team manage the impressions made on your patients and prospective patients.

In this section we will investigate how the team can present itself most positively to the public and what it will take to gain and retain patients in a challenging marketplace. The chapters in Part 2 address questions of prime importance to dental practices today including:

- How do patients choose a dental practice?
- What are the *do's* and *don'ts* of telephone protocol from the patient's perspective?
- How can the practice communicate positively on paper to the patient?
- What influences patients' perceptions in relation to decor and the facility?
- How do patients want to be communicated with by staff and doctor(s)?

- How can the practice maintain a balance between expectation and reality in the patient's mind?
- Most importantly, what does it really take to build good long-term patient relationships?

It is important that the entire dental team recognize that every one of these issues is manageable. It is up to the team to acknowledge that this is a group responsibility and the group must ensure that a positive message is sent out to patients in order to retain present patient base, gain new patients, develop relationships with patients, and increase the likelihood of treatment acceptance.

IMPRESSION MANAGEMENT AND SELF-PRESENTATION

We all manage the impressions we make on other people to varying degrees. Sometimes we do it with careful planning and with an eye on the desired outcome, such as in an interview situation or in giving a speech. Other times we may not realize that we are in the process of impression management because the actions are so deeply ingrained, such as in the giving of common courtesies, an automatic "thank you" offered in response. Even if there is no conscious concern for the impression being made on others, one cannot deny that, by way of our existence, others will have an impression of us—who and what we are. That impression can occur even if they have never met or seen us. It can come from hearing or reading about us.

With the understanding that you will be making an impression on others on an individual basis, it is critical to gain an understanding of the process that your patients go through in viewing you, your team, and your entire practice. One of the seminars we offer on this subject matter is "What Do You Say Before You Say Hello?" That question applies here. How are you communicating with your patients before you ever speak to them yourself? First, let's look at defining two very important terms: *Self-Presentation* and *Impression Management.*

The term *self-presentation* is used to describe how we present ourselves to others without consciously thinking about it.[1] When we "self present" we are communicating to others in a most natural and automatic manner. Self-presentation includes the elements of basic communication including the verbal, vocal, and visual. Social psychologists use the term *impression management* to describe the process by which we monitor our presentation to others. This is done on a conscious level and indicates a desire to control the image that is being projected to others. We are socialized to manage some aspects of impression on others. For example, polite manners, appropriate clothing, and grooming are often taught at an early age. Parents who attend to this recognize and value the greater acceptance of their children and themselves by society. These parents strive to manage the impressions the children might have on others.

Likewise, it is crucial for key elements of the dental practice to be managed. Throughout the following chapters you will find numerous ways the entire team can manage effectively and positively the experience patients will have in the practice. Remember this, if *you* don't manage the impressions of your practice, then someone or something else will! For example, if your patients hear a radio station playing when they are on hold, then you have given up management of the impression of your office to that radio station. Do you want a DJ, newscaster, or perhaps Howard Stern to be the arbiter of taste and quality in relation to your practice?!

The terms and concepts of *impression management* and *self-presentation* will be used throughout this book and it is important to understand the subtle differences between the two. As much as possible, all team members need to be aware of how they may be perceived by patients. This means taking the concept of *self-presentation* into a conscious mode and managing it, in other words, *impression management*. Awareness of how one is perceived is a first critical step towards communicating positively with patients. It is exceedingly important that the impressions made on the patient be managed.

There is a flip side to this, however. Patients could respond negatively if they thought every means of communication was being measured by the practice or the members of the team came across in a superficial, patronizing, or contrived manner. There is a delicate balance here. When you manage impressions of your office because you value your patients and want to provide only excellent quality service, your patients will respond positively.

THE THREE PHASES OF PATIENT PERCEPTIONS

From our patient surveys and interviews we have identified three phases that patients go through in viewing and understanding the dental practice. Let us look at this process through the eyes of a new patient.

The *Pre-Appointment Phase* includes any printed matter produced by the office that the patient sees. This means documents like letters, notes, brochures, newsletters, and any forms that you may send the patient. The type of paper you use, the colors, logo, typeface, all are communicating about you to your patients. This subject matter is addressed at length in chapter 10.

Also in the pre-appointment phase are patient perceptions of your practice based on phone contact with your office. This includes matters involving telephone protocol, telephone systems, and the vocal and verbal skills of your team. This subject matter is addressed at length in chapters 11 and 12. Patients also make judgments about your practice based on any phone book listings, particularly display ads in the Yellow Pages. Promotional materials which are sent via direct mail and/or any advertising items fall into the area of the pre-appointment phase as well.

The *Appointment Phase* starts with the impression the patient gets from your location. When patients view the complex or building where your office is located, they start to anticipate what your office will be like. The maintenance of the facility, the safety of the location, and the cosmetic features of the facility represent you even if you do not have the responsibility of maintaining these areas. The patient perceives that your choice of this location represents a certain level of acceptance of its appearance. The appointment phase includes then, everything from appearance of the facility on the outside, parking, decor, physical appearances of your office itself, and all of the team interactions that occur throughout the appointment.

The *Post-Appointment Phase* starts at the close of the clinical appointment. It is here where patients in our focus groups comment on how they viewed their overall experience with the practice. From the moment that patients leave the treatment room and walk to the counter, they are starting to judge whether the practice put more emphasis on them as a "case," an income source, or whether the patient is seen as a human being who is cared for and is a valued member of the practice family. What occurs during the final moments in the office is revealing for the patient. This is the point when patients reflect on their expectations and consider whether those expectations were met or whether they were let down. For the new patient this is a time-compressed process because they have had only one experience in the office. These issues are addressed in chapter 19 in relation to financial matters and in chapter 21 where you will learn how patients view their experiences following an appointment in your office.

Some might say that once the patient has reached the post appointment phase their perceptions are set, that you can no longer influence their thinking about your practice. This is not the case. The reality is that you are still in the position to improve relationships with the patient and increase positive perceptions of your practice based on your actions. In this section we will look at specific steps that you can take to help develop and maintain long-term relationships with patients.

In the final chapter of this book, Twenty-two Top Tips, you will learn the issues that are raised most frequently by patients in our focus groups. I strongly suggest that the practice give these areas very special consideration. In the on-going quest to gain and retain patients, these are issues that many of your patients will be highly sensitive to. In a staff meeting, rate your office on each of these areas. The areas that are the weakest need work first. Reference those chapters that are indicated at the conclusion of each tip. As you make changes, consider conducting a survey with your patients to ensure that you are moving in the right direction. You'll be able to use the results of the survey also to communicate back to patients your belief in them and your willingness to accommodate their preferences wherever possible.

PATIENT PERSPECTIVES: NEW PATIENTS VERSUS PATIENTS OF RECORD

In our focus groups, patients reflect on "expectation versus reality" when they compare their pre-appointment expectations to the actual appointment reality. If they had high levels of expectation prior to the appointment, and their expectations are not met during the appointment, they may be disappointed. This could result in the patient grazing from the practice and not returning. This thought process typically occurs during the post-appointment phase of the process, but where does this place the long-term patient of record? Their experiences with the practice extend over a much longer period of time. These are the patients who are looking for a measure of consistency and stability from the office. Has the practice maintained the same level of communication and contact throughout the relationship with the long-term patients of record? Most importantly, recognize that every day, with each patient, you are creating a part of that patient's history and view of your office.

In current continuing education programs, I see listed a number of seminars on how to attract new patients. Yes, this is important today, but often I see and hear more emphasis placed on the new patient than the patient of record. In reality, it is these patients of record who are most crucial to the lifeblood of the practice. The majority of referrals to the practice will come from satisfied, long-term patients of record. Those referrals are coming from patients who reflect on their history of experiences in the office in a positive way.

It is your long-term patients of record who are the most valuable to your office. They are also the ones who need to be monitored in terms of maintaining their degree of satisfaction. If these patients look back on their history with you and feel that they are taken for granted, are not appreciated, or that they are not receiving the value for the dollars spent, then they are at risk. In this challenging time of lack of loyalty by patients, you absolutely cannot afford to lose your key long-term patients.

ARE THEY OBSTACLES OR OPPORTUNITIES?

I love to go on dental appointments! It's because I always see opportunities that are there for the taking. The only problem is that often they are not taken! I truly believe it's because those opportunities aren't recognized; they aren't seen. I promise you that you are surrounded by opportunities—they just need to be seen and then appropriately acted on. Unfortunately, in many cases, I believe that problems are seen instead of opportunities.

In his book, *The Seven Habits of Highly Effective People* Steven Covey so wisely noted, "The way we see the problem *is* the problem." You have many challenges today; you can choose to look at them as obstacles or opportunities. I propose that in many cases, the situations which initially may appear to be obstacles often can be seen in another light, as opportunities.

I hope that between the covers of this book you will uncover some of the opportunities that present themselves to you sometimes veiled as obstacles. Here's a brain teaser to test your perspective and to start you on this journey. The following letters can be read in three different ways. What do you see and how do you choose to view this little challenge?

Opportunityisnowhere

Don't look for a key to this puzzle. It's in you. May you find opportunities here and now as well as in your practice daily!

REFERENCES

[1] Kleinke, Chris L.. *Meeting and Understanding People*, W.H. Freeman and Company, New York, NY, 1986.

9
Patient Selection of a Dentist

"My best friend recommended a dentist ... and I've gone to him for 13 years."
— F O C U S   G R O U P   P A R T I C I P A N T

How patients view doctors may be quite different from how doctors perceive themselves. Likewise, patient perceptions of how to choose a practitioner differ from those viewpoints of the practitioners themselves. In a dental patient survey that we conducted we asked patients what they believed were the most reliable ways to locate a quality dentist. Patients responded in the following manner:

"What is the best referral source for a high quality dentist?"[1] (Boswell/1994)

- 61.2% Friend/family referral
- 35.8% Doctor referral (physician or dentist)
- 3.0% No answer

Of the patient participants in the survey, none chose referral service, Yellow Pages, direct mail, advertisement, location, or managed care list.

When we asked these same patients how they selected dentists in the past, responses were more varied:

"How have you chosen a dentist in the past?"[1]

- 69.0% Friend/family referral
- 37.0% Doctor referral (physician or dentist)
- 25.0% Convenient location
- 7.0% Dentist is personal friend
- 6.0% Managed plan
- 2.0% Direct mail
- 1.5% Yellow Pages
- 1.0% Referral service
- 4.5% No response

Note: Multiple answers were accepted.
Percentages do not equal 100%.

In our focus group work, we've queried patients about their feelings on selecting a dentist: what is important, what is the order in which they choose a doctor, and what are the primary influences in staying with a specific practitioner? Focus group patients respond positively about referrals from friends and family. Their trust level is high with these referral sources. However, a primary concern to patients is the location of the practice. If they were given three practice names from three different relatives, the typical inclination would be to narrow down the list to one doctor by way of location. Obviously this is not the ideal way to select a healthcare provider, yet it weighs heavily in a patient's decision making process. We found that the upper income and more highly educated patients want more specific information on the practitioner's background and clinical experience.

Patients of all demographics expressed interest in knowing something about the practitioner's personal communication style. A common focus group comment is, "I want to go to someone who cares more about me than the money."

Patients often narrow their selection to one practice via a phone call to the office. The perceptions of the practice based on this initial phone call can mean the difference between making the appointment at that office or crossing the doctor's name off the list and going to the next one. Therefore, the telephone skills of the individuals representing your office are extremely important (See chapter 11).

As an undercover patient, I once visited a highly respected dental laboratory under the guise of having just moved into the area and searching for an excellent dental practice. The laboratory technician was extremely accommodating and very knowledgeable. He remarked, "We've never had a patient come in to look for a dentist ... but it's a great idea." I was given the name and address of a local doctor and the lab tech even called the dentist's office to make sure that they were open and would allow me to drop in for a visit. I did so, and was very impressed with this office. The idea of a patient going to a laboratory as a referral source is a great idea, but very, very few patients would think of this.

Another survey was conducted of dental patients to determine their methods of selecting a practitioner. Motes, Huhmann, and Hill reported interesting answers to their questions of practitioner selection.[2] Their research resulted in the following findings:

- Patients with household incomes less than $25,000 used referral services more than their wealthier counterparts;
- Males versus females had a decided preference for using family members as referral sources;
- Patients over the age of 40 were more likely to visit or call an office to gain information prior to appointing;
- Lower income households were more likely to resource information about the office by a direct visit or a phone call;
- Dental patients on the whole are more likely to use referral services than patients who are seeking a physician;
- Building signs, office locations, and print advertisements are used as secondary sources for information, not typically primary factors in decision-making.

ADVICE YOUR PATIENTS READ ON DOCTOR SELECTION

Consumer Reports Books published *Complete Guide To Dental Health: How To Avoid Being Overcharged And Overtreated.*"[3] In this book the author devoted a sizable chapter to help consumer readers understand what to look for in a dental practice. He defined the pros and cons of the solo practice, the group practice, and he offered perspectives on practices that advertise, and those that participate in managed care plans. Patients are even doing research on the Internet to gain professional advice on locating dentists with whom they feel confident and comfortable.

Consumers are learning from publications and/or periodicals and magazines about what to look for in caregivers. In an article, "Find A Great Doctor," practitioners offered insights to patients.[4] Panel members made suggestions to readers on the following topics:

- Check practitioner credentials
- Inspect the office
- Gauge doctor rapport

All three topic areas are certainly important ones. How the patient interprets these is another matter. Patients do not really know how to check credentials. One patient in a focus group commented, "I'll judge how good the dentist is by how many letters are after the doctor's name." Although this might be an indicator for some patients, it will not offer an absolutely accurate view of the level of clinical skills or expected excellence in results. It is in the other two areas of inspecting the office and gauging rapport where patients feel greater comfort. After all, they understand these two categories more than the first. When it comes to inspecting the office they will comprehend the messages of the non-clinical areas before they will be able to evaluate the clinical areas. What the office looks like in the reception area is going to send a message to patients and they know how to judge and qualify this. On either a conscious or subconscious level, they also make judgments based on the rapport that has been developed with the entire dental team.(Fig. 9-1)

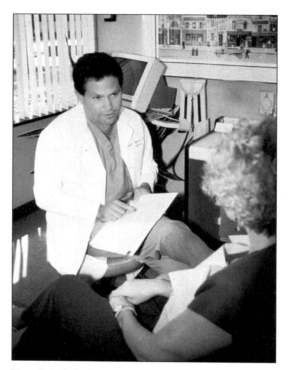

Fig. 9-1 Patients accept treatment, give referrals, and remain loyal when there are strong bonds of trust.

The issue of communications was mentioned numerous times by members of the clinician panel mentioned above. Some of their comments to patients/readers included:

- "You want to find someone with a generous dose of compassion, who is non-judgmental, and respects you and your culture."
- "Look for someone who ... takes a complete history, someone who treats the whole person, not just the disease."
- "A good dentist knows that there is a person behind that tooth."

- "In this high-tech, no-touch world, what really matters is finding someone who will take the time to listen to the patient."
- "Look for an accessible staff that calls you back when they say they will, and schedules appointments in a timely manner."
- "Look for someone who is willing to discuss issues and treatment options."

Research reported in the *Journal of the American Dental Association* found interesting results in patient concerns about practitioner competence and care.[5] This study explored dentist and patient views of the same topic areas in dentistry. Patients were asked about what they liked most about their current dentist. They were offered nine options to choose from. Results showed that "the qualities of professional competence and caring about patients received almost equal mention."

Patients and practitioners were asked to rate how important a particular quality was in relation to their own dentist, or in relation to themselves (for the practitioners). In comparing the responses, it is interesting to note that patients found "being friendly and cheerful with patients" to be a significantly more important quality in a dentist than the actual rating that dentists gave themselves in this same area.

The qualities that patients did find the most important to them and that they valued the most were the dentist's "caring attributes such as gentleness and friendliness, and their professional competence. Previous studies have found that these are traits patients would like to see in the ideal dentist."[6]

Viewpoints like these are corroborated consistently in our focus groups. Non-clinical issues related to communication, rapport, sense of caring, and trust are key factors in patients' minds.

A part of communication that is elementary to developing rapport with prospective patients and maintaining relationships with patients of record is your choice of words. Focus group participants verbalized discontent when any member of the team used terminology foreign to them or spoke over their heads. As a patient myself, I'm aware of what patients are talking about when a team member uses the word, 'prophy', for example, or if they ask if I've had a "Panorex" taken. These terms are so basic for the team that they've forgotten that many patients may not understand. If there is no rapport, some patients won't even feel comfortable asking what you mean. Know your patient's dental IQ so that you can communicate in a manner that the patient will feel comfortable with and understand.

How you handle patient complaints and concerns will affect your patient retention and patient referral rates. The most successful retailers and hoteliers have recognized for years that the "customer is always right." Of course you can find exceptions, but the erudite staff knows how to communicate so that the patient feels he/she is right, without feeling patronized. The complainers who are heard, acknowledged, and whose complaints are handled graciously often become the biggest fans of a business—even more committed to the business than they were prior to the problem. They know they will continue to be treated fairly by a team they respect and trust.

The following comments offer the perspectives of some patients relative to selection of a dentist:

"What criteria would you use to choose a dentist today?[1]

"Professionalism of the dentist."

"Their concern for my personal welfare and their attentiveness."

"Sterilization, atmosphere, and how comfortable they make me feel."

"Confidence that treatment is in my interest and not just the dentist's financial interest."

"High quality care, but friendly attitude is part of that."

"Modern and up-to-date equipment."

"I can generally assess competence by reputation and self-presentation."

"Whether the dentist is a nice guy."

"Up-to-date equipment and procedures."

MEANS TO POSITIVELY INFLUENCE PERCEPTIONS OF YOUR PRACTICE

We asked patients about specific factors that could positively influence their perceptions of the dental practice. Patients were given a list of items to choose from and were asked to select the top five items which would influence them positively. The results follow.

"Which of the following promotional items would most positively influence your perceptions of a dental practice?"[1]

- 46.0% Practice brochure
- 39.0% Dental practice newsletter
- 28.0% None*
- 15.0% Toothbrush
- 13.0% New patient packet
- 13.0% New patient video
- 9.0% Appointment gift (not toothbrush)
- 7.5% Referral gift
- 1.5% Other/comments
- 4.5% No answer

*We asked focus group patients to comment on the 28% response rate from the written patient survey. They interpreted this to mean patients who did not *consciously want* any type of promotional items to influence them.

In reference to the 1.5% on "comments", patients remarked they would be most positively influenced by "information on new procedures/services, clinical concerns, patient tips".

The 9% of "appointment gift" referred to an advertising specialty such as a magnet or promotional item of either a dental or non-dental nature.

*Note: *Percentages do not equal 100% because multiple answers were permitted.*

Patient Reasons For Changing Dentists

In our survey we asked respondents to rank the top five reasons why they would leave the care of their present dentists. Their responses are significant because reasons why a patient leaves the care of a practice will also be of concern to them when they seek a new doctor.

"Which of the following would cause you to leave one dentist to find another?"[1]

- 73%   Poor quality
- 68%   Poor doctor attitude
- 42%   Poor staff attitude
- 39%   Outdated technology
- 33%   Fees too high
- 19%   Insufficient services
- 10%   Hours inconvenient
- 4.5%   Poor insurance coverage
- 4.5%   Poor payment policies
- 4.5%   Other/comments
- 3%   No answer

*Note: *Figures above do not total 100%; multiple answers were accepted.*

The fact that 73% of the respondents indicated poor quality as the primary reason for leaving the care of a practitioner is significant. One might ask, "Why did not 100% of the respondents indicate that this would be a reason for leaving a dentist?" The answer might be that patients do not know how to judge quality in the dental practice and were making such judgments based on other criteria. Responses in relation to interpersonal issues such as doctor and staff attitude are consistently corroborated through feedback and/or focus groups. Regardless of the doctor's reputation or clinical skills, the interpersonal issue always comes into play: attitude and ability to communicate positively with patients can be and is a primary factor in a patient deciding to leave or to remain with a practice.

Patients want the office to be up-to-date. How can patients determine whether the technology within an office is outdated or not? We asked patients in focus groups this same question. A healthy 39% of the respondents to the written survey considered this a significant issue, and we found that focus group participants considered it important as well. However, the focus group patients often used non-technology criteria to judge the clinical equipment in the office. Some patients were able to make comparisons between a previous dental office they had visited and the equipment in the present dentist's office. In other words, they were comparing "apples to apples", but other patients still made judgments even if they could not make such comparisons. Some of the comments we heard were, "If the furniture in the reception area looks old and worn, then the clinical equipment probably is too;" "If I see paint chipped off of any equipment or if the cabinets and counters look old, then the equipment probably is too." Once again, patients make judgments based on parallels they can draw to a world which they *do* understand.

The survey response of 19%, "insufficient services," was a particularly interesting one. I frequently find as an undercover patient that practices do not communicate effectively on what they can do for patients. This is a delicate issue but a very important one. It relates to marketing, promotion, patient education and is all wrapped up within the communication skills of the team. The office that communicates well with the patient is able to educate the patient and help him/her understand what the practitioner can do and what services can be provided without coming across as if they are "pushing treatments".

For example, we conducted a survey of patients of a specific dental practice and we asked the patients about their attitudes and preferences in working with this office. We found that a very high percentage of the patients in the practice did not know about services that were offered by the practitioners, even though the patients expressed interest in these same treatments. The practice, in its desire to remain low key with its patients, was unwittingly withholding information that would have been received well by patients. Consequently, the issue of "insufficient services" is an important one as it relates to communications and marketing by the practice. It is here where a practice could effectively use the help of a marketing or practice management consultant to determine the best approach to take. A caveat is appropriate: be sure the consultant understands you, your practice, your locale and most importantly, maintains the delicate balance in offering patient-friendly information. If not handled well and with sensitivity, you could drive patients away.

REFERRALS

Doctors and staff members frequently express interest in how to gain referrals from their existing patients of record. This is an important issue and it is appropriate for the team to ask about the referral source. The best time to make such a request comes when a patient has complimented either the office or the treatment that was just received. That patient is in a positive and receptive frame of mind. This is the time to respond with something like,

> *Mr. Kent, we are all really pleased with the results of your treatment, but even more importantly, we're delighted that* you're *so happy with the results. It's been a real pleasure to have you as a patient in our practice, and we'd like to have more patients just like you. We'd appreciate the opportunity to help any of your friends or family who may be looking for excellent dental care.*

If you have just completed aesthetic treatment for a very satisfied patient, you could also add the following, "... and you know, your smile looks so great that you're going to get feedback from others. If you'd like, we'll give you some referral cards for those who compliment you on your great smile."

The important concept in relation to asking for referrals is this: make sure that the request is placed in a complimentary manner. It must be patient-centered first, and not come across as primarily practice-centered. In the patient's mind, the referral request should be more an issue of, "Here's what the doctor would like to do for my friends and family", rather than, "Here's what the doctor wants me to do for him/her." It's the flip side of the same coin. However, the approach you choose tells the patient something about you.

When you do receive a phone call from the referred patient, you certainly want to find out the name of the patient who gave the referral. Knowing about the referred patient prior to that patient's appointment is a definite plus for the entire team. You may be able to gauge some level of patient knowledge just by way of knowing who the referral source is. Dr. Tom McDougal puts it this way,

*We rely on axiom #7 from plane geome-
try: things equal to the same thing are
equal to each other. Knowing our referral
sources helps us to know the level of trust
pre-established with the new patient. It is
more difficult to build a relationship with
a patient selecting us by location, or
because they picked our name randomly
from the phone book.*

You are a step closer to building rapport with your new patient when you know the referral source.

Some offices strive to learn even more information by contacting the referral source. This approach must be handled very delicately. If not handled in an appropriate manner, it could be perceived as a failure to maintain the confidentiality of the new patient and could have legal overtones. However, if referral sources are contacted by phone with the intent of thanking them for the referral, this approach can be very effective. A statement like, "Mrs. Marks, Julie Bishop contacted us and made an appointment to see Dr. Kent. She mentioned that she had received Dr. Kent's name from you and we wanted to let you know how much we appreciate your confidence."

The confidentiality that is important to maintain in the discussion is the type of treatment that Ms. Bishop requested, or the nature of the office visit. It would also be inappropriate to ask a direct question of the referral source about the referred patient, "Could you tell us just a little bit about Ms. Bishop so that we could help her feel more comfortable when she arrives here?" This is requesting a subjective view of another individual and should have no relationship to the treatment that is going to be given.

Offering a statement to the referral source in a complimentary manner may elicit some information about the referred patient without asking for it, "We really appreciate receiving referrals from our patients. You've been with us for so many years that we feel like you're a member of the family and we want you to know that we will warmly welcome your friend." Insights that you may gain from such a statement can be valuable to you. But it is critical that the phone call not be perceived as one soliciting information about the new patient.

Any statements or questions which smack of soliciting information could be perceived as (1) "They want me to tell them something about my friend," (2) "I don't want the doctor's office to disclose any information about *me* to my friends," (3) "Next time I talk to my referred friend, I'll tell her that the office inquired about her." Any of these thoughts that may occur to the referral source could position the practice awkwardly in that patient's mind.

The sole purpose for that phone call should be to thank the referral source. In addition, any perspectives that might be offered by the referral source should be taken as possibilities, not necessarily probabilities. That is, make sure you gain your information about the patient's goals and desires from the patient, not from the referral source. What that referral source thinks is going to be important to the patient may *not* be the reality. The result could be your communicating to this new patient from the wrong point of view. If the referral source *does* give you an indication of what the new patient's goals may be, use this as a *starting place* to gather specific information from the patient.

TRUST VERSUS NEED

Patient trust is a precious concept. When strong bonds of trust are built between patients and the team, the practice is likely to experience increased referrals and a high patient retention rate. Trust is also an enormously important factor in influencing treatment acceptance.

We have surveyed patients to determine the primary reasons why they accept treatment. They were given a list of options from which to choose. A similar list was given to practitioners and they were asked, "On what basis do you think patients accept treatment?" In both cases, patients and practitioners chose the same top two factors: trust and need. However, there were marked differences in the frequency of responses (Fig. 9-2). Though dentists felt that trust was definitely a significant

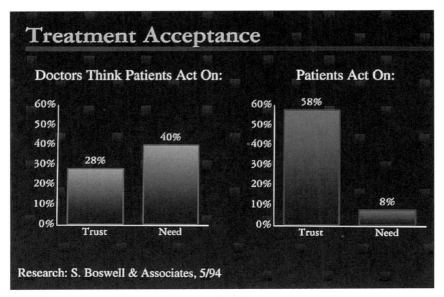

Fig.9-2 Patients, practitioners view trust differently.

factor, they thought patients placed greater significance on patients accepting treatment due to need.

It is crucial for practitioners to understand that patient perception of "need" is based on the patient's:

- presence of pain and a desire for relief, and/or
- perception of aesthetic need or desire, and/or
- a clear understanding of the clinical condition based on effective practitioner education of the patient

It is the third factor that may result in the high contrast between responses of patients and practitioners. If the practitioner has not educated the patient well, then the patient doesn't fully comprehend the need. Trust in the team is far more significant in gaining treatment acceptance than patient comprehension of clinical need. This same issue of trust is crucial in gaining and retaining patients. The entire team must put special emphasis on developing trusting relationships with new patients and maintaining the trust of patients of record.

HIGH TECH AND HIGH TOUCH: IMPACT ON PATIENT SELECTION OF DENTAL PRACTICE

As an undercover patient I have visited offices that are on the leading edge of technology and offices that are very traditional in terms of the technology used. What are the preferences of patients in comparing these two very different types of offices? We wanted to hear directly from patients about their preferences and so we took this subject into focus groups. We asked patients to consider the descriptions of two very different types of practices.

Then we asked them to make a selection of one office over the other. These are the two offices we described:

Practice A: This office was described as having cutting edge technology with the most advanced equipment available to dentistry today. The doctor provided high levels of patient education via sophisticated technology. The practitioner was formal and very business-like in approach. When he came into the office he proceeded with the clinical treatment or consultation promptly. His exhibited interest in the patient revolved solely around the clinical issues. The staff members in this office were of the same behavioral style as the doctor. They were more formal and operated the office in a strictly business manner.

Practice B: This office was very traditional in its use of equipment and technology. The office had maintained conventional equipment and decor, and did not use the advanced technology that was found in Practice A. Patient education was offered via use of models, books, and primarily verbal explanation by the practitioner. The practitioner was more informal than Doctor A and spent the first moments of the appointment chatting with the patient about the patient's interests, work, and/or family. His exhibited interest involved the patient in both interpersonal and clinical issues. The staff in this office was more informal than in office A. They showed sincere warmth and friendliness to patients and each other.

Three critical aspects of the comparison we stressed were:

1. The practitioners were both excellent clinically—their skills and results were comparable.

2. The fees in both offices were exactly the same and they offered the same payment plans.

3. Both offices operated in a time-sensitive manner. Patients were always seen within 15 minutes of their appointment time slots.

When we polled focus group participants about their preferences, overwhelmingly the patients opted for Practice B. However, in the discussions that followed, patients indicated that their real preference would be the blending of these concepts; they wanted the benefits of an office that was technologically advanced, but not at the expense of losing the personal touch. When the choice was forced on them, they strongly leaned toward the comfort that comes from a warm and caring relationship with the practice.

An interesting issue arose in the process of comparing these two offices. One male participant commented, "If the high-tech office has equipment that will lessen any pain I might have in a procedure, then there's no question, I'd opt for that, even at an increase in fee." His viewpoint brought forth additional commentary from others in this group. It became obvious that if new technology would reduce pain and shorten recuperation time, then that's what patients wanted ... regardless of their earlier stated preferences.

Based on patient responses, the ideal high tech-high touch office would be:

Practice C: This office would offer patients the benefits of up-to-date technology presented in a nurturing environment. The doctor would provide a high level of patient education through use of an intraoral camera, for example. The team would educate the patient as to all benefits afforded through use of the equipment, including communication with insurance companies for faster responses, and greater likelihood of coverage.

The doctor and the team would place more focus on the patient than on the technology. It would be clear to the patient that the technology was used as a tool to most effectively reach the patient's desired goal, and not an issue of "technology for technology's sake." The entire team would evaluate the best approach to take in discussing technology with the patient, on a patient by patient basis. The team would show special sensitivity to those patients who appeared to be technophobes. All patients of the practice would recognize that they were in a unique practice—one that had gained the desired balance of high-touch and high-tech.

Patients remarked that if an office had advanced technology and equipment they would reason that the practitioner was probably staying current on the latest treatments as well. It is true that, " ... a patient will assume that your high tech practice is also using the latest clinical techniques. This can help you position yourself in the ever-increasing battle being waged to lure your patients elsewhere."[7] This is an important issue to patients. Patients consistently communicate that they want the entire team to be "up-to-date". Many patients will deduce, right or wrong, that evidence of sophisticated technology means that the practitioner is also "up-to-date."

Dr. James Reisman of Dallas, TX, offered this: communicate to the patient that "the benefit of the technology is for the patient, not solely for the practice." A focus group patient expressed concern that, "an office might be buying sophisticated equipment that's really not necessary for the me and it's coming out of my pocket." Be sure to educate patients properly as to the benefits of the new equipment so they don't perceive it to be a knee jerk reaction to new technology.

One piece of equipment that received overwhelming acceptance by all focus groups, all demographics, was the intraoral camera. Regardless of gender, ethnicity, socioeconomic level, this wonderful tool was viewed favorably by all patients. If you currently have an intraoral camera, it would be wise to incorporate its use with patients as often as it is appropriate. This is a powerful internal marketing tool and the time you take to become adept in using it and teaching with it is a very worthwhile investment. It can be particularly meaningful to the new patient. If not used during a patient's appointment, at least inform the new patient briefly about it and possibly demonstrate its use.

One office I visited had an intraoral camera in each of the five treatment rooms. They had a policy of keeping an image on the screens at all times for promotional purposes. A patient walking through the office sees not blackened TV screens, but a series of impressive high-tech instruments.

We showed patients promotional pieces for all types of clinical technology from major suppliers. The most positive responses we received were in relation to the intraoral camera, and secondly, the laser. Patients were somewhat mixed on the laser, but indicated a responsiveness to this equipment in the dentist's office if they were going to have an invasive procedure and this instrument might eliminate pain and cut down on recuperation time. Patients who were fearful and/or had concerns about pain indicated that they would value use of the laser even if it meant a reasonable increase in treatment fee.

Dr. Arlen Lackey, a nationally recognized clinician on high-tech subjects, has integrated intraoral camera utilization into his Windows 95® computer network via imaging software. The digital signals of patients' treatment needs are transmitted to twin operatory monitor screens; one large screen for patient viewing in front of the chair and a second smaller screen behind the patient for his own use. Using software that permits on-screen viewing of drawn symbols, similar to the technology used by television football sportscasters, a highly effective visual communication system is created. This system permits rapid decision making by the patient in relation to conditions that are present and the solutions that may follow.

Focus group participants frequently raise the issue of education and its importance in relation to perceptions of value in a dental practice. When patient education combines with co-diagnosis, the results are positive for both parties. It is here when patients understand the benefits of technology to them. "Educated patients can make informed decisions regarding what they want. They become co-therapists," says Dr. David Garber of Atlanta, GA. "This is one of the major roles of technology...not for glitz and glamour, but to educate patients."[8]

Dr. Lackey reports that his patients are amazed and delighted by the benefits of advanced technology used in his office in Pacific Grove, CA. Intraoral cameras and digital X rays provide instant communication and benefit patients by a more rapid and clear understanding of their treatment needs.

The offices that are the most effective in using technology do so to increase patient education and build on a developing relationship. Dr. Robert Frazer of Austin, TX notes that, "The number one reason to have a computer is to allow extremely high touch. Important personal notes can be entered, when appropriate, by anyone and not forgotten. This office has been computerized for over 20 years and with computers at every chair connected via a local area network. We've used computers at all significant places of human interaction for 16 years."

Some patients are going to love any type of technology you incorporate into the clinical setting. These technophiles will be interested in how the equipment works and what it can do. You'll recognize them because they'll ask insightful questions about the technology and be excited about it. In the general U.S. population, technophobes outnumber technophiles by more than two to one.[9] Often these are the same folks who don't know, and don't want to know, how to set the clock on the VCR! Their apprehension relates primarily to their own operation of sophisticated technology, which is not the issue in your office! However, some people fear and resist the ever-advancing use of technology in place of human contact. These patients will respond strongly to high touch in a high-tech environment.

As technology becomes more and more a part of our everyday lives, we can expect this to change. For example, the public resisted using answering machines years ago and now telephone recorders are commonplace and accepted in most homes. Just don't try to engage the technophobes in long discussions of how the equipment works or how wonderful it is. Mainly they'll be interested in the end results ... how it will benefit them.

Approach the topic of technology in a patient-friendly manner. Don't talk about it in exactly the same way with all patients. You are dealing with individuals and the way you address the subject must be suited to the needs of each patient. The approach you take in communicating about technology with your patients must take into account two important issues:

- What is the behavioral style of the patient? (See chapter 15.) Communicate about the technology in a manner that will help the patient feel at ease.
- Are you talking with a technophile or a technophobe? Seek out the patient's comfort level with technology and proceed appropriately.

Based on our focus group discussions related to technology and dentist selection, patients prefer an office which:

- Has up-to-date technology that aids in providing patients with high quality, painless treatment;

• Uses technology to aid in patient education but not in place of interpersonal communication and explanation to the patient;

• Balances high tech and high touch: maintains the human connect and develops a warm relationship while using modern technology in a patient friendly manner.

A final word on this subject comes from a patient, one who has an enlightened perspective and understands the subtleties involved in maintaining the delicate balance. Dr. Ronald Goldstein's patient, Dr. Johnnetta Cole, President of Spelman College in Atlanta, GA, put it this way:

> *When I come to this extraordinary dental practice, I always have the feeling that I am in the presence of technology that is at least one step ahead of where everyone else is. It is a very reassuring feeling, because I don't think this technology is here for its own sake. It really goes to the heart of the mission of whatever is being done. If the mission is to give me the best oral health possible, to give me the best look possible, then I want Dr. Ronald and his colleagues to cart in every piece of high-tech equipment they can find.*

She then acknowledged the sensitivity of the team and made a request, one that might be made by all patients to all practices.

> *My hope is that in bringing in all of this high technology, this office will never lose its sensitivity. I also hope that it will not become the kind of place driven by machinery, where it takes human interaction to explain what that machine just told you. It takes a caring doctor who says to you, 'This is what we are going to do,*

this is why, this is our goal ... ' So again, I love technology, but I want us to remain profoundly sensitive to each other as human beings.[10]

TOP TIPS:

1. Determine the dental IQ of the prospective or new patient as soon as possible and communicate in a manner appropriate for that patient.
2. Find out from new patients why they left their last dental practice. Address this issue to the patient—what they can expect from your office in relation to this topic.
3. Find out what the patient wants. Patients respond to those practitioners who show a genuine interest in them and help them meet their personal goals.
4. Conduct a survey of patients to find out the strengths and weaknesses of your office. Then get to work *immediately* on strengthening those weaknesses. Communicate to your patients the steps that you are taking.
5. Make yourself available to meet prospective patients. Even a brief but warm "human connect" between patient and practitioner can be very powerful in influencing the patient positively about the practice.
6. When prospective patients call the office for information, make sure the staff greets them warmly, thanks them for their inquiry and provides information specific to the caller's areas of interest.

7. Ensure that there is a patient-centered balance between use of technology and development of interpersonal relations with patients.

8. Reestablish a strong message of appreciation with your patients of record. This cannot be understated. Your patients *must* know that they are sincerely appreciated and valued by the team.

9. Loosen up! Patients like it when the practitioner takes his/her profession seriously, but not himself/herself too seriously. Staff members respond to this too!

REFERENCES

[1] Survey of dental patients, conducted by Suzanne Boswell & Associates, Dallas, TX, 1994 (Refer to Appendix A).

[2] Motes, William; Huhmann, Bruce A..; Hill, C. Jeanne. "Following the Drill: The Search For a Dentist," *Journal of Health Care Marketing*, Summer 1995, Volume 15, No. 2.

[3] Friedman, Jay W. *Complete Guide to Dental Health: How to Avoid Being Overcharged and Overtreated*, Consumer Reports Books, Yonkers, NY, 1991.

[4] Barnett, Robert A. *Find a Great Doctor, First Magazine*, Englewood Cliffs, NJ, October, 1994.

[5] Gerbert, Ph.D., Barbara; Bleecker, Ph.D., Thomas; Saub, Edward. "Dentists and The Patients Who Love Them; Professional and Patient Views of Dentistry," *Journal of the American Dental Association*, March, 1994.

[6] Gerbert, Ph.D., Barbara; Bleecker, Ph.D., Thomas; Saub, Edward. "Dentists and The Patients Who Love Them; Professional and Patient Views of Dentistry," *Journal of the American Dental Association*, March, 1994.

[7] Freydberg, DDS, Barry. "Plugging into Computers," *Journal of the American Dental Association*, July, 1996.

[8] Bonner, DDS, Phillip. "Equipping the Complete Dental Practice," *Dentistry Today*, January, 1994.

[9] Mitchell, Susan. "Technophiles and Technophobes," *American Demographics*, February, 1994.

[10] Dr. Johnnetta Cole made these comments on video as part of Dr. Goldstein's presentation on High Technology at the Thomas P. Hinman Dental Meeting in Atlanta, GA on March 21, 1996.

10

Your Practice Identity: Patient Perceptions of the Practice on Paper

"This brochure looks too cheap and this one looks too expensive!"

—F O C U S   G R O U P   P A R T I C I P A N T

T he words above were spoken by a focus group participant as she and the rest of the group evaluated about 25 promotional pieces collected from different dental practices. Attitudes and preferences of patients do vary based on the demographics of the focus group, but there are certain truths which are basic to every group queried. Those truths are:

- If the brochure or collateral piece looks "cheap" then the patient questions the clinical skills of the practitioner and patient protection (infection control) in the office.

• If the piece looks highly sophisticated or elitist, patients express concern that they would feel uncomfortable in this office and that it would be too expensive.

• If the piece looks like it was very expensive to produce, patients equate this with a very expensive practice.

Interestingly, the focus groups which represented higher income socioeconomic groups, and/or highly educated groups frequently indicated that the more expensive looking pieces did not necessarily equate with high quality services. In addition, they stated that they would have higher expectations in relation to the value offered for the price paid. In other words, they would expect to get a good bit more for the dollar spent in this office though they recognized that this might not be the reality.

Any time you produce and print materials that will be seen by patients, you are influencing their perceptions of your practice. In this chapter we investigate an area of your image referred to by Madison Avenue as "corporate identity." In relation to the dental office, we will refer to this as practice identity.

PRACTICE IDENTITY

You already have a practice identity whether you realize it or not. Your identity is what your practice looks like on paper, plus, it's the name you have given your practice. The identity which you have established may be working for you or it may be working against you. The choices you have made throughout the existence of your practice have helped to communicate who you are to your patients and your community. What is the composition of this practice identity? Sometimes these elements are so basic that it's easy to overlook them and yet these same basics are influencing your patients. Let's look at the most elementary items to begin with, your letterhead, envelope, and business card. Your practice identity in these elements is based on:

- Paper and paper color
- Color ink
- Type face
- Design and layout on the page
- Graphics, logo or design elements

These are very basic elements. But if we go beyond that into the larger picture that makes up your total practice identity, we also must consider these same elements in relation to your:

- Newsletter
- Brochure
- Educational materials generated by your office and promoted or produced for patients

A most important point in looking at your total image on paper is the congruence and cohesion among all pieces. Gather together all the printed matter or promotional pieces which your patients see and spread them out in front of you. Do they look alike? Do they look like they belong together?

If you elect to use a professional design firm to assist in development of practice identity, make sure you select one that has experience in creating materials for the dental profession. Companies like Solutions By Design in Fresno, California, have extensive experience with development of practice identities for dental groups. The firm president, William A. Poss, indicates that, "By creating a cohesive series of communications from letterhead to referral slips, the practice is able to communicate to the patient in a manner that results in increased trust and confidence." Considering the investment in time and money, it is all important that you select an organization that truly understands your issues. If you combine these collateral pieces and they look like a mish-mash of styles, colors, papers, fonts and graphics, that's the message you are sending about your practice to your patients. This is a key aspect of impression management and in this situation you have not effectively managed the impression you're making on patients.

It is extremely easy, particularly after a number of years in a practice, to have accumulated numerous differing styles of collateral pieces. It is perhaps easiest for the new doctor to conceptually produce a cohesive package of collateral materials, but because they're starting "from scratch" their budget may be tighter than that of the practiced professional. Having different "looks" in promotional pieces isn't necessarily bad. However, it does not present the practice as a stable, solid office in the same way that a well designed and well thought out practice identity does.

Think about Coca Cola® or Kodak®. Most people can very quickly recall the colors and some of the design elements and concepts used in establishing the corporate identities of these two companies. You can bet that they would think very long and very hard before changing their logos or colors. Chances are good, you can envision the script of Coca Cola® and the yellow-red-black distinctive color combination of Kodak®. The consistency of use of these elements tends to make a statement to the public of stability. Your practice identity is probably not going to attain the renown or recognition of a Fortune 500 company, but with consistency in practice identity you will be sending your patients a message of stability (Fig. 10-1).

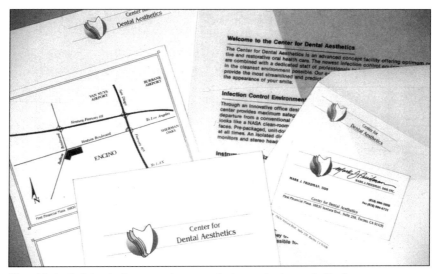

Fig. 10-1 Collateral pieces must communicate a cohesive and effective message. (Courtesy Mark J. Friedman, D.D.S.)

WHAT'S IN A NAME?

Part of your practice identity is what you call yourself. Patient perceptions indicate that a practice that has a name other than that of the doctor is any one of the following items or a combination of several:

- Larger office than that of a sole practitioner
- A more established practice
- A clinic
- A group practice, possibly incorporating specialties
- Specialty practice

Interpretation depends largely on the name that you have chosen and printed text that may accompany the name. For example, a practice that has a name of Smile Design Center may be interpreted as an office which offers primarily aesthetic treatments. The patient doesn't know, however, whether this is the office of one doctor or several. Conclusions about this will be based on what else may be printed on the business card or appears in letterhead or other collateral materials.

The quality and sophistication of any logos which are also used in the practice identity will influence patient perceptions of quality, as well as practice size. An office name, such as, Desert Valley Dental Center offers the patient little information in terms of the type of practice. Patient clues will be derived from other elements and the collateral materials. Anything which points toward the concept of "clinic", right or wrong, is frequently seen in a negative light in focus groups. Patients tend to interpret a clinic setting as one which is less personal and may not offer the quality that might be found in a traditional dental practice environment.

If you choose a name for your practice other than your own name, make sure that your choice is one that you can live with for a long time. It needs to be a name that you can "aspire to and not outgrow."[1] In addition, if it is not a clinic environment, make sure that there is nothing in the name which might lead unknowing patients to misunderstand.

If yours is a group practice you have options as to the name of the practice. Some offices opt for the use of each doctor's name, such as Beckman, Travis, and Larson. However, as patients have noted, this sounds like a legal firm. An office name that uses no surname eliminates this problem, such as Park Forest Dental Care. Another alternative is to combine the principals' names with a group modifier, such as Randall-Erickson Dental Group.

There are several important considerations in relation to the naming of a group office. One of them as stated above is ensuring clear public understanding relative to the type of practice. This is particularly important for those patients who seek fee-for-service environment. Secondly, there is the issue to be considered relative to the practitioners involved in the practice. If there is any possibility of a staff change in the practitioners involved, then a generic group name would be preferred. In addition, associates may feel more comfortable with a practice that has a generic name, rather than a doctor-specific name. To ensure patient acceptance and understanding you might consider proposing practice names to a focus group of your own patients for feedback.

PATIENT PREFERENCES IN COLLATERAL MATERIALS

Throughout the balance of this chapter you will gain insight into patient preferences related to specific elements within the practice identity and you will be offered tips on how to communicate most effectively with patients.

It is important to acknowledge that as community and societal issues are changing and evolving, patient attitudes and your responses to patients must change as well. This was discussed at length in Part 1 of this book. Accommodating the needs and awareness of your changing patient base is important. This is one of the reasons that you may find you have very different styles in some of your collateral pieces; you have changed, your practice has changed, and your patients have changed. As much as possible, it's advisable that the practice not make drastic changes in the practice identity. From a practical point of view it's very costly. But even more importantly, it is confusing to patients. If you must change an element in your practice identity to adjust to societal or marketing trends, then try to maintain some continuity in design elements. For example, if you change your graphic design or logo, try to keep the same paper or ink colors you have used before.

PAPER, COLOR, AND INK CHOICES

Your choices of paper, colors, and ink are very basic elements of the practice identity. These should be chosen with great care and the uniformity should be reflected among all collateral pieces if at all possible.

There is an important societal trend today and a significant movement toward using recycled and recyclable paper in business. Recycled papers are frequently recognized by a fleck-like visual texture. There is mounting responsiveness to use of this type of paper in letterhead, business cards, brochures, and newsletters.

The quality of the paper you use will strongly influence your patients. A very heavy, highly textured paper may be perceived as high quality and perhaps more expensive as well. There is also a growing trend towards a very slick, smooth surfaced paper. An important difference between these two is that the smoother the surface of the paper, the fewer problems you're going to have in ink saturation during photocopying or printing. If it's a photocopied document the ink may actually rub off the surface of the rough paper because the toner has not saturated into the paper texture. You've probably seen this in letters you've received when toner from one page transfers to another page, resulting in a shadowed or smudged appearance.

In selecting colors of paper, stay with neutral, soft shades, or white. Avoid any color which may be trendy and may outdate itself in a couple of years. Patients tend to prefer classic white or light shades of blue or gray.

Consider carefully the colors you'll use in the typeface for your letterhead and business cards. Stay with the classic colors as much as possible; they won't outdate themselves. As in paper colors, avoid any shade that may be trendy. Use of metallics, gold or silver, can produce a strong, very attractive appearance. It also can look very expensive to the patient and depending upon your patient base, may work for you or against you. Evaluate this carefully before selecting a metallic ink.

LOGOS

Any visual element you incorporate into your practice identity becomes an important part of the patient's understanding of who you are. Patients respond well to a strong and professional logo or design element incorporated into a promotional piece. Regardless of group demographics, patients expect the logo for a dental practice to be "professional" in appearance. This does not mean that the logo needs to look "stuffy." It should not, however, look home-made or haphazard. Addition of a graphic or logo can add appreciably to the aesthetic appeal of any collateral materials. (Fig. 10-2.) As soon as you place a graphic on a piece of paper you are starting to tell the reader much more about you. The quality of the design, the sophistication level, the visual message you are conveying can be very powerful. The graphic alone can communicate to the patient who you are.

When we showed patients sample graphics on brochures or letterheads they typically had very strong reactions to them. The more highly educated and higher income focus group participants leaned toward very conservative and/or sophisticated looks. This same demographic did not care for cartoon-like or "cute" graphics if they were considering the practice for their own adult services. If looking at the office as a family practice, they agreed that the more informal approach could work, but even in that instance they communicated a dislike for those graphics that depicted the patient as a coward. In showing the same graphics to patients of lower education or middle to lower income levels, there was more receptivity to the cartoon-like quality graphics.

LAYOUT AND DESIGN

In evaluating patient responses to layout and design of brochures and newsletters, there were many similarities among the different demographic groups.

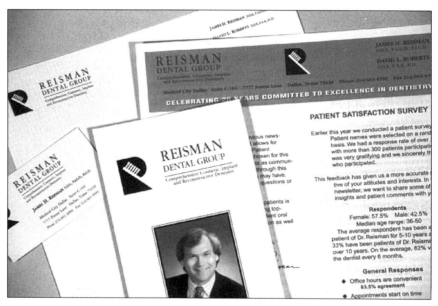

Fig. 10-2 This newsletter incorporates a strong practice logo that is repeated in all the practice's collateral pieces. (Courtesy James Reisman, D.D.S., F.A.G.D)

PATIENTS LIKE:

- Sufficient "white space" so that the piece looks easy to read.
- Headings and bulleted or numbered lists that increase ease of reading.

• Pictures of doctor and staff, with a slight preference towards clinicians working with a patient either in the treatment room or greeting the patient in the reception area.

• Inclusion of graphic elements that make the piece easier to read and more interesting to the eye.

• Topics of interest to the patient should be at the beginning of the brochure or newsletter; promotional items or issues relating to finances/insurance positioned at the close of the piece.

• Information specific to the doctor's educational background and credentials. Many patients also respond to some personal information such as marital status, children and a few interests.

PATIENTS DISLIKE:

• Scary "before" pictures; include only pictures of "happy, satisfied" people.

• Text-heavy copy with little white space.

• "Business" issues listed at the beginning of the promotional piece, including finances, insurance, or anything that relates to "rules" of the office.

• A picture of the doctor who looks stiff or overly formal.

• Quotes from unknown patients. Patients in focus groups tend not to believe quotes that do not show a patient's name or at least initials. The only acceptable exception is when quoting survey responses which should be anonymous.

• Avoid printing photographs in colored ink. If you're trying to save money by using only one ink color, think about what your face will look like when it's blue! This is a common mistake.

In your promotional piece consider the issues that are discussed in Part 1 of this book. If your goal is to reach a broad-based market, you will be more effective by addressing some of these societal issues. For example:

- If you use pictures of patients, be sure that you address a range of ages and cultures. If your staff is multicultural, including a photograph of your staff is particularly helpful in reaching different ethnic groups.
- Communicate your accessibility to those who may be physically challenged. This is a major issue today, and if your office has been designed in such a way to ensure ease of accommodation, let your patients know this.
- If you are using recycled or recyclable paper, indicate this with the appropriate recycle logo on the rear or at the bottom of the promotional piece.
- If your office is equipped with advanced technology, let your patients know how this can help them or how it can help them feel more comfortable in your office.
- Ensure that the words you use are positive in approach. Avoid negative terminology like "we do not process insurance forms", instead let the patients know what you *will* do for them in relation to insurance.

BROCHURE CONCEPTS

It is doubtful that a patient is going to sit down and read a lengthy treatise about your practice. If you are designing a brochure, you must ask yourself what are the most important facts patients need to know about your practice. If you give them too much information they're probably not going to read it all and they may never read the most important points if they are lost in the text of your tome.[2]

Instead, write your piece so that it is patient friendly, short, to the point, and pared down to the most important information. That way, they will more likely read the entire piece and your important points will not be overlooked. If you are set on giving the patient additional information, put it in the form of a brochure insert. This way you could opt to include the insert or not. This also affords greater flexibility because you can keep your more expensive brochure piece intact and easily change and update the insert. However, if you take this approach make sure that you're using the same types of paper, ink and typeface. Consistency is crucial.

Graphic artist, Wanda Bedford, who also created the illustrations in this book, has many years experience in creating commercial graphic design pieces, as well as teaching the subject matter to young designers. She suggests that in determining what content and how much information to include, start with a list of all the data you feel is important. Get everything down on paper. Then back up and cross off the items that may be least important to patients. Remove text until what remains is the cleanest and most direct visual presentation of your material. When text is surrounded by a significant amount of white space, the text increases in perceived importance. As a result, we are more likely to read it. When there is little white space and the promotional piece is text-heavy it can produce a negative response and the reader may be resistant to reading the material.

Ms. Bedford also makes the following suggestions:
• Use strong contrast in color.
• Crisp, clear color differentiation will be responded to more positively; it is more pleasing visually and more likely to be read.
• Make sure that any photographs you use can stand alone and that the photo tells the story whether there is a caption or not. If your photo requires extensive explanation or more than one picture to explain the story, then it is counter-productive.
• Never use more than three type faces within the same document. Sophistication of personal computers and myriad fonts available encourage experimentation. This can be very dangerous in that a page can look poorly designed and difficult to read. Using two fonts is better than three and one font, used in different weights and sizes, is perhaps easiest to read and the most pleasing to the eye.
• Unless designed by a professional artist, avoid using type that reads over any texture. This technique is best handled by a professional who understands and can manage its complexities. Attempted by the novice, this can result in text that is not read, and/or is visually distracting.

Bear this in mind, if the reader has to work to find and understand the meaning in your promotional piece, it has lost its purpose. Simplify. Simplify. What follows is a list of elements to consider including in your brochure. These are items that are important to patients and help to market your practice:

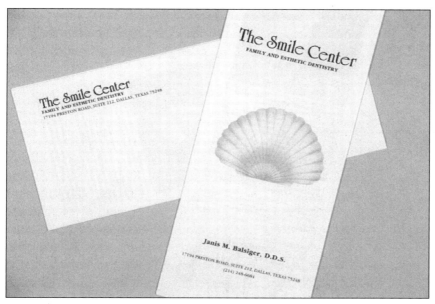

Fig. 10-3 Patients respond well to brochures which tie design to dental aesthetics. (Courtesy Jan Balsiger, D.D.S., F.A.G.D.)

BROCHURE ELEMENTS THAT BUILD PATIENT CONFIDENCE

- **Doctor biography:** Address education, credentials, affiliations, and some personal information. Patients are interested to know if the doctor is married and/or has a family. Include outside interests that are health related, like jogging or sports activities which communicate well about you. Be careful about including information which may be perceived as elitist by some patients. This information should highlight the doctor's professional career and it should promote distinctions, honors, and areas of expertise.[3]

- **Staff information:** Include credentials and affiliations. Patients like it when staff members have been employees of the practice for a long time. If applicable, include either the average tenure of staff members, or the combined years of staff tenure.

- **Patient protection:** Address infection control procedures in your office. Use the term "patient protection," as it is caring and less alarming than "infection control." Be specific in this area and site compliance with ADA, CDC, and OSHA regulations or guidelines.

- **How you are different:** This is a very important topic, for you want to differentiate yourself from other practices. First *you* must know how you are different, then that must be communicated to your patients. (See chapter 20 on marketing). Address issues like technology, continuing education, specialized services; patients must know why they should choose your office or stay with your practice.

- **Emergencies:** Let patients know how to reach you and how you typically respond in emergencies. Let them know what to expect. If you give patients your home phone number for emergencies, be sure to include this in your brochure. Patients are very impressed when they have that kind of access to the practitioner.

- **Map:** Include a map of your office location and indicate major thoroughfares that lead to your immediate locale. A map with only your closest streets is not as helpful to the patient who is driving a long distance as a map that also indicates major thoroughfares. Written directions are not important so long as you have graphics that include landmarks to help the patient locate you.

- **Mission statement:** Tell patients your mission statement or practice philosophy. If you have any difficulty in fitting this item into your brochure it can also be positioned in a brochure insert. If your mission statement may change, it would be wise to place this item in the insert. If you have a formal mission statement that was scripted by the entire team, let the patient know that. Patients like to know that the entire team was a part of your process in developing this statement. However, there are some patients who will be skeptical. If you present this statement to your patients, you'd better walk your talk. Business people who are familiar with the significance of a written mission statement will be those most likely to observe if you are congruent or not.

Items above are *musts* to include in your brochure. You may be surprised that some of the following elements are considered optional. It's strongly suggested that this information be provided to your patients but these items do not need to be printed in the brochure itself. They could also be placed in a brochure insert which affords you more flexibility in making changes and updating information.

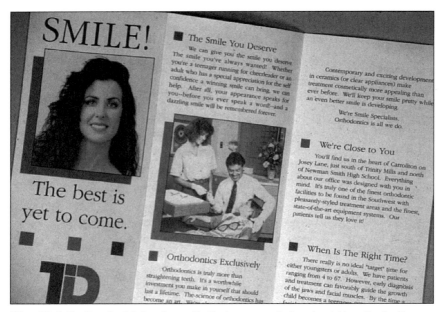

Fig. 10-4 Dr. Daugherty's brochure effectively communicates about his orthodontic practice. Colors are high-energy and an inside photo shows the doctor and team member with a patient. The photo's friendly informality helps a prospective patient feel at ease with the practice. (Courtesy Terry Daugherty, D.D.S.)

OPTIONAL BROCHURE ITEMS

• **Hours:** If it's possible that your office hours may change, or if your office hours vary by season, placing this item in an insert simplifies your brochure and allows you to make changes easily.

• **Services:** As with hours, you may feel that this is a *must* to include in the body of the brochure itself. Clearly, the information is important and vital to the practice. However, the services that you promote and the way that you promote them may change. You may add services or delete them. You may want to reformat the way you're promoting your services. Putting these items in an insert gives you that flexibility. Make sure that the terminology you use is patient friendly. For example, patients do not like the word *bleaching*, they far prefer the term *whitening*. The term *aesthetic* may be responded to more positively by some men and women than the word *cosmetic*.

• **New Patient Process:** Welcome the new patient and provide information on what the new patient can expect during the first office visit.

• **Societal issues:** Sociotrends is the topic of Part 1 of this book. Depending upon where your office is located and the demographics of your client base, you may want to consider including some of the elements that address these societal concerns. Doing this means truly understanding your *customers*, what is important to them, and your ability to communicate an understanding and appreciation for their issues. For example, if your office is located in the Pacific Northwest, where there is a high awareness and sensitivity to ecological issues, you may want to address the subject of recycling and disposal of sharps and plastics.

Congruence is so important in every manner of communication from the practice to the patient. In designing your brochure make sure that it looks like who you are. If you offer extensive treatment in aesthetics or if you actively promote aesthetic dentistry, patients will be judging your *aesthetic eye* in relation to the design of your brochure as well as any collateral pieces from your office. If you actively promote your office as a family practice, your collateral materials must reflect this as well. The design, and/or colors that you choose must speak well to the entire family.

PUTTING IT ALL TOGETHER

Where do you start putting together your practice identity on paper? To communicate most effectively it's best to gain professional assistance in this project. Design of a logo and assistance or guidance in selecting paper and typeface that will really stand the test of time is best done by those who have experience. However, you don't need to spend a fortune in the process of doing this either. Here are some options:

• **Advertising agency or design firm:** This is the most professional and frequently most expensive option. However, poorly designed materials that don't work for you or that you scrap are certainly more expensive. If you go with a professional firm make *sure* they have experience with dental practices, they understand your profession, and have a good grasp of who you are as a practice, who your patients are and where you want to be in five or 10 years. If the firm you start working with doesn't seek out this information, cut your losses and find somebody else, fast!

• **Graphics designer:** Instead of working with a team, or a firm, you may be able to locate an individual artist who works on a freelance basis. This person will probably be less expensive than working with a company. This individual should be able to design a graphic element, or logo for you as well as give you direction on paper and typeface. Working with an individual like this means that you will be giving this person direction as to who you are and where you want to go, so you must feel confident and prepared to do this.

• **Art School:** If you are in a metropolitan area another cost-effective alternative can be to contact an art school in your city. Frequently, universities that offer courses in commercial design or art schools that instruct in commercial art will take on "company projects" from the real world. In cases like this, you may present your practice to a class who then develops a practice identity for you. The benefit is that you might have many options from which to choose and typically the class is instructed by a professional artist who oversees all work and directs the project.

• **References from practice management consultants:** If you work with a practice consultant from your area or know consultants in your area, contact them for possible references. They may be familiar with brochures that have been well done for other clients. They can save you much time, effort, and money in directing you to the right people. In addition, some consultants include logo and practice identity services in their portfolios. For example, McKenzie Management in Dublin, OH offers a service of assistance with logos and brochures. The benefit of this approach is that the practice consultant will understand the profession and how best to present you in your market.

• **Preprinted collateral materials:** You also may consider purchasing preprinted practice identity items from catalogue companies or suppliers, items like letterhead, business cards, and matching envelopes. You provide to the company the imprinted information that you want to appear on their stock paper products. Companies like Smart Practice offer an excellent choice of high quality, dentistry-specific options at reasonable rates.[4] If you produce a newsletter or brochure, you will need to locate a supplier who will provide similar paper in the appropriate size you need and you will also need to ensure that the design of those items are cohesive and consistent with the balance of your practice identity. Specialty paper supply companies, like PaperDirect offer a wide range of coordinated papers and envelopes in various sizes and weights.[5]

TOP TIPS:

1. Ensure that all collateral materials look similar: same paper, colors, typeface, and graphics.
2. Make sure the perceived cost of the brochure and newsletter are appropriate for your client base. What may look reasonable to one demographic group, may appear unprofessional to another. Present yourself appropriately to your patients.
3. Before making important practice identity changes, ask for patient opinions. Take a poll of patients in-office, or invite a select group of long-term patients to give feedback and aid in decision-making.
4. Try to print different collateral pieces at the same time. If at all possible, print your business cards, envelopes, letterhead, and newsletters in the same press run.
5. Be conservative in how many pieces you initially print of any new collateral piece. After using them for a short time, you'll find additions and modifications you'll want to make. Print a larger quantity on the second press run.

6. Put your full telephone area code, and postal code on all collateral pieces. Don't assume you'll only receive calls from local areas! Depending on your locale and particularly for those practices near an international border, consider adding your country to your address.

REFERENCES

[1] Maynard, Roberta. "What's In A Name," *Nations Business,* September, 1994.

[2] The ADA booklet, *How to Develop a Practice Brochure,* offers excellent guidelines and checklists for brochure creation. This booklet, Item M041, is available through the ADA's catalog department.

[3] Levin, Roger Paul DDS, MBA. "Welcome Your New Patients Properly," *Ultimate Dental Marketing and Management,* Vol. 2, No. 2, The Levin Group, Baltimore, MA.

[4] Smart Practice, Phoenix, AZ; (800) 522-0800 offers specialty papers and products created specifically for the dental profession. Their catalog includes many other products for the dental practice.

[5] PaperDirect, Secaucus, NJ; (800) 272-7377 offers a wide range of high quality, specialty papers and business paper supplies in coordinated sizes and styles.

11

Tele-Talk: Lifeline to Your Patients

*"I was on hold so long I forgot why I was calling ...
and I never called them again!"*

—FOCUS GROUP PARTICIPANT

The phone rang seven times when it was answered breathlessly by the dental office receptionist. She had obviously raced to the phone anticipating that I would hang up. She immediately put me on hold without asking permission to do so, then returned to the line after about 90 seconds.

"Things are really crazy around here today," she confided. Despite her apology, she was clueless as to how patients might respond to this incident. It was a moment of truth that lost credibility for her and for the practice.

;ly, she cast doubt on the entire team. There's no
the fact that each member of the team wields
s power in influencing the patient's view of the
ictice. In less than two minutes from the first ring
phone, the office had presented itself as a
ized and unprofessional one.

The doctor may not have been aware that his
receptionist handled my call, and presumably others, in
this manner. But in this brief interaction the practice might
well have lost a prospective patient. Of greater
importance, the doctor may have lost a number of patients
over time due to the way they were treated on the phone.

AN INTERRUPTION OR AN OPPORTUNITY?

The front desk and the phone lines offer
wonderful opportunities for building long-term
relationships with patients. They also can present real
challenges in maintaining office equilibrium. Before we
address the challenges it's important to reevaluate the
benefits of the phone. It's truly your lifeline to the world.
The vast majority of your business comes through those
lines. Without the phone, it's likely you and most other
businesses would be *out of business.* Though it's the most
important business tool in your office, the phone is often
viewed as an interruption not an opportunity.

I recognize that many seminar audience members
think, "Oh, but you've never worked in a dental office,
patients don't know how hard it really is." It's true, I have
not worked in a dental office and neither have the majority
of your patients. Patients *don't* know about the stresses
and challenges you face, and frankly, they don't care. That
is not meant to be flippant; it is a reality! Patients are
calling the office for a purpose and they want help. It's not

the patient's role to accommodate the staff, it's the other way around, if the practice wishes to remain in business.

The scenario: There is a hygienist out sick, there were two emergencies that morning, there's a patient at the counter who is in a hurry, there's a patient on hold, and the phone rings again! I'd say that's a stress-producing situation. When you lift that receiver, the caller has no idea about your scene. The sound of your voice and the words you say, communicate a tremendous amount to the caller about the practice. Here is where impression management is crucial.

If you're the one who answers the phone in your office, before you pick up that phone to present the practice to the world, be sure that you take a breath, put a smile on your face, inject some energy in your voice and recognize that with lifting the receiver, "It's Showtime." You are literally and figuratively putting your practice on the line.

Here's what patients respond to in telephone communication—a staff member who:

- has a friendly voice that is warm and reassuring,
- communicates a caring attitude that accurately represents a caring team,
- is knowledgeable about the practice and treatments,
- answers questions knowledgeably and competently,
- recognizes and acknowledges the strengths of the entire team,
- has confidence in self and the practice and communicates it verbally and vocally,
- acknowledges the value and importance of the patient to the practice, and
- communicates pride to be a part of the practice.

THE TELEPHONE, THE PRACTICE AND THE PATIENT'S PERSPECTIVE

Before looking at your telephone service through the patient's eyes, let's take a look at your own view of telephone service. How well do you understand your patients' attitudes? Take this brief quiz and then evaluate your own telephone service in light of patient preferences.

Telephone Quiz

1. What is the maximum "acceptable" number of telephone rings to patients, before they become concerned that the office might not be open?

a) 2

b) 3

c) 4

d) 5

e) 6

2. What type of service/system do patients prefer after office hours?

a) Answering service

b) Answer machine/system

3. What is the patient's maximum acceptable on-hold wait time?

a) 15-30 seconds

b) 30-45 seconds

c) 45-60 seconds

d) 60-75 seconds

---

4. If put on-hold, what do patients prefer to hear?

a) Music

b) Information/education tape

c) Nothing

5. Which of the following is the most reassuring for a prospective patient to hear when calling the office for the very first time?

a) Information about the doctor's background

b) Infection control measures taken

c) Specifics as to why other patients like the office

d) Other

6. Who has priority in service, the person at the counter or the person on the phone?

a) Person at counter

b) Person on phone

c) Other

7. A prospective patient has just told you her full name on the phone. Which is the preferred way to address her during the conversation?

a) First name

b) Last name and honorific (Miss, Mrs., or Ms.)

The quiz above would be a good one to conduct as part of a staff meeting. Every staff member is also a patient, whether at a dental office or a medical office, and all of us experience some frustrations as customers of other businesses.

PATIENT RESPONSES

Here's how patients in our focus groups responded to the issues above:

1. Patients are consistent on this—when an office phone rings more than three times, patients start to get concerned, "The office isn't open? They're understaffed? I've got an emergency, what am I going to do?" Any business phone should be answered by the third ring. If the phone must be left unattended, it is better to put it on your answering machine or answering service rather than let it ring too long.

2. There is a good bit of controversy surrounding this issue. Patients in surveys identified a preference for an answering service. Why? They wanted to talk to a "real human being." However, quality is an issue here. If you use an answering service that does not adequately represent your practice, then that is not providing adequate "service"! It could be working against you. This is an important element in impression management.

In a survey we conducted of practitioners, we found that the majority of practices used answering machines after hours. (Fig. 11-1.) With an answering machine or system, you are able to control the quality of image presented to your patients. If you have a wonderful answering service that accurately and *consistently* represents you well to your patients, don't change

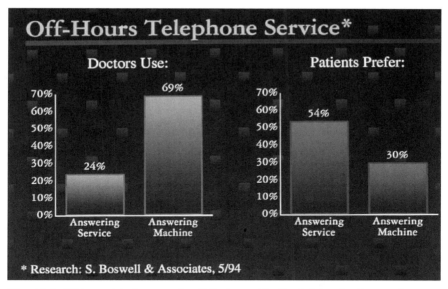

Fig. 11-1 Off-hours telephone service: Patients would rather talk to a "real person."

anything. If you get any complaints at all, there are probably more problems that you just haven't been told about. Either find a truly service-minded service or get a reliable answering system so you can manage the impression being made on the public.

3. In focus groups, patients state that 30-45 seconds is the maximum "acceptable" on-hold time. If you must keep patients on-hold longer than that, be sure to touch base with them intermittently to let them know that they haven't been forgotten.

4. This is an issue presently in flux. Our patient focus groups indicate almost an even preference for music and "nothing". The on-hold, informational tape was a new concept for many dental patients; most had not yet experienced this in relation to their dental offices. They were open to the idea with stipulations on the content of the tapes and the approach taken.

5. The most appropriate response is *other* because answers a-b-c are *all* important to patients. Which one is the *most* important depends on the patient. Knowing what is the most important, and what to talk about in general with prospective patients takes finely tuned interpersonal skills.

6. Like question 5, the most appropriate response here is *other*, it all depends on who reached the receptionist first. If the call came in first, then the person at the counter is second in line. If the person at the counter was already talking with the receptionist when the call came in, the caller should be advised of the situation and the patient at the counter should be helped first.

7. The correct answer is *(b)*. Until you are given permission to use a person's first name, it is appropriate to take the more formal approach. If you're going to err, it is better to err on the side of formality. Using a person's first name may be perceived as presumptive and overly familiar. This can be an especially sensitive issue when talking with a person who is a generation or more older than you!

Let's take a look at some of the top issues that are influencing public perceptions of your practice on the phone:

THE TELEPHONE GREETING

Before prospective patients set one foot through the door, they hear a voice and words over the phone. They start to envision the person who answers the phone and they may anticipate the quality of clinical care and service provided by you and your team. The receptionist is in an extremely important position in influencing patient perceptions. This cannot be understated.

Patients in focus groups have discussed at length their impressions of offices based on the individual who answers the phone. As a result of patient feedback, we have identified three elements of the greeting that patients respond well to. They are:

1. The name of the practice. You may use the doctor's name as in, "Dr. Smith's office ... ", or the business name of the practice, for example, "Mission Valley Dental Center ... " Avoid using, "Doctor's office ... " It is not specific to the practice, does not clarify that the patient reached the right number, and it lacks importance; this could be any healthcare office—medical or dental. The practice identity must not be very important if it isn't even announced!

2. Announce your own name. For example, "This is Sally ... " Patients like to know who they are talking with. If it's the first time a caller has contacted your office, this is a first step in building a personal connect with the prospective patient.

3. The third element is optional. You could conclude the greeting with the two elements listed above or you could add one of the four suggested below:

a) "Good Morning (afternoon, evening)." This phrase would precede the practice name and the receptionist's name. It is a friendly introduction and softens the greeting just a bit.

b) "Thank you for calling ..." This phrase would precede the practice name and would be spoken in conjunction with the practice name, as in, "Thank you for calling Dr. Smith's office." With this phrase you are making the introduction to the greeting a little longer, however, the concept of thanking the patient is important today and certainly appropriate to communicate to your callers.

c) "How may I help you?" This element follows elements 1 and 2 above and helps to jump start callers and move them toward expressing the purpose of the call.

d) "How may I direct your call?" This phrase would follow the receptionist's name. This third element is most appropriate in an office that typically transfers calls from a central system. This phrase tells the caller that the call will be forwarded. It aids in keeping the caller from starting a conversation unnecessarily. This phrase typically would not be used in a smaller dental practice.

Patients have indicated that when the greeting goes beyond three elements it can seem too long. A longer greeting may be appropriate the first time a caller contacts your office, but for patients of record this is unnecessary.

Imagine this, you call a dental practice and the receptionist answers the phone with, "Thank you for calling Dr. Jones and Dr. Smith's office. This is Rebecca. How may I help you?" Reading this greeting is quite different from hearing it spoken. If Rebecca has a patient at the counter and another on hold, she may be in a hurry when she answers this call and so she rattles off the greeting with an unfeeling monotone. If it's the first time a prospective patient has contacted the office, Rebecca may come across as almost robotic in tone. This is experienced not only by the caller, but also by the patient who is standing in front of Rebecca and hears the greeting as well. The practice would do well to increase Rebecca's awareness of the power of her voice in every phone call to the office.

I was doing some field research in comparing the perceptions of offices by phone versus the reality of what the office was really like. I'd called the office of "Dr. Larson", and "Bev" answered. She sounded hurried and abrupt. She answered my questions, but offered no additional insights or information about the office. Had I been the average caller seeking a new dentist, I probably would have eliminated this office from likely candidates. However, I wanted to see if my "pre-appointment" vision matched reality.

What a surprise! On an unscheduled drop-in visit, I found Bev to be very cordial and helpful. She offered to show me the office, gave me a brochure on the practice, and encouraged me to make an appointment for a new patient exam. This was a shock. The woman on the phone did not match the woman I met in person. Though there was a definite improvement, these issues came to mind:

- What could I expect *next* time—who was she really?
- Would the non-clinical inconsistency point toward clinical inconsistency?

She may have been pressured when I called the first time; maybe there were patients at the counter; maybe other patients were on hold. The caller doesn't know. The caller only knows that in that brief "window on reality" she seemed uncaring. For the patient it was a moment of truth. And the crucial matter here is that a significant number of patients never would have made an appointment, never would have seen her as I did. Nevertheless, there was an issue of inconsistency that would place doubts in patients' minds.

THE IMPACT OF VOCAL TONE

If you're about to skip this segment because you're thinking to yourself, "How can vocal tone be such a significant element in relation to perceptions of the practice by patients?" let me assure you, it plays a huge part in how your office is perceived. Callers will come to very rapid conclusions about the practice, right or wrong, based on the perception of the receptionist's vocal tone in those fleeting moments on the phone.

If we don't have an actual image of the person we're talking to, we create our own based on perceptions by voice. We also create an image of the person's mood, style, and service attitude. We meet someone we've talked with several times on the phone and either they fit our "vision" or they don't. How does all of this affect your practice?

I contacted an office that had hired me as an undercover patient. The staff member who answered on each of the three phone calls I made to this office spoke in a flat monotone. Each time, this receptionist was vocally lacking in any kind of warmth or feeling. It would be likely that many callers would interpret the behavior to be acceptable to the doctor/owner of the practice. Likely response by patients might be, "This is the way the office is, unfeeling, uncaring." If the patient has nothing else to go on, then they make judgments based on their own experiences and their own version of reality.

Knowing that vocal quality will affect another's perception, a pleasing, confident voice will produce a positive response, so long as it's matched by a congruent verbal message.[1] When people call your office who don't know you, or never have visited your office before, they have only the verbal message and the vocal quality to judge your competence—right or wrong. In a highly competitive marketplace, and dentistry *is* a marketplace to patients today, those few fleeting moments on the phone can result in an appointment, a referral, or in disillusionment!

Listen actively to how the caller communicates. If he/she speaks much more slowly than you, then slow down to match the speed. If the caller speaks faster, speed it up just a bit. Don't try to copy, but adjust your pacing to theirs.[2] If you hear a quick, hurried vocal pacing, pick up your speed! One patient noted, "I'm from New Jersey and it drives me nuts when I call an office and it takes them forever to make a point." Likewise, if you have a slow talking caller, and you are ripping right along vocally, this can be off-putting to the caller. Slow down a little. That commonality will help the caller feel more comfortable with you. Speaking slowly doesn't mean you can't communicate with enthusiasm. Your energy and enthusiasm is heard in your inflection, not necessarily the speed.

In addition, matching the tone of speech can be very effective. If the caller has a very soft voice and you tend to sound gruff, you may be sabotaging yourself. Softening your voice just a bit will help the caller feel more comfortable with you. This is not imitating, but adjusting to a softer level within your own natural vocal range. People feel comfortable with those who sound like them. The exception to this is if the caller is angry or anxious. Obviously, you would not want to duplicate these moods! In those circumstances, soften the voice, slow down just a little, and include verbal indications of support or concern that may help to calm the caller.

At a seminar I conducted on self-presentation, a member of the audience posed an interesting question. He said, "I live in a part of the country where there are many different ethnic groups. Sometimes the accent is so strong that I have trouble understanding what the caller is saying." In such a situation, it becomes even more important to create a feedback loop. Communicating back to the caller what you understood was said will enhance your relationship and ensure that you heard correctly. Remember, the caller is probably accustomed to being asked to repeat what he/she has said and will appreciate your concern for accuracy.

Smile as you speak. Just as you may visualize a radio DJ, your callers see you. Your voice is a wonderful instrument and a powerful tool to help build rapport with patients. Think of your voice like the packaging that can make your words more interesting, compelling, and credible. Positive vocal quality will enhance your face-to-face presentations and certainly increase your competence in communicating on the phone.

USING THE PATIENT'S NAME

Be judicious in how you address the patient on the phone. Do not be arbitrary or overly familiar with patients.[3] You won't go wrong taking a formal approach, you could go wrong by being too informal. Use the patient's last name until given permission to use the first name. This applies to the entire team including the doctor. Any doctor who has been corrected by a patient understands the sensitivity of this issue. The greater the age difference between the team member and patient the more important this is!

TAKING MESSAGES: FINISHING THE FEEDBACK LOOP

If the caller wishes to leave a message for someone, then it becomes very important how the message is taken. The caller wants to be assured that the message is taken accurately and that it will be delivered to the party in question. Most callers will appreciate a feedback loop. In the effective feedback loop the listener paraphrases the message taken. This offers two benefits: (1) The caller knows that the message was actually written down. (2) If there was any misunderstanding it can be cleared up immediately. For example, the person taking the message might paraphrase a communication in this way: "As I understand, Mr. Jones, you'd like Dr. Thomas to return your call after 5 p.m. on Thursday, and just to be sure that I got your phone number right, it's (214) 555-1234. Is that correct?"

In a situation where you are taking a phone number, always repeat the phone number to the caller. Many times, the patient wants to know that you got it right, but may feel awkward about asking you to repeat it. Therefore, it's really a reassurance and a courtesy to do so without the caller having to ask. It also ensures that he/she has given the right number to you! [4]

Staff members should avoid making any statements like, "I'll be *sure* to have Dr. Jones call you just as soon as she gets in." Can you really ensure that Dr. Jones will call as soon as she gets in? Though it might sound good, making a statement like that can backfire on you. You may hear from that caller later and he may be upset with either you or Dr. Jones when the call wasn't returned promptly. The best response in a situation like this is, "I'm going to put this note on Dr. Jones' desk so she'll see it when she does get in." Or if in fact you'll see Dr. Jones and hand it to her personally, then let the caller know that. But refrain from telling the caller when the call will be returned, unless it is truly in your control.

ACTIVE LISTENING

I hear it over and over again in patient focus groups: the most common complaint by patients today is they don't feel "listened to." One of the most powerful things you can do in talking to patients is to acknowledge what they are saying; let them know you heard and understand their needs. The very best way to do this is through verbal feedback. Let them state their concerns, let them *hear* that you're listening with comments like "yes, I see", "tell me more about that." Then most importantly, when they are through, paraphrase back to them what you understand they are looking for and what end results they desire. Let them hear that you understand before you offer comments or suggestions.[5] They'll be more likely to listen to your ideas once they know you really heard their concerns. This is unquestionably the most powerful verbal message you can give them. They'll want to be a patient in a practice where they feel heard and understood. If there were a miscommunication, it would come out at this point. Of course, that is only to benefit both of you. Some ways to ensure comprehension and communicate that you're really listening is to:

- tell the caller that you're taking notes, "Mr. Smith, I'm making some notes on this as you're talking;"
- give verbal acknowledgment, "I see", "yes", "I understand;"
- give verbal feedback, "Let me make sure that I got this right ... " Then offer a brief synopsis of what the caller said.

"CHATTY" PHONE CALLS

On occasion you'll get phone calls from patients, colleagues, suppliers, or friends who'll want to chat. Maybe you're swamped, or on a deadline, and maybe you know from experience that this is the person who'll talk on and on and on and you won't be able to get off the phone. You want to manage the situation with some delicacy. One way to handle this is to sandwich your key statement between two softening statements. For example, you might say something like: " Oh Jack, it's always good to hear from you. My challenge is that I'm on a project right now with a tight deadline. Unless it's something you need an answer on immediately, can I give you a call back after 3 p.m. I'll be past my deadline then and I can talk with you more comfortably."

In this situation, you've made your predicament clear, but you've softened it with statements that are friendly and indicate an interest in the individual who's calling. The other important point is that when you close this communication, make sure you leave the ball in your court. In other words, don't ask Jack to call you back. It's much better for you to call when *you're* ready to talk. The only concern here is don't forget to call him back. Make a note to yourself; otherwise he may feel like you really are putting him off indefinitely.

The Complaint or Objection Call

If you're given an objection or complaint, do not disregard it, and do not minimize it. If someone has taken the time to make a complaint, then it's serious to that person. Minimizing it, or not addressing the issue will only leave a very bad taste in the caller's mouth. Besides, it's important to know what objections or complaints there are about your practice or about a service. Actually, the patient is providing valuable information and should be thanked for taking the time to do so. If objections or complaints are not handled adequately, from the viewpoint of the patient, then one of two things is going to happen: either they'll get angry and repeat the complaint, or worse, they won't say anything else—they'll be dissatisfied and they'll spread the word. This is the worst word-of-mouth a practice can get.

Let's say that a patient makes a complaint: "Jane, I called last week for an explanation about my last statement. Someone was supposed to call me back. What's going on there?" First of all don't interrupt what the caller is saying or try to cut him short. It's best that he vent his emotions, and get them all out—then you can work toward a solution. Trying to stop him will only make matters worse.[6] Besides the words, you can hear in the inflection that the caller is upset and this must be addressed. One patient in a focus group said, "I called the office about a statement error. The bookkeeper kept interrupting me. I couldn't even finish my point. It just infuriated me."

The staff member who has the ability to empathize will find the going much easier. This has even been proven by fewer malpractice suits against physicians who listen to patients complaints and show sincere care. A New York attorney specializing in personal injury suits said: "I get a lot of people saying that if the doctor had just said he was sorry, I wouldn't be here suing him."[7]

Sometimes a team member's attitude can increase the patient's anger and in a brief moment, one that can never be retrieved, a flash of anger, annoyance, or a lack of courtesy can ruin a practice's reputation in the patient's mind. The converse is also true. A team member who has an excellent manner of responding to the concerns and needs of the patient is going to be a great good-will ambassador.

Here's a tip if you find yourself getting frustrated at a patient on the telephone. Slow your mind down and reduce tension by doing the following:

- Close your eyes.
- Keep the telephone earpiece against your ear, but move the mouthpiece by pivoting it in an arc away from your mouth.

- Inhale deeply and exhale very slowly while counting to [10].

This can help to reduce your tension and get you back in control. The technique of deep breathing is helpful in reducing tension whether you're on the phone or not. Bear in mind, it's best not to do this in view of patients; they may become concerned!

Let's investigate that patient's complaint about the statement. How should the receptionist address this problem? She might say something like: "I can certainly understand your distress over this situation, let me look into it right now and find the answer for you. Can I ask you to hold for just a moment while I get the records on this? I am going to put you on hold briefly and I'll be right back with you."

It's important to acknowledge the feelings of the caller and to avoid discounting or belittling their concerns. The patient wants to know that the receptionist is on the patient's side and wants to help. That must be addressed verbally and the vocal quality must back up and be congruent with the words. The receptionist may then come back on the line with, "Mr. Smith, I have your file in front of me. I understand your question and concern. I'm going to talk with our bookkeeper, Mary Jones. You'll hear back from me by 4 p.m. today."

By Jane's saying that she'll call back by 4 p.m., doesn't really ensure that she'll have the final answer then. Does this mean that she should delay calling until she has the details requested? No. Most importantly, patients say they want to know that the problem is being addressed. If they are kept waiting with no idea of what's happening, it only causes more concern. What's important here is that the patient knows that Jane is working on the problem and the patient is not forgotten.

"Hello, Mr. Smith. I told you I'd call back by 4 p.m. Mary and I are working on resolving the issue on your last statement. We should have it all settled with the insurance company by mid-day tomorrow. You'll be pleased to know that we *did* find the cause of the problem and it's one that can be remedied easily. I recognize how frustrating this has been for you and we sincerely apologize. You'll hear from me by 2 p.m. tomorrow at the very latest. Please know that we're all working on it, and I will get an answer for you. Thank you for being so patient."

Make sure that the words you use are positive words. Avoid using negative words. You don't want to place additional negative thoughts in the mind of the caller and you want to indicate you're a positive person working on the patient's behalf.

Sometimes there's a tendency in handling complaints to add a lot of unnecessary information. This is something that the team needs to be aware of. Patients don't really care about how the problem is solved. They *don't* want to hear about internal problems. They just want the problem solved. The point is—get to the point. Eliminate unnecessary information that may confuse or irritate the patient.

In handling a complaint call, here's what patients want:

• Let the caller air the complaint fully before taking any position. Not letting the caller vent his anger will only add fuel to the fire.

• Communicate a concern about the situation. This does not necessarily mean agreement, but empathy for the caller's predicament or irritation.

• Let the patient know that you want to find a way to make the situation right. This statement must be handled judiciously. Be sure you're not misunderstood and that the patient interprets the statement to mean that you're complying with whatever the patient wants!

• Ensure that you've understood the patient accurately by creating a feedback loop and succinctly reiterating what was said. *Do not* repeat any negative words used by the patient.

 • Be aware of your own vocal tone and pacing of your speech. Slow down and soften the voice a bit to help defuse the patient.

PUTTING PATIENTS ON HOLD

Sometimes there's no way around it, you have to put a caller on hold. In the ideal world this wouldn't happen. You'd be able to talk with each patient as the call comes in, and with no interruptions. However, we don't live in a perfect world, and so we must find the very best way to place a call on hold.

"The worst thing is if they put you on hold and don't even ask permission. If the receptionist answers the phone and immediately says, 'hold please.' I just hang up." This patient was talking in a focus group about how she felt about being put on hold in some situations.

If you must put a patient on hold, ask permission first! If the caller is on hold more than one minute chances are good that he/she thinks he/she has been forgotten. Being forgotten is unpardonable today; it means the patient is unimportant and not valued by the practice. This is one of the reasons that patients move from one practice to another—they don't feel valued.

Managing public perceptions at the front desk is a challenge and an art. It's also an opportunity to show real service skills and interpersonal savvy under pressure. This doesn't typically come naturally, it's most often learned. However, some people learn the skills and gravitate to this art more readily than others.

If you foresee that getting back to the patient quickly is going to be a challenge, let the patient know and give the patient an option of what to do, "Mrs. Jones, I'm presently assisting a patient at the counter and I have another caller on hold. I can call you back within 15 minutes or you may hold if you prefer—it will be at least two or three minutes."

Consider that you have a queue, or line, of patients in front of you. Some of the patients enter the queue in person and others enter the same queue by phone. It's important that patients be assisted in a "first come-first served" manner and that callers, who aren't cognizant of your situation, be made aware. The receptionist needs to make the situation visual for the caller. The person who is standing at the counter can see what's happening. This person will appreciate when you recognize that they were "in line" first. When you state to a caller, "I'm presently assisting a patient at the counter " you're really speaking to the person at the counter as well as the caller!

Let's face it. Once in a while, you'll have a caller who says, "No, I can't hold." What do you do? The worst thing would be to put the patient on hold anyway without acknowledging his statement. At this point it is especially important to give a visual cue to the patient at the counter. The cue should be an indication that you must address the phone call for a moment, it should show absolutely no irritation toward the caller on the line. The best way to handle this is to make direct eye contact with the patient in front of you, smile, lift the index finger in the "just a moment" gesture and respond verbally to the caller so that the standing patient understands your predicament. Saying to the caller something like, "I'm just finishing with a patient at the counter and I'd be able to be with you within one minute!" Use a questioning tone that is also friendly, then wait for a response. If the caller still says that he can't hold, ask for assistance from another business staff person who may be able to either complete the transaction with the counter patient, or assist the caller.

The worst case scenario is when you are by yourself at the front desk and cannot enlist assistance; the caller will not be put on hold and demands your attention. In this situation, you must make the standing patient aware through your verbal message to the caller. As you speak to the caller, look directly at the patient in front of you. Maintain professional composure and address the caller in a manner succinct as possible.

This is a difficult situation to say the least. The person at the counter needs to see and hear that you've been presented with a predicament, but you are handling it in a professional and gracious manner. Most people who view your dilemma and see that you handle it well will admire your ability to do so and be understanding about it. Most importantly, on concluding the call *do not* say anything disparaging about the caller or the situation to the patient in front of you.

Some of the phone systems available today have timers on them that will indicate exactly how long a person has been on hold. If you must leave your station to check on something for a patient on hold, ask another staff member at the front desk to monitor the counter to ensure that the patient is cared for. Key points here are:

- Ask permission before putting a caller on hold, "Would you be able to hold? I'll be back in just a moment."

- Wait for patient response. *Never* zap the hold button before receiving a response from the patient.

- Touch base intermittently, *at least* every 60 seconds, "Mrs. Smith, we haven't forgotten you, Cindy is checking on your records right now." Remember beyond 30-45 seconds, patients start to feel forgotten.

- On return to the phone, apologize for having put the patient on hold and thank them for their patience.

What does the patient hear when on hold and what do they prefer to hear? There are basically three choices: Music, an "on-hold" informational tape, or nothing. What are the patient preferences? We asked patients about this in focus groups. The responses were divided almost evenly between *music* and *nothing*. A very small percentage of the patients chose *informational, on hold tapes* because very few patients were aware of this medium in relation to dental offices. They were certainly aware of the concept, but since they hadn't experienced hearing dental practice tapes, they didn't know how they'd feel about them.

So we played demos from several different *on hold* companies in the focus groups. Responses were quite interesting. Those tapes that interspersed music with information were perceived to be higher quality and more patient friendly. They also liked the concept of using both male and female voices on the tapes. Patients had very strong feelings about the content of the tapes. Anything that smacked of aggressive marketing was responded to negatively. However, when the tape was patient friendly and educational in nature, patients responded positively. More on this subject as well as appropriate topics for tape inclusion is in chapter 20 on marketing.

Any music you play over the phone must be managed. If you access a radio station, you are allowing the station to manage the impression callers will have of your office. What if it's the Howard Stern program that your patients hear when on hold?! You are affording him the opportunity to influence your patients. Choose your own music and make it appropriate for your patient base. You control the mood of the moments that your patients are on hold.

Caveat: Be aware that there are legal implications in playing copyrighted music on hold or in your office. You could be violating the copyright laws.[8] This is a complex issue and it is wise for the practitioner to investigate the legal obligation on a local, state, and/or national level.

CONFIRMATION CALLS

To confirm or not to confirm, that is the question. I've heard both sides of this issue. Some say, "Don't place confirmation calls to patients; it only trains them to be reliant on you; they should be responsible for their own commitments." The flip side of this issue is, "You've got to place the confirmation calls. If you're concerned that the patient is going to cancel when you call to confirm, it's better to know that ahead of time than to have *no-shows*. At least you're given a chance to fill that time slot." Both points of view are valid. So what is truly the best action for the practice to take?

We took this question to the patients. In focus groups we asked patients, "Do you want a confirmation call or not?" Most patients indicated that they did want confirmation calls. More than 75% of patients indicated an appreciation for the reminder call. The balance of the patients indicated that they don't want or need a confirmation call and may find it even irritating if they get one.

From the patient's perspective, the ideal solution is to ask new patients how they want this handled. It's always a good idea to place a confirming call prior to the first appointment with a new patient. However, when that patient is in the office, the business staff could ask the patients their preference. "Would you like a confirmation call prior to your next appointment?" By taking this approach, you're giving the patient options. Patients like this and perceive the office to be a caring one that wants to accommodate patient preferences. In other words, the patient perceives that you are customizing your service as a part of a unique relationship with this patient.

Should the confirmation call be placed one or two days before the appointment? Again, we posed this question in focus groups. Patients responded with a slight preference for one day prior to the appointment. The ideal situation is to ask the patient what he/she wants. Pose questions to new patients like, "Would you like a confirmation call before your next appointment. Would you like to be called one or two days before the appointment? At what number should we contact you?" These questions offer patients options and are both patient-friendly and service oriented. These same questions can be asked when a patient is scheduling an appointment. Getting answers to these questions in advance can save you time, money, and frustration!

What you say in the confirmation call is very important, particularly when first working with a new patient. As an undercover patient, I receive many confirmation calls, some good and some not so good! The least effective one I received was a message left on my recorder. It went like this, "We hope you'll be able to make the appointment on Tuesday at 2 p.m. If there's any problem, please give us a call." Needless to say, I was shocked! After all, the appointment wasn't optional! What you say in a confirmation call is communicating to patients what you find to be acceptable patient behavior; you're training the patient. That message was telling the patient that it's okay to cancel or even possibly "no-show".

The best confirmation call I received was also a message on my recorder. It went like this, "We're really looking forward to seeing you Tuesday at 2:00." It was stated in an upbeat, friendly but confident voice. The underlying message was, 'we expect to see you!' Other effective approaches I've heard include, "We have Tuesday at 2 p.m. reserved for you." This adds importance to the appointment and implies a commitment on the part of the patient.

The incidence of reaching a recorder on a confirmation call has increased. As a result, in seminars I conduct many staff members have inquired about asking patients to call the office regarding the confirmation message that was left on the recorder. This is perfectly acceptable to patients, but don't expect to get a 100% response from them! You might add to your message, "We would greatly appreciate a return call from you acknowledging that you did receive this message. Our number is _____."

Emergency Calls

One of the most powerful forms of "advertising" you can get from your patients is word-of-mouth about your handling of a patient's emergency. Focus group participants consistently use this as a barometer for the amount of caring and responsiveness by the entire dental team.

In one of our groups a female patient related an incident that had caused her extreme distress. She chipped a central incisor the night before a very important meeting with the board of directors of her company. She was distraught about appearing before this powerful group with a "snaggle tooth". The focus group was very impressed that the doctor had given his patient his home phone number in case of an emergency. This patient noted that her concern was getting the problem fixed prior to her morning meeting.

She contacted the doctor at home and he met her at the office at 10:30 that night, about three hours after her phone call to him. The problem was resolved and she returned to her home that same night, the tooth repaired. She could smile with confidence!

At the close of this focus group, two patients approached her and asked for the name of the dentist.

How you handle emergencies, how accessible you are, and how responsive you are will go a long way to keeping patients in your practice and gaining referrals from them. As in the case above, many times patients' concerns are, can they even reach you? Then if they reach an answering service or recorder, how long will it be before you get the message and return the call?

Doctors Fred Aurbach and Norton Bicoll both of Dallas, TX use pagers and cellular phones for patient contact. Their patients remark about their accessibility and the comfort that brings. Dr. Aurbach who frequently travels uses a national pager and returns calls from wherever he is. Though he may not be in the same city as his patient, he is accessible and able to ensure that the patient gets help. The patients of these doctors are certainly reassured of feeling valued, cared for, and important.

Patients are reassured when they know that they can reach the practitioner at any time of the day or night. Even if they've never had a dental emergency themselves, when they are presented with the prospect of such, they state that the "caring dentist" is one who will be available to them. Dr. Tom McDougal, who lectures   nationwide to dental teams on developing and maintaining high standards of service to patients, confirms this, "Twenty-four hour availability is essential in delivering ultra-service to patients."

Here are some issues that are important to patients as they relate to emergencies. As you review this list, ask yourself, "How would our patients rate us?"
Outside of regular office hours patients want:
- (in a perfect world) to reach the doctor directly,
- (ideally) to hear back from the doctor within one hour of their emergency call,
- (acceptable) to receive a call from a staff member or on-call colleague within two hours.

During regular office hours patients want:

- (in a perfect world) to be told to come to the office right away,
- (ideally) to be seen by the office on the same day the phone call is placed

Naomi Rhode, RDH, CPAE, confirmed that opportunities can come from assisting callers in emergency situations. She related to me a dramatic illustration concerning a dentist friend. This dentist's name in the phone book was shown at the bottom of the listing because his last name began with the letter "R". He received an emergency call from an individual who indicated that he was not a patient of the practice. However, "Dr. R." agreed to treat the man. The patient who arrived at the office for emergency treatment was Richard Nixon! The offices that turned down this patient because he was not a patient of record, lost the opportunity to treat a whole family and a lot of secret service members as well!

After Hours Calls

In conducting some "real world" research on answering systems and emergency messages, I placed about 50 calls to offices one weekend. There was a significant range in quality of messages and information offered. But there were two calls that stood out from the others. One office had its calls forwarded to the doctor's home line and the doctor actually answered the phone! The second call caused me some concern about this office. The staff member who recorded the message said, "We accept emergencies for patients of record, only." What was jarring about this was the vocal tone in conjunction with the verbal message. It was brittle, cold, and abrupt. She presented the office as one that was uncaring and strictly business. Emergencies are frequently opportunities to develop new patients and reinforce existing relationships. Refusing to treat some emergencies is one issue, but the way that it is stated is another issue entirely. If you must make a statement like this, make sure it doesn't sound rigid or cold.

If you use a recording system after hours, ensure that the quality of the message is good. Listen to the tape after recording it. It should:
- be free from static and background noise,
- present the practice in a warm, friendly, and upbeat manner,
- avoid negative words, phrase the message using positive words.

Patients want to hear on the tape:
- office hours,
- what to do in an emergency,

Information on the recorder that is optional, yet helpful includes:
- fax number,
- location.

When we discuss emergency contact in focus groups, patients strongly indicate that there is a great deal of reassurance that comes by way of knowing the emergency number is the doctor's home phone. This courtesy communicates a feeling of importance and a message of being valued by this practitioner.

An ideal way for you to manage this is to use a telephone company feature called, "Distinctive Ring." This feature can be ordered through the telephone company at a slight add-on cost per month. It requires no equipment changes at all on your home phone line. You are given a second phone number different from your home phone number. This number can then be given to your patients for use in emergency calls. Should a patient contact you by that number, your telephone will give a distinctive ring. In many cases, this will be a double ring. Consequently, when you hear this type of ring, it is an indication that a patient is calling you on an emergency basis. If you opt to do so, you can allow a home recording device to answer this call; this could then be monitored and the call returned to the patient. In order for this concept to work, *only* give this number to patients for emergency calls. If you are concerned about electronic devices which can reveal your primary home phone number, you can request that the phone company block your own phone number on any outgoing calls you make.

Patients are reassured and feel greater confidence in the practice when they know that the entire team is involved in the continuing education process. Therefore, if your office is closed due to attendance at continuing education programs, be sure to let your patients know this. Make a special audio tape for the days of the meeting. Then be sure that you switch back to your original tape after the meeting is over. I have called offices where the after-hours tape indicates, "We are at our state dental association continuing education meeting from the third to the fifth . . . " However the date that I called the office was the eighth and they had not switched back to their original tape. This can actually cause more concern in the patient's mind. The office is not paying attention to details.

Patients want to be able to leave a message on your office recorder and this raises a legitimate concern regarding appointment cancellations left on your recorder. In a seminar I conducted, one audience member suggested, "On the recording tell callers, 'this recorder does not accept cancellations!'" Another audience member noted that the office had cut down on recorder cancellations by requesting that patients, "contact the doctor at home if you are calling to cancel your appointment!"

As in the issue of patients who cancel their appointment when they receive the confirmation call, at least you know about it in advance. The patient is not a "no-show". It gives you an opportunity to fill the time slot.

In using an answering service you must monitor it frequently. After all, you are giving up the management of your image to an outside company. There are problems that can be experienced through use of an answering service. If you've found one that is very reliable and presents your practice consistently and positively to the public, count your blessings and stay with them. But don't give up monitoring them; have others call at odd hours and pose the kind of questions that patients ask. Pay attention to any complaints you receive from patients about your service. Any single complaint you receive about service represents ten people who have problems but say nothing. These are the calls you need to be concerned about. How do they perceive your practice? The same information that is available from an office recorder should also be available from your answering service.

I do have a bias toward a well scripted answering system over which you have control. You are able to manage the quality, the tone, and the biggest advantage is the consistency that is produced through use of a recording system. Two issues are crucial in your recording:

• Patients *must* feel assured that they will be able to reach you in an emergency. Ensure that you handle this well in your recording and that you promptly respond to patient emergency calls.

• Because technology is taking the place of a "real person", the recorded voice *must* be warm, caring and welcoming.

VOICE MAIL

Voice mail is sometimes said to be a sophisticated relative of the answering machine. In reality it can provide far more options for callers and the practice. This does not necessarily mean that it is the best option of communication for your patients! A sizable portion of the public today rails against the cold anonymity of this technology and real care must be taken in relation to patient perceptions. This technology is still in its infancy.

Business and the public is struggling with how to handle it, evidenced by consultants who work with clients on how to approach and manage the technology. Likewise, equipment providers even have formed an association to ensure that user frustration doesn't lead to backlash. The "Voice Messaging Educational Committee promotes correct use of their products" and assists companies in making the technology more user-friendly.[9] There are many advantages to a sophisticated system and voice mail can be particularly advantageous for the larger office with many team members.

In the dental practice, voice mail is most effective when it remains "in the background" working for the benefit of both patients and the team. For example, "message mail boxes" can be accessed by patients *if* the patient has been given the number in advance. Patients could opt to leave a voice message for the doctor or team member and ask the phone receptionist to "connect the call to Dr. Jones' voice mailbox." This can also be helpful for colleagues leaving messages for specific team members. The key concept here is that the doctor or team members must determine if the "mailbox" number is to be given to a patient or not. Also the patient is given the choice of whether to use the mailbox during office hours or to leave the message with a "real person."

One of the benefits of some systems after hours is patient access to mailboxes that provide patient-friendly information like hours, directions to office, and even educational information about the practice or services. This approach to voice mail is somewhat of a cousin to *on hold* concepts. However, its key difference is that the information is accessed when, and only if, the patient elects to hear it.

Caveat: Although voice mail technology can be effective after hours for messages, the automated voice should *not* be the first voice that greets the patient during regular office hours. The public currently has an adverse reaction to any health care provider that separates itself from its patients to this extent during regular hours.

NEW OR PROSPECTIVE PATIENTS

The following items are those that are important to new or prospective patients in learning about your practice. They also help to promote the practice. Bear in mind that when a new or prospective patient calls your office, it's his ballgame. Issues that are important to the patient should be addressed first; issues that are important to the practice should be addressed second. Sometimes these concepts can overlap as in providing answers to patient's questions that also help to promote the practice.

As soon as you have learned that this is a perspective patient, or a new patient calling, make every attempt to avoid putting this individual on hold. If this is a serious inquiry from a prospective patient, and you offer to call the individual back, you most likely have lost your opportunity with this caller. If need be, forward the call to another individual who can answer the prospective patient's questions.

I was making inquiry calls to numerous dental offices to determine how well they were promoting their practices. One office did an exceptional job of helping this caller feel important and valued. The individual who answered the phone indicated to me that she could answer my questions more readily at another phone—that she was at a very busy front desk and she was going to move to another office where it was a little quieter. At that point, she switched to another office and another line where she seemed more relaxed during the conversation. This action communicated to this caller that she valued and appreciated the inquiry; her demeanor was likely to encourage any patient or any caller to feel special.

Consider the following list as ways to present your office positively to the public.

• Find out what is important to the caller. If the caller says, "tell me about the doctor." Find out the patient's specific interest area, as in, "I'll be happy to. Tell me about your interests; did you want to know about our office specifically, about the doctor's background, or about our services?" Once you know what the patient is interested in, you'll be marketing the practice in a way that is the most valuable to the patient.

• Make positive statements. Whatever you are discussing with any patient, take a positive approach even if it is an unusual request that is being made. A statement like, "let's see what we *can* do" versus "We *can't* do that." No patient wants to go to an office that takes a negative approach.

• Speak well of the dentist and the team members. This is very powerful and confidence-building for patients, they like to hear when the staff communicates pride and enthusiasm for the entire practice.

• If the patient is new in your area and makes an appointment, be sure to offer directions to your office as well as where to park and what door to enter, if that is an issue in relation to your building. Also be sure to welcome the patient to the area!

• When responding to patient questions about the team or your office, quote other patients. "Our patients say they really appreciate how gentle the doctor is." If the patient had previously communicated a concern about pain or expressed anxiety, this kind of statement can be very powerful.

Caveat: Express reality only! If the patient is let down, or if you have exaggerated reality, patient trust in the practice will be shaken.

• Listen for subtle insights as to what is important to the patient, whether it's clinical or non-clinical. A statement like, "My husband has been transferred and the family will be here next month," offers opportunities. Inherent in this statement are numerous chances to build a connect and develop a relationship with the family. Asking about dental care for the balance of the family is appropriate as well as verbalizing an affirmation that the office is responsive to children.

• Posing questions to the caller like, "What other information can I provide you about the office." "Is there any other way we can help you?" These statements indicate an office that is sensitive to, and wants to meet the needs of the patient.

• Be sure to thank these callers, "Thank you for calling our office and giving us the opportunity to see how we might be of service to you." "Mrs. Smith, thank you for selecting our office. It's going to be a pleasure to meet you next week." This is an absolute given; patients *must* be acknowledged today. They must know that you value them. The words, "thank you" are crucial in gaining and retaining your patients. This can not be understated.

Patients discuss this at length in focus groups; if they feel unappreciated, if they feel undervalued, if they are not acknowledged, they are at risk of leaving your practice. Every team member must understand the significance of this.

PROFESSIONAL PROTOCOL TIPS

The following concepts for professional telephone protocol, when used collectively, will send a message of efficiency, credibility, and service to your callers. These concepts will enhance your telephone image.

1. Always have writing materials near the phone—paper and pen or pencil, as well as message pads. If necessary, attach chained pens to the phone. Searching for pen or note paper sends visions of a disorganized individual.

2. Introduce any calls you transfer—stay on the line to ensure proper transfer and introduce the caller. Patients don't like having to explain a second time why they're calling.

3. Use positive words in all communication. Avoid using the word "no," especially at the beginning of a sentence. Challenge yourselves to rethink communication in positive terms.

4. Consider carefully how you close each call. Close the call with an indication of what will happen—will you call him back, if so, when? Will she be sending you information, if so when should you be expecting it? Explain what is to happen next as a result of the call. Thank your patients and prospective patients for calling if it is appropriate for the type of call placed. They are the lifeblood of your organization. In a competitive marketplace, the consumer needs to be told that his

business is valued and appreciated. Help him *know* he is truly important to you and the practice.

5. Realize that each person who answers the phone represents far more than himself or herself. It is a powerful role which affects the perception of the entire practice. This concept goes beyond communicating with patients; it also affects perceptions of different departments within the same office. Besides serving the patient, you also serve each other within the same practice, and the respect given to the patient hopefully transcends to all peers and team members as well.

6. Develop and print your own telephone procedures for the team. I find it is a rare office that has written instructions. Consistency is crucial and without written procedures it is easy to have inconsistency. Write out a list of procedures staff should follow in answering all calls—both external and interoffice. Make sure the list is understood by all employees and posted by every telephone. Periodically call in to your office and experience these procedures as the patient does.

Fax Technology

It's hard to talk about communicating in business today without addressing the facsimile machine. A few years ago callers would ask, "Do you have a fax machine?" Today they ask, "What is your fax number?" These machines have changed the way we do business and have made the world a lot smaller. If you don't have a fax machine, you need one! Once you have it, you'll wonder how you managed before. Spend just a little more money and get a plain paper fax instead of the thermal paper variety, it's well worth the difference in cost.

Be sure to include your fax number on all collateral materials, letterhead, business cards, brochures, and newsletters. Add the number to your outgoing *after hours* message, or provide it to your answering service. Here are some fax facts:

• Keep your fax message as short as possible. Don't use a full page cover sheet when a smaller one will do. The 3-M company produces several types of "stick-on" notes which act as the leader for the fax.

• It's a good idea to phone the patient or colleague before you send the fax to alert them it's coming. If you accidentally fax it to the wrong number or if there is a transmission error at the other end, you may not know that they haven't received it. Or call following transmission to ensure that they know it was sent.

Top Tips:

1. Remind yourself that you're not there to schedule patients, but to help people and to build relationships.
2. Preventing objections is more pleasant than overcoming them; anticipate patient concerns and address them up front.
3. Be specific on the phone; the success of follow up calls and patient compliance is in direct proportion to how specific you are.
4. Only trained people should answer the phone; better to put the phones on an answering system than to have patients think that the team member is unprepared, uninformed, untrained. Manage the impressions you make!
5. Have something of value to offer on every call you make; make sure patients hang up from the call feeling valued.

6. At the close of every call either thank the caller for the inquiry, or summarize the discussion, whichever is appropriate for the type of call received or made.

REFERENCES

[1] Decker, Bert. *The Art of Communicating*, Crisp Publications, Inc, Los Gatos, CA, 1988.

[2] Moine, Donald J.; Herd, John H. *Modern Persuasion Strategies: The Hidden Advantage in Selling*, Prentice Hall, Inc., Englewood Cliffs, NJ, 1984.

[3] Caplan, Carl Michael. *Dental Practice Encyclopedia*, PennWell Publishing Co., Tulsa, OK 1985.

[4] Jameson, Cathy, *Great Communication=Great Production*, PennWell Publishing Company, Tulsa, OK, 1994.

[5] Elgin, Suzette Haden. *The Last Word on the Gentle Art of Verbal Self-Defense*, Prentice Hall Press, New York, NY, 1987.

[6] Jameson, Cathy. *Great Communication=Great Production*, PennWell Publishing Company, Tulsa, OK, 1994.

[7] _____. "Trying to Be Nice is No Labor of Love," *Wall Street Journal*, New York, NY, November 29, 1990.

[8] McAndrew, Tara. "Paying for Playing," *Illinois Dental News*, Chicago, IL, February, 1996.

[9] Keates, Nancy. "After the Beep . . . Please Mind Your Manners," *Wall Street Journal*, New York, NY, May 29, 1996.

12

Dental Office Decor: Picture Perfect for Patients

"Either this wallpaper goes, or I do."
— OSCAR WILDE

How important is the appearance of your office and the availability of amenities to your patients? Do they really notice the details and if so, how does your office decor influence patients? Here are some comments patients have made about these topics:

- "The office is beautiful and it's a soothing environment. I've got three kids under 10, I like being in an environment that's calm, quiet, and pleasant!"

- "This office has two reclining chairs in the waiting room, I've never seen that in a doctor's office before."

- "There's a TV in the ceiling and it helps me get my mind off of what's happening."
- "If they've got old magazines in reception, then they're probably not taking care of other details either."
- "I look at the cleanliness of the furniture and the carpet to determine if the clinical areas are clean."
- "There's a phone in the waiting room and I like knowing I can check in with my office if I need to."

Because patients do not know how to judge clinical matters, they use other criteria they do understand. The appearance of your office and the amenities that you offer to patients communicate a great deal to them. There is also a delicate balance. It is crucial that practitioners understand the mind-sets of their patients and prospective patients. As one patient commented, "As soon as I walked in that office and I saw the furniture I just knew I was going to be hit with a big bill." Your office must be consistent with the overall image of the practice and it must be consistent in both design and in maintenance. Let's look at some of the key elements in relation to decor and how patients may respond.

As patients enter the office, impressions have already started to influence them about your practice. The first time that a patient pays a visit to your office, your location, the building maintenance, the accessibility to the building, and the safety of the surroundings, all influence patients. This is a parallel to what realtors refer to as "curb" appeal. What a house looks like on the outside as a prospective buyer approaches will influence their expectations and their mood as they prepare to enter the house. If it looks great on the outside, then they are expecting good things upon entering. If it doesn't look so great on the outside, they may not even want to see the house.

Even the appearance of your doorway can represent to patients what may be on the other side of that door. One office I visited was located in a medical park where the grounds were beautifully maintained. The walkway to the front door was bordered by beautiful plants and ground cover, but when I reached the front door, my positive first impression dropped several notches. The light tan doorway was covered with fingerprints. I couldn't imagine how long it had been since the door had last been cleaned. That was the first physical impression of the practice. If you were the patient what might you think about infection control measures in this office? If you were one of the patients who had concerns about this issue, imagine your thoughts as you walked through the doorway!

LOCATION AND PARKING

The maintenance of the building and the grounds communicate something about you regardless of whether you own the property or not. You might say, "I have no control over the maintenance of the grounds or of the building manager!" However, that's not the point for your patients. Their feeling is, "Well, the doctor chose this location and so its appearance must be acceptable to him or her." Sometimes, patients can be attracted to a certain office or practice solely because of the outside appearance or location.

I was an undercover patient for the office of a general practitioner. I had made the preliminary calls to the office and was given directions to the location. However, when I arrived, the signage for the office indicated that there were two doctors in the same suite. They were partners in the sense that they were sharing office space, but each had his own independent practice. That had not been made clear in the initial phone calls to the office, and it was therefore, confusing to drive up and see the partner's name listed first. I was initially unsure that I was at the right office. This should have been communicated on the phone so that patients wouldn't be surprised.

Signage is extremely important. The sign needs to be clear and easily readable from primary access areas. Make sure that shrubs and foliage do not obstruct the view of your sign. If appropriate to your location a spotlight on your sign can be attractive and brings attention to your practice. A sign that is well designed aids in communicating a quality message.

One office that I visited was located in a high foot-traffic area frequented by middle-income adults. The office had affixed to their front door a business card holder, which contained a supply of business cards for passers-by. In addition, office hours and phone number were listed on the door making it easy for patients to know when to call.

Ease of accessibility is becoming more and more important. Patients would prefer to drive right up in front of your building and park instead of having to go to a parking garage. Frequently, offices that are located in dental or medical complexes require patient use of a parking garage. As addressed in chapter 1 on the Aging of our Society, many patients are expressing appreciation for a less complicated way of doing things. If an older patient is required to park in a parking garage and then pay for parking, this can be considered an inconvenience by some patients. Offering a token or covering the patient's cost of parking will help to alleviate some aggravation that can be caused by the inconvenience.

Make sure that regardless of the type of facility you are in, patient safety is ensured. Adequate lighting during winter months or on inclement days is becoming more of an issue for the public due to increased crime. Also important for colder climates is adequate sanding or de-icing during winter months.

Accessibility to your office for the physically challenged is very important and becoming more so. Adequate ramps allowing patient entrance to your facility can help to communicate a message of value to, and importance of, wheelchair users. One patient noted, "The ramp was located at the far end of the strip office center. It was very inconvenient and awkward especially during our rainy season."

RECEPTION AREA

What does your patient see upon entering your office? How welcoming does the environment appear even without a smiling staff member to offer a warm greeting?

On entering the office of Dr. Tom McDougal, patients see a spectacular display of live plants and greenery. A self-service beverage area invites patients to feel at home. The reception area looks much like a comfortable living room. Beautiful atrium windows extend over the seating area and bring a sense of nature inside. This backdrop offers a soothing environment for patient-centered service that is congruent with the quality of care provided by the practice. The likely interpretation by patients is, "We are important and we will receive exceptional service and clinical treatment here."

There are many visual factors that will affect how patients interpret your office and the care they think they will receive. Colors, textures, furniture styles, and room arrangement all combine to affect your patients in different ways. The decor of your office can influence:

• the patient's perception of the clinical skills and treatments provided by the office,

• the perception of fees charged by the office,

- the patient's mood prior to entering the treatment areas, and
- the patient's likelihood of returning to the office and/or making referrals to the office.

Important design issues like functional zoning and traffic flow are critical to production and efficiency within the office. Though they will influence the patient, most patients are not as aware of these factors as they are of the basic aesthetic elements of decor.

LIGHTING

Patients remark that they want the lighting in the office to be bright enough so they can read easily. However, they do not want it so bright that it is distracting or seems "hospital-like", as one patient put it. In asking patients in a focus group to describe what the ideal office looks like, they frequently indicated "soft overhead lighting in reception and table lamps or standing lamps in the seating and reading areas."

Just as patients do not care for a "too bright" room, they also dislike seating areas that are too dark. A patient in one group commented, "If the room is too dark it starts to look depressing and almost scary." If they were forced to choose between too bright or too dark, too bright was preferred.

Patients are less likely to describe clinical areas with any degree of confidence. They are less sure of what they like and are more apt to describe what they do *not* like in clinical areas. In one focus group, patients remarked that unpleasant lighting in the treatment room would be that which is glaring or harsh on the eyes when the patient is in the supine position.

FURNISHINGS AND THE APPOINTMENT COUNTER

When shown photographs of different styles of furniture for the reception area, patients indicated a strong preference for individual seating rather than couches. This preference may relate to issues of territory and control. When the patient is in an individual seat, the patient does not have to interact and is not required to "share" space as when seated on a couch next to a stranger.[1]

The reception counter at the appointment area is one patients do have strong feelings about. They frequently comment they do not like the windows or, a "hole in the wall". Patients far prefer an open counter. The reason and preference for this is that they can more readily monitor the team and know what is happening. They have stated that if they have questions, they feel far more comfortable approaching an open counter than a small window. As one patient said, "If I have a question, I'm going to feel okay about going up to a counter, but if there's a patient already standing at a window, I'm not going to feel comfortable standing in line."

Patients also indicate that they think the team is more aware and understanding of what is going on in the reception area when there is a counter rather than a small window. For example, one patient noted, "At my last appointment, a young mother had two children in the waiting room. They were spreading toys all over the floor and their mother didn't supervise them. I don't think the staff knew what was happening because they were behind that wall and they couldn't see through the little window."

Also, when shown illustrations of different offices, patients indicated a preference for the open counters which were designed in an arc or flowing line. They commented that it appeared more patient-friendly and more visually attractive, not as "hard-edged". This counter design is one that is advocated by T.H.E. Design in Austin, TX. An underlying message to patients in relation to this type of design is that the dental team is open to patients. Patients see this and the interpretation is that you are accessible to them.

The following items are optional in the reception area. However, we have learned from focus groups that they are highly appreciated.

- **Patient telephone:** A telephone in the reception area that uses a line specifically designated for patient use. Avoid signage with this phone unless you find flagrant misuse by patients, that is, patients using it for extended conversations that may interfere with the use by, or comfort of, other patients.

- **Refreshments:** Patients really appreciate it when an office has refreshments available such as coffee, other beverages, or appropriate food. What food is appropriate? Fruit or light, healthy snacks. I visited the office of an orthodontist where an office member brought homemade coffee cake that had caramel and nuts drizzled across the top! This is not the best choice of snack, particularly in the office of an orthodontist.

Another office I visited offered healthy juices and bagels in the morning. Patients who arrived for early morning appointments were particularly appreciative.

- **Writing desk:** Though this was not at the top of the list of patients' preferred amenities, those patients who liked the idea felt very strongly about it. One saleswoman noted, "My dental appointments are usually slotted between sales calls and I can sit down at the desk and take a few minutes to prepare for my next meeting while I'm waiting." If you do include a desk in your reception area, decide whether it's to be used for decoration or whether it will be functional for patients' use.

COLORS AND TEXTURES

Patients are most responsive to colors and textures that help them feel relaxed in the dental office. When we ask their preferences, they frequently cite soft colors and pastels. Many also like soft neutrals that are accented with cheerful, bright colors, as long as the accents are not jarring.

Soft textures are preferable to hard-edged finishes. Just as carpeting helps to absorb sound, it also gives a softer, "home-like" feeling to the office. Area rugs can add visual texture to a room, but care must be taken as they can result in hazards and possible falls. Walls covered with fabric offer a lot of patient-friendly benefits because they absorb sound, add visual appeal to the walls, and a side benefit is that they can also cover cracks or wall imperfections! In addition, this kind of wall treatment provides a comforting, insulated feeling to a room. Most importantly, patients like the idea of fabric on the walls. In discussing decor with focus group participants, the majority of participants perceived this to be a quality design treatment that seemed "softer" and more soothing than "hard" walls.

PRIVACY ISSUES

Patient privacy is particularly important in the dental practice. Any location where there is likely to be a discussion related to financial matters, patients must be afforded privacy. They talk about this in focus groups and very much dislike discussions of their bills or payment plans to occur in front of other patients.

A patient only has to overhear a financial discussion in the next treatment room, and their concerns are, "If I can hear that patient's discussion about finances then other people can hear my discussion and my concerns as well." Make sure that you afford the patient the opportunity to discuss these matters in private. If your treatment areas are in an open-bay design or if it's possible to hear from one treatment room to another, then it is strongly suggested that a consultation room or private office be utilized for financial discussions. This also relates to matters at the counter. There needs to be sufficient distance between the patient who is handling a closing financial matter and other patients in the vicinity.

READING MATERIAL

The reading matter that you provide in the reception area is frequently a matter of discussion by patients in relation to decor, patient amenities, and even perceptions of cleanliness and infection control.

There are certain publications and types of publications that patients like to see in reception. The two most frequently mentioned popular publications are *Life* magazine and *People* magazine. Other frequently voiced preferences include: a sports publication (like *Sports Illustrated*, but not the swimsuit issue please!), a news publication (*Time, Newsweek,* etc.), a mainstream women's publication (*Ladies Home Journal, McCalls, Redbook*). The breadth of selection offered depends in a large part on the demographics of your practice. If you have a high percentage of baby boomers, then including publications that would appeal to them is important. This is also a significant factor in addressing the interests of different cultural groups. Focus group participants of various ethnic groups affirm that this variety would be welcomed.

Patients also comment on the unusual magazines they find in some offices. One patient said, "I like it because my dentist has some really interesting ones that I would not normally see, so it's stimulating. I like the ones with travel photographs and articles about resorts, and some of the high tech and science magazines. I started subscribing to *Omni* when I found it in his office!"

It's also strongly suggested that you include at least one publication of a health nature. *American Health* magazine is an excellent selection. The publication itself is very supportive of the dental profession, with a regular column on oral hygiene. By having a publication like this in your office you are making a statement that you recognize the importance of overall health and that you do see the patient as a "whole person".

I also have been in offices that include books on health. I've even seen heart healthy cookbooks in offices with blank recipe cards that are preprinted with the practice name on it. Patients could copy recipes on the cards and use them in home cooking. Each time they'd look at the cards, there would be positive associations of health with that dental practice! Any of these options sends a positive message to your patients.

In evaluating the mix of reading material, I suggest that the office include 50% consumer publications and 50% dental-related, patient education items. Additional items to be considered for inclusion are collateral materials about your practice, practice newsletter, and brochure. (See chapter 20 on marketing.)

In addition to collateral pieces that promote your practice, seriously consider including photographs of your work. This may be best presented in the form of photograph albums. Many patients are impressed by seeing before and after pictures of treatments offered by your practice. However, I am amazed that many of the offices have these albums unlabeled and tucked away on the shelf where patients don't even see them. Get them out on a coffee table or in an area where patients will see the books. Have the albums marked clearly on the outside so patients recognize what the book includes; frequently, patients will not open an album like this if there is no indication on the outside what it is. Include typewritten comments under the photos that explain what treatment the photo illustrates.

Caveat: Though patients find these before and after pictures fascinating, avoid using any before pictures that show bloody detail or that might look painful. Patients of all ages consistently comment on their distaste for seeing "scary" photographs in a dental office.

You may consider including purchased books of professional photographs illustrating before and after treatments. However, if these books are used, make sure the patient understands that you are *not* intending to imply that this is your work. A book like, *Change Your Smile* dramatically illustrates before and after treatments without any likely misattributions implied or inferred.[2]

DECORATIONS

One of the most pleasant decorations that can greet patients when they arrive in your office is fresh flowers. Patients do like to see plants and silk floral arrangements in tasteful colors that coordinate with the office decor. However, it is fresh flowers which typically gain the most points with patients. We're not considering the issue of practicality here as much as patient preference!

If you promote aesthetic procedures, recognize that many of the patients who visit your office in search of aesthetic treatment may have greater sensitivity and awareness to the appearance and furnishings of your office. Congruence and consistency, once again is crucial here. I visited one office undercover and was shocked by what I saw. This office presented itself as offering "high-quality cosmetic care for the aware and discerning patient." The text in the promotional piece read well but the office did not look as good as the advertisement did! The chairs in the reception area had been bumped against the wall so many times that there was a line of chipped paint running horizontally across the room. There were spots on the floor and the toilet paper holder was broken in the bathroom. How could this office possibly promote aesthetic procedures when it couldn't keep its own office in presentable order?

Not long after that visit, I saw another office that provided a dramatic contrast to the first. I visited the office of Dr. Jeffrey Shapiro in New York City, NY. I was impressed with the subtlety of decor, the fine artwork and the furnishings that complimented the image of a finely tuned practice of aesthetic dentistry. What I found particularly significant with this office was the congruence and consistency of the image with that of the practice brochure. The promotional piece had design elements reminiscent of art deco style. The reception area of the office had similar design lines in the wall, lamps, and ceiling treatment. The ambiance of the office duplicated the feeling experienced in reading the brochure. This kind of congruence is rare and highly desirable.

Dr. Shapiro suggests that when designing the office, "first set the image you want to portray and make sure it is an extension of yourself and your philosophies." This philosophy was evidenced in the congruence seen between the brochure and the office design. Another important point is appropriate here—that the practitioner must be comfortable with the environment in which he/she is working. The decor must work for *both* the patient and the practitioner! When the practitioner is comfortable and at ease in the environment, the patient is likely to share these feelings.

The details in the decorations you use tell a great deal more about you and how you feel about patients. A well designed reception area will help them understand that the same attention to detail and quality here is what might be expected in your care of them as well. What elements you use in your reception area decor also depends largely upon the demographics of your patient base. Obviously, the more sophisticated and urbane your patient base is, the more important that your artwork or decoration be of a sophisticated and high quality level. Regardless of whether you are using original artwork or museum prints, the subjects and selections should be appropriate for the dental practice.

I visited one office that reminded me of a SoHo gallery in New York. The doctor was a modern art aficionado and he enjoyed "trying out" his new purchases in the reception area and hallways of his office. It was like a revolving gallery. Each time patients came in they would see a new piece. However, his tastes were so eclectic that it was likely that a good percentage of his patient base may not have related to many of these pieces. They were primarily non-objective and abstract lithographs. Some of them were very large pieces, extremely bold and dramatic with broad slashes of brightly contrasting colors.

This doctor was creating a space which he enjoyed. The patient doesn't need to understand your preferences, but your decor should not result in the patient feeling uneasy. Research in intensive care units have shown that some abstract art can increase anxiety in patients whereas subjects of nature are responded to by patients with greater regularity. [3]

The Art Research Institute of Atlanta, GA takes a unique approach in offering healthcare organizations artwork that combines photography, nature, and window concepts to increase patient sense of wellness and aid in reducing patient anxiety. Owner Joey Fischer's artificial windows are created with transparencies of nature subjects and are set into what appears to be windows. The "windows" can help to bring the image of the outdoors to windowless rooms and a computer driven light box can offer endless options and views of a soothing and strikingly beautiful outside world.

The importance of windows to dental patients cannot be understated. In a focus group discussion on decor one patient remarked, "I was having my teeth cleaned at a new dental office and the room that I was in had no windows. I felt trapped and the room felt really small." Another patient commented, "I sat in the chair staring out the window at the roof of the building next door. It was in the middle of summer and it was about 101 degrees outside. All I could see was gray concrete and it looked hot. I sat in that chair for two hours and it seemed like four hours." When patients have nothing positive to view, when everything in their immediate surroundings of the treatment room is clinical, then patients are more likely to focus on their own internal issues, worries, or stressful thoughts. If you don't have windows in the treatment room(s) then use some type of artwork to aid in patient distraction.

The office of Dr. Susan Hollar of Arlington, TX is such a model of beauty, her office design won a city award for beautification of the area. I was delighted with the facility when I saw it the first time. The first view of the office as I approached the parking area was naturalized plants and flowers artfully sculpted to surround the free-standing building. (Fig. 12-1)

The reception area was professionally decorated in soothing colors with a sophisticated southwestern theme. But what really made me recognize the unique atmosphere of the practice was the treatment areas. What

I'd seen from the front of the building was even more spectacular in the back. Sitting in the treatment chair, I faced a wall of glass that looked out on a beautifully designed landscape that included squirrel and bird feeders.

During my treatment, I had the pleasure of watching squirrels dashing about eating the wildlife food left for them. I saw several varieties of birds and there was an Audubon bird book available in the room for patients. The property was landscaped yet looked entirely natural. Although the office was located in a highly populated area, I felt like I'd been transported to a lush oasis. This is a decor that would undoubtedly provide soothing and pleasant distractions for patients. (Fig. 12-2)

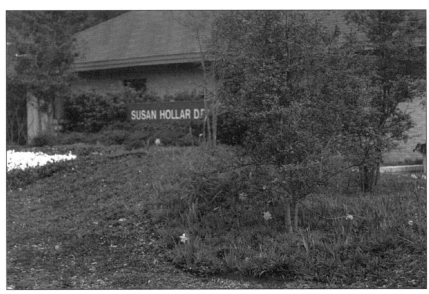

Fig. 12-1 The exterior of Dr. Susan Hollar's office welcomes patients and visitors with beautiful landscaping. (Courtesy Susan Hollar, D.D.S., F.A.G.D.)

Patients really do want some kind of softening in decor whether it is in the reception area or in the treatment

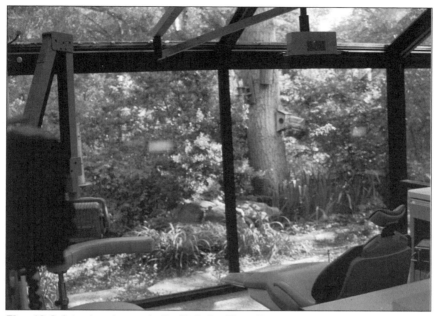

Fig. 12-2 A treatment room in Dr. Hollar's office offers a peaceful view of nature. (Courtesy Susan Hollar, D.D.S., F.A.G.D.)

room. Listed below are items that patients indicate they like to see in the dental practice:

RECEPTION

- **Art:** Artwork, prints, or photographs that are soothing and comforting in subject matter and in artistic approach.
- **"After" photographs:** Save the *before* photographs for the coffee table album and place only photographs of smiling, attractive people on the wall. These photographs are perhaps best placed in hallways, leaving the reception area to have a living-room feel to it.
- **Freestanding artwork:** Sculpture, mobiles, or stabiles send a message of uniqueness to your patients.

These pieces of artwork are more unusual to see in a dental practice and tend to communicate to the patient that you are different.

- **Degrees and certificates:** Patients *do* notice these. They might not read them, but as with the number of initials after your name, they do send a message to patients! Get them out of your personal office and into an area where patients can see them, the reception area, the hallway, or treatment rooms. Handsome frames and a grouping of certificates or degrees can make an attractive presentation all on its own. These are also very appropriate for presentation in a consultation room. If you do place them in the consultation room, position them so that the patient will be facing them during discussion.

- **Fish tanks:** Patients *really* like these. They find them very soothing and remark that watching the fish helps to reduce their anxiety.

- **Children's amusements:** If you promote your office as one which treats children, make sure that is apparent in the reception area. Children's books, magazines, and toys, are most appreciated when there is a specific area within the reception room for children. The possibility of this of course, depends upon the size of your reception room. Many adult patients, particularly older adults, appreciate a separation from the children's play area. (Fig. 12-3)

- **Patient education equipment:** There is much to be said for the benefits of technology in helping to educate the dental patient. It must remain patient friendly and the patient must have some ability to control it, not vice versa. We have learned from patients in focus groups that they prefer video or computer patient education technology to be positioned in an area away from the main reception room. This is addressed in greater depth in a later section of this chapter.

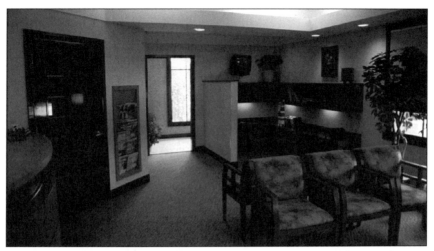

Fig. 12-3 This reception room includes a designated children's area and a magazine rack to reduce clutter. Muted colors give a relaxed feeling. (Courtesy T.H.E. Design, Inc., Austin, TX)

TREATMENT AND HYGIENE ROOMS

- **Windows/pictures:** This is a top priority for patients in clinical areas. They want to either look out a window *at* something or *into* something such as a photograph or piece of artwork. In one office I visited, the treatment room had no window. None was needed; a patient of the practice was a very talented professional artist and painted a wonderful, very large and fanciful picture of a fish tank filled with all manner of tropical and exotic fish. A patient could get lost in the intricacies of that painting! The treatment room next door had an oddly placed window in a corner, facing a large tree. The same artist painted branches along two walls in this treatment room to appear as if the outside tree branches extended across the room. Both of these were clever solutions to challenging situations.

- **Certificates:** Patients *do* like to see certificates and degrees in treatment rooms. Place them in the visual field of the seated patient; they increase patient confidence in the practitioner(s).

- **Intraoral camera:** If you use an intraoral camera make sure that it is positioned so that the patient can view the monitor while he/she is seated. I was a patient in one office where the doctor had the monitor positioned *behind* my chair. The doctor could see the monitor but I could not!

- **Instruments:** Patients would prefer that your clinical instruments remain behind their line of vision as much as possible. Patients have stated that not only does this *clean* look appear more sterile but it's more comforting for them to *not* see instruments or equipment until they really have to.

REST ROOM

The rest room is an area that is much discussed in continuing education programs and frequently noted as an area where patients make judgments about the entire practice based on cleanliness, orderliness, and attention to detail. This is certainly true.

There is yet another issue that patients sometimes raise in focus groups that relates to the location of the rest room. Patients have stated that they do not like rest rooms that open immediately to the reception area. They would prefer to exit the reception area and go through a short hallway or pass by the business area to access the rest room. There is a sense of greater privacy when the rest room is slightly separated from the reception room area.

For the same reason, patients appreciate the privacy that is afforded them when there is an audible fan in the rest room. The sound of the fan helps to build a greater sense of separation and privacy. Other elements that are important to patients in a rest room are as follows:

- **Adequate lighting:** Patients appreciate a rest room that is quite bright. It is perceived as cleaner and it is easier for the patient to check personal appearance in the mirror.

- **Oral hygiene amenities:** Patients appreciate availability of mouthwash, toothpaste, disposable toothbrushes, and dental floss. Inclusion of these items makes a statement to your patients of their importance and enables the patient to feel more prepared and comfortable prior to treatment. Bulk dispensers, or individual packaging of these items ensures that the patient is using fresh and clean supplies.

- **Facial tissues**

Needless to say, the rest room needs continual monitoring by the staff in terms of neatness and cleanliness. This area must be immaculate. It is a prime factor in a patient's determination as to whether the office is clean and safe. So many factors can negatively influence this perception including full wastebaskets, burned out or missing light bulbs, old or empty toothpaste or mouthwash containers, broken or missing tiles, chipped porcelain, peeling wallpaper, and broken or ill-repaired hardware. As a mystery patient I have seen all of these and more in various offices.

Some practices promote and sell oral hygiene supplies, like toothpaste, mouthwash, etc. If you promote such products, you are making a statement of endorsement and quality. Therefore, you must make sure that these are the products used as amenities for patients in the rest room. One office I visited actively promoted oral hygiene supplies to their patients. They had displays and counter cards with product information in the reception area and treatment rooms. However, in the rest room they used over-the-counter products such as a patient might buy in a drugstore. Mixed messages were being sent here. If these pharmacy-brand products were appropriate for use in the dental office then why should patients invest in more expensive products being promoted by the practice? This was a matter of mixed messages that could make the patient question the practice in other areas as well.

CONSULTATION ROOM

It is important for the office to have an area that affords privacy for discussions with patients whether discussing payment plans, treatment plans, or any other subject matter of a confidential nature. As addressed throughout this book, privacy for the patient is a very important matter. A consultation room offers the and the team this privacy in a professional area free from distraction. (Fig. 12-4)

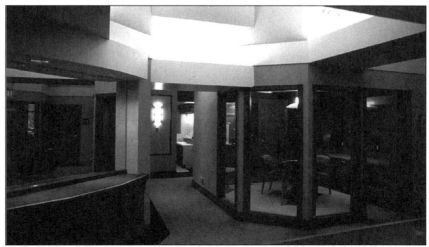

Fig. 12-4 The consultation room provides comfort and privacy. (Courtesy T.H.E. Design, Inc., Austin, TX)

Patients have indicated that the following elements are particularly effective in a consultation room:

- **Windows:** Because you're discussing treatment plans and finances in this room, the patient does not want to have a sense of being "trapped." Windows on an exterior wall can help in this respect as does a window in the doorway to this room.
- **A round table** that comfortably allows more than one person to be seated.
- **Comfortable padded chairs** with casters so that the patient can easily pull up to or leave the table.
- **Degrees and certificates:** As mentioned earlier, if they are included in this room, position them on the wall the patient will face during discussion.
- **Technical equipment:** This is an ideal room in which to conduct patient education using videos or computers. Inclusion of this type of equipment in the consultation room also increases the patient's perception of the practice; the office is seen as one that is up-to-date.
- **Reference items:** This is an excellent area in which to include books and visuals that may be used for patient education and/or case presentation.

The most comfortable and patient-friendly consultation room I have seen was decorated in soothing pastel colors. The wall next to the hallway was covered with padding and fabric which aided in noise reduction. There was a round table in the center of the room and one of the walls formed a half circle that was both pleasing to the eye and increased a sense of comfort for the patient; one did not feel cornered. In addition, there was a window in the doorway which looked out on the hallway and a portion of the reception area. The consultation room included a computer and an intraoral camera monitor. There was also a TV and videotape player as well as a self-contained 35mm slide projection unit and x-ray light board. This room also included a corner seating area with two comfortable chairs, a corner table, and a lamp. There was a silk flower arrangement on the table and a photograph album opened to examples of the doctor's treatments.

The most ineffective consultation room I personally experienced was one that was exceptionally small. It was like a large closet. There were no windows. The treatment coordinator positioned herself at a large desk between me and the door. A consultation room like this is counterproductive; I felt trapped and almost suffocated by the tight space and the furniture that was too big for the room.

THE SENSES AND THE DENTAL PRACTICE

When patients first enter the office, they are influenced by sensory factors. Music, room temperature, odor, and visual stimuli such as decor and furnishings, all combine with many other elements to make up the environment. These elements will influence the patient's perceptions of the practice as well as the patient's mood and behavior during the appointment.

Patients frequently discuss how they feel about the office in terms of the sounds they hear and the smells they notice as they enter reception or the treatment areas. "The thing I don't like about my dentist's office is the smell; it smells clean but unappealing!" This patient was talking about her feelings on entering the dental office and she described it as, "like walking into a brick wall of medical odor." Some patients have indicated that the overpowering medicinal smell has brought back bad memories for them and increased their anxiety in the office. Whatever you can do to decrease patient awareness of medicinal odor will be appreciated. What process you use to do that is important. "Odor control is an extremely important aspect to consider in office design." Harry Demaree, DDS, of T.H.E. Design, Inc. of Austin, TX, indicates that his firm, "designs proper ventilation so that offices do not smell like a dental office." Certainly, ventilation is the primary issue relating to odor control.

Aromatherapy is also making inroads in dental and medical environments. Having been used in retail environments for some time, the concept has received public acceptance. Perhaps the most effective use of aromatherapy is in the background when patients are unaware of it. It can aid in "texturing" the air without imposing a strong or cloying, sweet scent often associated with aerosol sprays or room deodorizers. These units can be unobtrusive and can be controlled in terms of the amount of scent that is used. In addition, there are many fragrances from which to choose.[4]

The sounds experienced in the dental practice can be soothing or unsettling. I was seated in the reception area of a dental office, awaiting my clinical exam. The doorway which led from the reception area into the clinical areas was open. Even though there was music playing softly, I could still hear the whirring sound of equipment from the closest treatment room. I also could hear the hygienist talking with the patient and the garbled mumbling of patient response.

As is probably the situation with some of your patients, I too had some nightmare experiences as a child in a dental office. Those frightening experiences are burned into my brain and all it takes is the sound of that equipment combined with a medicinal odor to send me right off the edge! Here I was, sitting in the reception area, calmly flipping through a magazine when those sounds entered my awareness. It would have been a simple matter to close the door and spare patient anxiety. As it was, for patients who had a similar history to mine, those sounds would influence our behavior and mood as we moved into the treatment room. The hygienist might now be dealing with a patient who might be exhibiting edgy behavior.

In reality, the situation was more complicated than it first appeared. In talking with the doctor later, she explained that there was an airflow problem in this office and that the reception room door was kept open in order to allow for sufficient air movement. Interestingly, this situation involved two senses, that of hearing and that of feeling. With the door closed, patients were comfortable in the reception area because there were fans overhead. However, the staff became uncomfortable in the office because there was now no air flow to that area. The opened door was for the benefit of staff comfort and this resulted in patient discomfort. We discussed the option of placing quiet, portable fans in the staff area during the warm summer months in order to spare the patients' awareness of equipment sounds emanating from the clinical areas.

MUSIC TO SOOTHE THE SAVAGE BEAST

Music and the level at which it is played is also extremely important and certainly influences the patient's mood. Your choice of music in the office needs to be guided by the demographics of your patients. Music preferences also can be regional as in the popularity of country-western music in the southwestern United States. There are many variations of music preferences also based on socioeconomic and education factors. Most importantly, the music must be appropriate to the image of the practice. If you are presenting your practice to the public through collateral materials and promotional pieces that say yours is a highly refined and very sophisticated office, then patients expect that the environment, including the music being played, will support that message. Likewise, if you present the practice as relaxed, informal, and very upbeat, then patients expect music in that same vein.

A woman in one focus group related an incident that I found most unusual. She stated that every time she went to her general dentist, he had a sports, talk-radio station playing. This was a station which was totally sports all day. The doctor was a sports fanatic and treated a number of high profile sports personalities locally. Though this doctor was known for high clinical skills, the patient found herself becoming irritated in the office because she was not a sports fan and found the incessant radio chattering to be grating on her nerves.

To make matters worse, the dentist actively was listening to the radio discussions and would periodically voice his own commentary aloud in response to what was being said. The patient found this highly idiosyncratic and ultimately it became so irritating that she asked him if he would at least change to a music station during her appointment. It was his response which surprised me even more than the unusual situation itself. He said, "Well, I really can't do that. Knowing what's going on in sports is part of my business. I have to be aware of these things for my patients who are involved in sports professionally."

This patient said she left the office and never went back again. Her interpretation was that if the dentist didn't care about her as a person, then her best interests clinically were not taken to heart either. Her husband had been a patient of the practice as well. He enjoyed the entire environment, but he also left the practice to support his wife's viewpoint. It was clear from the situation, that what was important to the dentist was his *other* patients and his own enjoyment.

There are several significant issues to be evaluated here. Is the office one that is tightly focused on specific demographics of sports enthusiasts or participants? If so, and particularly if the patient was a non-sports, "difficult" type person, then releasing the patient might be an appropriate recourse for the practice. However, if the practice actively courted a more mainstream patient base, then the practitioner might need to take a closer look at his priorities. If these were reasonable patients who were an asset to the practice, whose needs was he meeting—his own or his patients? There are times when it is best for the team and the practice to have a patient leave the practice; there are also times when it is wise for the practice to accommodate the interests of the patient. This is a subjective issue and must be managed case by case.

Here's what patients say they like in relation to music in the dental office:

- Easy-listening to soft rock.
- Classical musical
- Instrumentals
- Country-western
- Soft jazz and soft rhythm and blues

There are risks in posting a list like this because the categories listed above are top preferences that patients like nationwide. This does not mean that each of these categories is going to be acceptable to *your* patient base. Again, we come back to knowing who *your* patients are and understanding what *they* deem appropriate. You will never find one style of music that suits every patient. You're never going to please all of the patients all of the time. It is possible however, to find a style or styles that will be found acceptable by the majority of your patients.

Music styles which are not as popular with the mainstream public and will not be as well received in the office as those above are:

- Hard rock
- Opera
- New age

Within each demographic group there are very different preferences. For example, patients who are in a higher income bracket or have higher levels of education may respond more positively to new age and classical music.[5] There are numerous other categories of music including Spanish/Latino, black, urban adult contemporary, religious music, big band sound, top forty, oldies, and the issue of talk radio. Whatever mix you choose for your office must reflect the interests and preferences of your specific client base.

One point on sound, and that relates to the amount of sound you're allowing to influence the patient. No matter how sweet the music may be, if the patient cannot hear what you're saying, then it's working against you and the patient. I am hard of hearing and I have been in numerous offices where the music interferes with the ability to understand the clinician. I have asked team members if it's possible for them to reduce the sound in the treatment room so I could hear them better. Most of the time this is done. However, I have become aware that not all sound controls can be adjusted by room, but instead require a single master switch, controlling all speakers. This can be a detriment to patient comfort and compliance. If at all possible, evaluate the options of individually controlled sound levels within each room if you are considering updating your office.

A caveat: Bear in mind, when you choose music style you are "texturing the air" around the patient. You will be influencing the patient's mood. You can pick up those moods or you can slow them down. Most importantly, don't unnerve them! Help them feel comfortable and relaxed in your office. (This obviously precludes blaring the music of Kiss or Guns'n Roses!)

A final caveat on public playing of copyrighted music: Make sure that you are within your rights locally and nationally in relation to the latest regulations on "public performance." When you are "broadcasting" copyrighted music, your right to do so may depend upon the kind of equipment over which the music is being played and/or the venue within which it is being played.

TEMPERATURE AND PATIENT PERCEPTIONS OF CARING

The temperature of your office also is influencing your patients. Many a time I have sat in the treatment room chair and felt chilled. I recall on one occasion when I commented on this to the assistant, she responded, "I guess it is a little chilly. We just don't feel it because we're moving around so much." And that was that! Here was a young woman who was not able to put herself in the position of the patient or relate to what the patient was saying. Make sure there are blankets available to help patients feel comfortable in your office. This is one of the "nurturing concepts" that helps patients feel that they are in a cocoon of comfort and safety in your office.

Dr. Tom McDougal notes that when a patient requests a blanket during treatment, the patient should "be handed one that is freshly laundered and wrapped in cellophane. We unwrap the blanket in from of him/her and tell about our commitment to patient safety." In winter months, patients often feel cold and have colds or flu more often. Especially at those times this can be a very significant and caring gesture for a patient. It is here where you start communicating to the patient incorporating several sociotrends indicated in Part 1 of this book, such as cocooning, patient concerns about infection control, and patient comfort in general.

ATTRACTIONS AND DISTRACTIONS

More often than not I hear the term "distractions" used in a positive way to describe a process of helping the patient remove himself psychologically from focusing on clinical matters. T.H.E. Design offers a different take on this same concept. They use the term "attractions" to define design details and equipment which might help to minimize patient concerns. I far prefer the idea of being attracted to something positive rather than distracted from something negative.

Research has shown, "the most positive distractions are mainly elements that have been important to humans throughout millions of years of evolution:"[6]

1. happy, laughing or caring faces,
2. animals, and
3. nature elements such as trees, plants and water. What follows are possible positive "attractions" for patients:

• Visual architectural design details that encourage the patient to think about positive elements of the environment within the clinical setting.

• Artwork such as paintings, prints or sculpture.

• Windows through which the patient views a pleasant scene and obviously, nature is most appealing to the patient.

• Headsets for radio or audio tapes wherein the patient has control over the music and can elevate the sound level as desired.

• Television that the patient controls. Offer a variety of tapes which will help to reduce patient anxiety and soothe the spirit. Movies such as "Die Hard 2," "Speed," and the "Godfather" may be exciting but they certainly won't reduce the patient's blood pressure!

• Virtual reality glasses that take patients out of the environment psychologically but allow them to interact with the practitioner. These are very powerful in that they give patients control and allow as much patient involvement as the patient desires.

TECHNOLOGY IN THE OFFICE

As discussed in chapter 9, technology is an extremely important and valuable tool in dental practices. Its value is to both the practitioners and the patients. We have taken the concept of technology into patient focus groups and asked preferences on where and how they would like patient-controlled technology to be utilized in the practice. Specifically, we've asked patients if they prefer patient education or promotional equipment to be in reception areas or in clinical or consultation areas. There were mixed responses to this issue. What we did learn was:

• Patients don't like uncontrollable sound other than music. For example, they did not want to be in a reception area where a videotape was playing and the voice-over could be heard in the room.

• Related to the item above, many patients did not like the idea of a television playing in the reception area. Some said they preferred to read, others said they didn't feel comfortable changing the channel when other patients were in the room. Other patients noted that the quality of television programming is so bad, they didn't want to be subjected to it!

• A significant number of patients did not like the concept of promotional pieces on video or computer in the reception area. The negative response increased appreciably when there was sound. However, they did feel that there was appropriate application for these concepts in another, more private, area of the office.

• Patients responded very positively to technology used to educate the patient when it was used in a private area. They indicated a preference for seeing videos and computer information relative to their conditions or proposed treatment when viewed in an office or consultation room. In other words, patients preferred for this concept to be customized to their own interests, to be offered in privacy, and for them to elect to view and control the medium. Those patients who responded negatively to the same technology in the reception area felt more positively about these items as they related to patient education in private areas.

• Imaging: Patients responded very positively to the concept of computer imaging. However, they wanted the process to be one which was private and viewed only by the patient in question.

I experienced something similar to this as a patient. I was having imaging done in an area where patients in the adjacent reception room had partial view of the computer photographs being taken of me. This felt awkward and I was ill at ease knowing that the two patients in the reception area could watch the process if they wanted to. My back was to them so I had no idea if they were observing or not. This room arrangement was designed with the intent for patients in the reception area to be able to view the computer equipment when it was not in use. The monitor could be left on with an image of "before" and "after" pictures on it. For those seated in reception, there would be a dramatic message of what could be achieved by this office. However, when that area was used for photography purposes, it worked against the patient.

(See technology in the office, chapter 9—Patient Selection of a Dentist; and chapter 17—Patient Perception of Service.)

THE DENTAL PRACTICE COCOON

Part of gaining and retaining patients as well as increasing treatment acceptance requires the development of an environment in which patients can feel comfortable and secure. Recognize the significance of developing the most effective *cocoon* possible for your patients; design and maintenance combine to speak to your patients about you. Items 7-10 following can help you gain a more objective viewpoint of your office as your patients might see it.

TOP TIPS:

1. Patients *love* radio or cassette tape headsets. These are inexpensive and your patients will appreciate your having them.
2. Check for *any* spots on the carpet or furnishings, marred furniture, or equipment. Get these fixed immediately. Your patients notice this but won't tell you, yet it's affecting their perceptions of you!
3. Make sure the bathroom lighting is bright, that any fan is in working order, fixtures are all functional, and that wallpaper, flooring and counters are presentable.
4. Ensure that oral hygiene products are available to patients in the rest room (in order of importance to patients): toothpaste, disposable brushes, mouthwash, and dental floss.
5. Ensure that the rest room is "freshened" several times a day and that supplies are checked including items above as well as facial tissues, hand cloths/towels. It is also crucial to check the cleanliness of the sink, mirror, and empty the wastebasket if necessary.

6. Light systems for interoffice communication is far favorable to other systems, particularly those that involve sound. Keep these light systems behind the patient. Patients notice when you're watching the lights, and if you're focusing on the lights, then you're not focusing on the patient.

Suggestions to Facilitate Gaining the Patient's Perspective:

7. Have each member of the team enter the office in the way that a patient might and view the office from this perspective. Compare what each person saw— negative and positive. Sit in the dental chair and look at the levels that patients see, higher than the counters, and lower than the counters. Observe the equipment and look for items that may need some cosmetic repairs.

8. Compare your brochure and any promotional pieces to the image of the office itself. Are the office and the brochure congruent? Is a consistent message being sent by both? If not, which is more accurate to the reality of the practice and which may need to be changed?

9. Have several non-dental professionals give objective feedback on the sounds and smells of your office. You may not be aware of any prevalent odor, because you are so accustomed to it.

10. Sit in reception during regular office hours and pay attention to sounds of the office. Can you hear equipment or patient discussions? Is the sound level of the music appropriate for the majority of your patients?

11. If you were in a wheelchair, where would you position your chair in reception? Would you be able to maneuver through the hallway and could you enter the treatment areas?

REFERENCES

[1] Goffman, Erving. *Behavior in Public Places*, Macmillan Publishers, New York, NY, 1963.

[2] Goldstein, DDS, Ronald H.. *Change Your Smile*, Quintessence Books, Chicago, IL. 1988.

[3] Ulrich, Roger S. "Effects of Interior Design on Wellness: Theory and Recent Scientific Research." This paper was presented at the Third Symposium on Health Care Interior Design, San Francisco, 1990.

[4] Reasonably priced aromatherapy units are available for purchase, as well as a wide variety of fragrances. One such source is JoCare International, Inc., (404) 262-7733.

[5] Piirto, Rebecca, "Why Radio Thrives," *American Demographics*, Sept. 19, 1994.

[6] Ulrich, Roger S. "Effects of Interior Design on Wellness: Theory and Recent Scientific Research." This paper was presented at the Third Symposium on Health Care Interior Design, San Francisco, 1990.

13

Patient Protection and the "Unspoken Question"

"I knew it wasn't clean when I saw the spots on the rug and the ragged magazines."

—F O C U S   G R O U P   P A R T I C I P A N T

I was addressing the topics of patient protection and patient perceptions at a conference of dentists and the handout material of this section was, "The Unspoken Question." At the morning break a dentist in the audience asked me, "Well, what *is* the patient's 'unspoken question'?" Although I thought the answer was self-evident, I realized that his query was valid. I had been thinking like a patient, not like a member of the clinical team. I knew the question, just hadn't verbalized it. I thought the audience knew also, but perhaps it had not been entirely clear to some practitioners present.

WHAT *IS* THE UNSPOKEN QUESTION?

The patient question I was addressing was, "Am I safe in your office, or am I at risk of contracting infection?" It's what patients think, but what they most often don't ask you. You hear the direct question very seldom, yet it hovers above the patient's mind as he or she experiences treatment in your office. You're seldom presented with this tough question, but what would happen in your office if you were?

Here's one situation that occurred when I entered an office undercover. I was at the front counter inquiring about the general dentist's practice. I'd asked a few questions about the doctor's background and then switched the direction of the conversation to see how well the young woman at the reception desk would handle this question, "Do you treat any AIDS patients?" This staff member gave me a blank expression for just a moment and then responded with, "No, we don't have any AIDS patients." I was surprised by her statement and asked her how she could be so sure. She told me, "Well, we ask patients on the patient history form!" Needless to say, I was surprised by what she apparently thought was a logical response.

You are probably not faced with too many patients who are this direct. I have no doubt that you *do* have patients that pose questions on the subject of infection control, but I also recognize that a very significant number of your patients are not talking to you about the issue of their safety in your office or about related topics that concern them.

The scenario above was an opportunity to effectively market the practice, but it was an opportunity unrecognized. It would have been far better for this young woman to have explained universal precautions and addressed the levels of infection control practiced in this office. She could have increased patient confidence and trust in the practice: She also could have offered a tour of the office and an explanation of the infection control area. If she didn't have the knowledge to do this herself, she could have offered to have another team member handle it.

You may be saying to yourself, "Well, that just takes too much time and we are not staffed or equipped to handle spur-of-the-moment tours for drop-in patients." However, the reality is that the vast majority of prospective patients in this type of situation would turn down the tour. Just the fact that the receptionist offered to do so would make a statement to the patient that the office is confident about its patient protection procedures, proud to take a patient through the office, and that it is a service-oriented office.

In fact, what initially what might appear to be an argumentative-type question from a prospective patient is actually an opportunity to promote the practice in a manner that builds credibility and meets patient needs. Instead, her cavalier comment would more likely result in a lack of confidence on the part of the patient.

PATIENT CONCERNS ABOUT INFECTION CONTROL IN THE DENTAL PRACTICE

In focus groups I do not raise the subjects of patient safety, sterilization, infection control, AIDS/HIV. I don't have to. When I ask, "Tell me what's important to

.n a dental practice?" The group participants invariably
; up this subject matter themselves. They discuss
mstances and situations that might cause concern on
)art of the patient. Some of these include:

- Reception areas that are unclean or disorganized.
- Spots on the floor, old furnishings, furniture and equipment that is in ill-repair.
- Magazines that are out-of-date (more than three months old) or have torn ragged appearance.
- Rest rooms that are dark, messy, or in need of repair or updating.
- Equipment in treatment areas that appears outdated or is showing signs of wear.
- Dust on anything.
- Dirty coffee cups or food in the business areas.

You might say, "None of these factors has anything to do with infection control in the clinical areas" and of course, you'd be right. However, patients know very little about how to judge clinical cleanliness, so they use more familiar concepts by which to judge the clinical. Unfair? Perhaps, but a reality that must be dealt with? Absolutely.

WHY PATIENTS DON'T POSE THE "UNSPOKEN QUESTION"

We've asked patients, "Given your concerns, have you talked to any member of the team about these issues?" Most commonly, patients respond, "No". Among the reasons that patients frequently are *not* talking to you about patient safety or sterilization:

- If the patient has been with the practice for a long time, the patient frequently feels disloyal by bringing this up, as if questioning the standards or ethics of the office.

- Patients don't know how to phrase the questions to avoid sounding argumentative.
- Many patients feel it inappropriate to pose questions like this of professionals.
- Patients know what their concerns are but do not feel confidence in expressing those concerns in the dental office.

CLUES PATIENTS USE TO EVALUATE OFFICE CLEANLINESS

In discussing office cleanliness and sterilization, we've asked patients, "How do you know when the office *is* clean?" These are some of the most common responses we hear from patients:

- The reception area and rest room is immaculate, no dust, no spots on the rug, and the furnishings are in good condition.
- The entire office area is neat and well organized. If the business area is visible to patients, it is kept orderly and staff food or beverage is not visible to patients.
- Team members are personally well-groomed and neat. (This is a very frequent comment and each team member should recognize the importance of personal appearance as it relates to patient perceptions.)
- Team members wash their hands in front of patients.
- In the treatment room and in view of patients, team members open bags that protect the sterilized instruments. (Make sure that the patient can see you do this; it is significant to them.)

- Team members take new gloves directly from the dispensers. Patients also notice when gloves are disposed of in front of them.
- Masks are worn during exam and treatment. Patients also observe when you are using disposable gowns and jackets.
- (For new patients) A tour of the office is given and the patient is educated about the infection control area.
- Signs and/or printed materials that address the issue of sterilization and patient safety in your office are available and visible.

FALSE SENSE OF SECURITY IN THE DENTAL PROFESSION

As a researcher of patients and as a seminar leader on patient relations, I am absolutely convinced that there is a false sense of security in the dental profession today about patient attitudes and patient protection. We hear about this consistently from patients. They are concerned. They want to know if they are safe. They don't feel at ease in bringing up the subject and so the question remains unspoken.

Since the team doesn't hear the questions, they may feel the patient doesn't have any concerns. It's easy to understand how this thinking could occur. Yet as often as I relate this in seminars, I'm confident that a high percentage of team members still leave the session thinking, "Well that's *other* offices, not ours!"

We've asked patients, "What would help you feel more comfortable in the office? What *should* the dental office do to help you feel more at ease and secure?" They respond openly about this. There's one concept that wins hands down. Patients put it this way, "If *you* will bring up the subject, we'll feel more at ease. We'll know it's okay to talk about it, and then if we have questions we'll ask!" How simple! It is almost so simple that it can go unrealized and more often than not it does.

So from the patient's perspective the responsibility is yours. *You* need to initiate the subject in a manner that is confident and credible. *You* need to elicit patient questions in a manner that communicates openness and banishes patient concerns.

THE FEARFUL PATIENT

What about the patients that have an exceptionally high fear level in relation to patient protection in the dental practice? How do they feel and what do they want in communication from the clinical team? On a number of occasions I've visited offices as a patient of this mind set. Having heard many of them talk in focus groups, I understand the issues that are important to them and the attitudes they carry into the office.

There are many approaches that can be taken, but the biggest challenge is recognizing this type of patient. Sometimes they "reveal" themselves openly by expressing their feelings. Other times, you're working in the dark and may not realize that you are treating a patient with these concerns. This places more responsibility on the part of the team to look for and recognize clues in patient behavior. Beyond being given direct questions from the patient, other clues are these:

• A new patient who hasn't visited the dentist for a long time and who closely observes clinical team members in relation to their use of personal protective equipment and their actions in treatment areas.

- Patients who ask questions about plastic that may cover equipment, about gloves or personal protective equipment.
- Patients who ask questions about Kimberly Bergalis, Doctor Acer, or anything of a related nature.
- Patients who pose questions or comment on any news item or media story about infectious diseases or infection control.
- Patients who closely observe you as you wash your hands and put on gloves.
- Patients who closely observe instruments before the treatment or exam.
- New patients who ask for a tour of the office or ask to see the sterilization area.
- Patients in the reception area who are seen reading printed matter you have provided about sterilization and patient protection.
- Patients in the reception area who seem highly observant about the decor. They seem to spend time looking around instead of focusing on patient distractions.
- Patients who choose not to sit in reception, but prefer to stand or pace.

This list includes behaviors that are also indicative of other concerns, such as general fear of the dental experience or anxiety in anticipation of treatment. Therefore, these cannot be considered a primary gauge for determining patient attitudes. They are, however, behaviors that patients in focus groups have stated they have exhibited in trying to determine their safety in the office. The very apprehensive patient may exhibit several of these behaviors.

Since this is an uncomfortable topic for patients to initiate, it becomes more important for the team to communicate openly about the subject. If team members feel that a patient is possibly one with a high sensitivity about safety in the dental office, it is wise to initiate the subject and to address concerns directly. This is especially important with patients new to the practice.

A POSITIVE EXPERIENCE

I visited an office which did a superb job in not only alleviating patient concerns, but also in promoting the practice. In visiting this office I told the receptionist I was moving into the area and I was trying to find an office where my husband would accept treatment. I explained that he had not been to a dentist for several years and had a phobia about contracting AIDS in dental treatment. I explained that he had agreed to make a dental appointment if I could find an office where he would feel absolutely confident that he was in a safe environment.

It is important to mention here that I had presented myself as an individual with a high dental IQ. I explained that I had completed orthodontic treatment in another state and also had been very pleased with the cosmetic treatments following removal of the braces. This receptionist was savvy enough to recognize the opportunity here. She had before her a patient who recognized the value of excellent dental care and was willing to invest in it. Consequently, the time that she was about to spend with me was an investment on her part. In addition, I had arrived in the office at a time outside of their regular patient hours. Her day was actually behind her and she was very kind in taking the time to educate this patient and promote the office as well. One other important note, which I did not realize until later, was that the receptionist was also the wife of the dentist. That is an observation only, although it may influence your interpretation of the following incident. That is *not* to say that a spouse is more likely to recognize these opportunities or manage them in a more positive manner than other team members. Every office is unique, every team mix is unique.

In this case the receptionist recognized and seized this opportunity in a most effective manner. She first showed me the autoclave and explained heat levels of sterilization equipment. She made a photocopy of the post card from Emory University that indicated the appropriate heat levels that had been registered for the sterilization units. She took me on a tour through the office and explained the sterilization methods used and briefly educated me as to the ADA and CDC guidelines on sterilization and infection control. I was given a disposal prophy angle. She even suggested that if my husband felt extremely strongly about this that it is possible for a patient to purchase his own hand piece that would be kept by him and only used for him.

She then took me into a treatment room and explained the barriers that are in place for patient protection. Back at the front desk, I was given a one page flyer that explained what the office did in infection control and how patients were protected in this office. In closing, she reiterated the importance of regular dental care for my husband. At this time, she expressed in a genuinely caring manner her empathy for my husband's concerns. She suggested that even before scheduling any appointment with my husband that he call and come by the office for a visit, to meet the doctor, and give him the opportunity to see the office and ask questions. She suggested that this kind of acclimation to an office can help ease the anxious patient into a more comfortable place.

This entire transaction took approximately 15 minutes, but by the end of that fifteen minutes I was absolutely sold on this practice. If the situation posed had been a real one, I *would* have gone home to my husband and suggested that I had found the ideal office for him.

Not only did this receptionist do a marvelous job, but in my brief minutes there, she introduced me to the doctor, who also came across in a very caring manner. The office itself was beautiful in design and offered amenities to increase the patient's comfort. This was certainly a rare experience. I've not had another visit where this question was handled so adeptly.

My message to you is not that this is the manner in which you should always communicate with these patients, but rather here is an office that presented itself in a unique manner, recognized what was truly an opportunity, and promoted the practice in a way that was very patient friendly.

A NEGATIVE EXPERIENCE

I've also had experiences where I've been concerned about my own safety in the dental office. One office in particular stood out as presenting concerns for me. I had selected this office based on an advertisement in the Yellow Pages. I was intrigued by the large, "glamour shot" of the female dentist. The advertisement text indicated that this was a very caring and gentle office. I wanted to see how congruent the office actually was with the image presented on paper. I had made an appointment for an exam and cleaning. When I arrived at the office, I asked the young man who worked at the front desk about how they sterilized their hand pieces. The "20/20" TV show on this subject matter was still much in the public's mind and I was curious how they were going to handle it. He laughed as he responded, "Oh, don't pay attention to all that stuff. It's just the news media trying to scare everybody." This was far from a caring attitude. It was belittling. It was making light of a patient's concerns. I hadn't even entered the clinical areas and my impressions had already dropped from what was an inauspicious start!

The clinical exam and prophy did not constitute a stellar experience for me. But what shook me the most occurred at the close of the exam, as I was about to exit the treatment room. The doctor removed her mask and placed it on the counter. The inside of the mask was smeared with face makeup and lipstick. I found it extremely unappealing and it made me question the judgment of the practitioner as well as the cleanliness of the entire office.

What did this say about the congruence of the office? The picture of the dentist in the Yellow Pages had been taken years earlier, and she seemed to be in a time warp. The makeup was an attempt to retain that earlier image. That is a statement in itself about the practitioner. The office was fairly congruent, but congruence does not imply that the office presents a positive image, just a consistent one. Yes, the office was consistent. No, it was not presenting itself consistently well.

Patient's Request for Reassurance: "Here's What We'd Like!"

In our focus groups, patients consistently remark that they have a high discomfort level with the idea of posing questions to team members about sterilization. Many of the focus group participants say, "Sure, I'd like to ask questions, but it would sound like I was questioning the ethics or professionalism of the office. That feels really uncomfortable to me. The office of any doctor is *supposed* to be clean and I shouldn't even have to think about it. But . . . ."

If patients don't want to bring up the subject matter, but are concerned, what's the best way for the team to handle this? That's the very question we have asked patients in focus groups. Their responses were resounding and collective, "The office should bring it up first." They want you to raise the subject matter to them in a reassuring way. They want you to educate them. By doing so, it is a strong indication to the patient that they are safe in your office. After all, you wouldn't bring the subject up yourself, if you weren't completely confident, would you? Based on responses from numerous focus groups here are the ways with which patients would like to be communicated on this subject matter:

• Create a one-page flyer on how infection control is handled in your office. This does not have to be an expensive piece. It could be on an 8 1/2 x 11 sheet of paper and photocopied. Address your office philosophy in relation to patient safety and infection control as well as the sterilization methods used. In this piece encourage patient questions and communicate an attitude that it is appropriate for patients to raise questions and that questions are welcomed. (Fig. 13-1)

• Purchase printed brochures on the subject of infection control and patient safety.[1] (Fig. 13-2)

• In any marketing or promotional materials sent to a prospective patient or a new patient prior to a first appointment, include each of the above pieces. Before the patient ever walks through the door you've already initiated an openness about this subject matter.

• For any patient of record who inquires about infection control, offer these same two pieces and encourage their questions.

• For any visitors to the office or for new patients who have not received this information by mail, make sure that they receive these pieces during their first visit to your office.

• Include signage in the business area and treatment rooms addressing the issue of infection control and the fact that you welcome questions of the subject matter. One office I visited had a tastefully framed sign on the wall in the reception area that related to infection control. This office had invited OSHA to visit them for inspection purposes and the signage indicted that the office had passed all requirements. This was a very positive statement for any patients visiting this office.

• With a very critical and objective eye view your office for any details that may unwittingly cast doubt on office cleanliness. A list of possible offenders is provided earlier in this chapter.

• Make sure that patients are able to see you wash your hands in the treatment room. Be sure that they can see you remove new gloves from the glove container and that gloves and masks are worn during all clinical exams and treatments by attending team members. Patients are extremely attentive about this matter.

• Be sure that patients see you open instruments. If you are working with a new patient, make sure that you educate the patient as to *your* procedures; they may be different than what patients may have seen in previous offices.

• If it is a new patient, make sure that you explain any other barriers that are used for protections purposes, such as plastic wraps on equipment.

• Make a point of showing new patients your infection control area, perhaps as a part of a general office tour.

• If you produce a newsletter or brochure, be sure to address this issue in a patient-friendly, educational manner.

• If you use patient education equipment in your reception area (video or computer), ensure that it is silent.

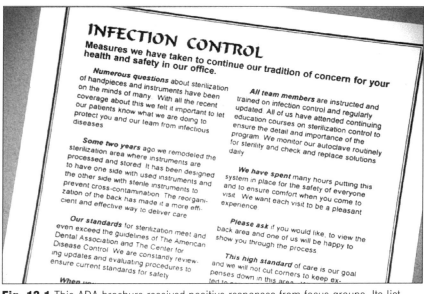

Fig. 13-1 This ADA brochure received positive responses from focus groups. Its list of "things to look for" in the dental office helps educate patients and increases patient confidence in the practice. (Courtesy American Dental Association)

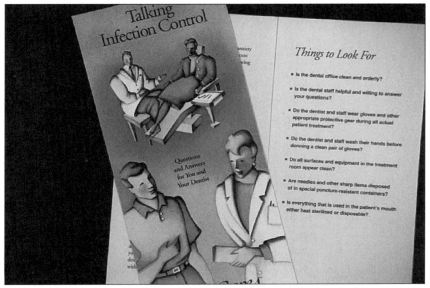

Fig. 13-2 Patients also liked a one-page flyer which describes the steps taken to ensure patient protection (Courtesy Frazer & Busch D.D.S., Inc.)

Several years ago, I saw an article about a dentist who was fighting a battle that affected the survival of his practice. The article detailed the journey this man had taken to recapture the reins of his practice and regain patient trust and confidence. A spiteful and totally untrue rumor was being circulated in his tight-knit community. That rumor would have a disastrous impact on his practice. But rather than allow his practice to wither, he opted to fight, and he did it in a forthright and courageous manner.

Here was a doctor who triumphed over a rumor about his having AIDS. The rumor was injurious overall and seriously threatened his practice. He fought it through numerous means. After his efforts and those of his family, friends, and colleagues, and after means that included a series of posters and advertisements, he rewon, and rightly so, the trust and confidence of his patients. He faced the demon directly and spoken openly and honestly with the public. His approach was direct. His patients returned. Trust and confidence, so vital to the life of the practice was once again instilled.

After reading the phenomenal story of his fight and his victory, I called him and discussed this challenge he had faced. I found a remarkable man who had grown stronger through this process and who had found the way to gain patient trust: address the topic directly.

MAINTAINING RAPPORT WITH BARRIERS INTACT

As addressed in earlier chapters, a significant matter for patients today is their comfort level within the dental practice. Patients do seek that warm, nurturing cocoon than can increase the likelihood of their returning to your care. However, by design OSHA regulations require that protective barriers exist between patients and practitioners. It is these same barriers that can sometimes send a message of cold and unfeeling sterility to patients. This is a narrow path to walk! It doesn't mean that building the appropriate barriers for safety will by default interfere with a warm and caring relationship. It only means that team members need to be more aware of this challenge.

Imagine for example, the fearful patient entering a treatment room that might be seen as barrenly sterile. In an effort to make surfaces and equipment easy to clean and sterile, the environment may look forbidding. The practitioner is clothed in a paper gown, is gloved, has on a mask and a wrap-around eye shield. All we need now is a head wrap and paper booties over the shoes and the patient might expect R2-D2® to enter the room next! This scenario comes close to reality in some offices. The patient's desire for a warm, nurturing care-giver is tested here. What this means is that the interpersonal skills of the practitioners become even more important. Many different kinds of barriers can be hurdled when team members know how to connect with a patient heart-to-heart. But if you place a cold and unyielding team member within the scenario described above, those barriers may be insurmountable.

When you are not in the process of treating the patient clinically, it is important that the barriers of personal protective equipment be removed. As much as possible, outside of the actual exam or procedure, communicate with the patient without the gloves or mask on.

For some patients, the very words, "infection control" may invite concern. The term, "patient protection" will be responded to more positively by these patients. It is a positive, caring approach to what some might say is a negative subject matter.

AN IMPORTANT CAVEAT

In one focus group when we were discussing sterilization and what patients look for in an office a patient brought up a very important perspective. She said, "My dentist used to have the chair and the equipment covered with plastic. Even the handles on the light were covered. This last time I went in, there was no plastic and it worried me. If it was important to do it in the first place, why did they stop?" This raises a very key point. Be very judicious about making changes in your infection control procedures—most particularly when it is something that patients might notice. If you start a new procedure, be sure you're committed to it, for once you've instituted it, a change back to earlier methods may present concern to highly observant patients.

PATIENT PROTECTION AND THE OFFICE OF THE FUTURE

The situation is not going to go away. On the contrary, although Dr. Acer is no longer front-page news, patients continue to be presented with different perspectives on the subject of patient safety and infection control. We read about it in magazines. *Time* magazine produced a major spread on their cover story about exotic world-wide infectious diseases, "Revenge of the Killer Microbes."[2] With diagrams and maps they plotted the plague locations worldwide. "Killers all around" the two-page headline shouted. Hollywood has not missed a beat and has provided the public with movies like, "Outbreak." Audiences saw a terrifying view of modern day plague in America.

Awareness and concern has become more mainstream as television news magazines like, "20/20," "60 Minutes" and "Dateline" continue to bring related topics to the forefront. Travelers are now more aware of airborne bacteria and infection likely to occur in flight. I even stayed in a hotel where there were pre-packaged alcohol wipes placed next to the phone with a "for your safety" sign!

Patients may not be talking to your about it, but you can be sure that they are far more aware and observant than they have been in the past. It is crucial for the practice to recognize this and not only to take the steps necessary to protect patients, but also to communicate and educate the patient.

Dr. Mark Friedman of Encino, CA is highly aware of the seriousness and significance of this issue. He has developed a cutting-edge approach to patient safety and infection control in his office. New patients to the practice are educated by a professionally prepared video tape that demonstrates the exceptional procedures, equipment, environment, and staff training that ensures patient protection in this unique office.

Dr. Friedman has designed his treatment areas to provide patients with the ultimate levels of safety. He refers to the concept as infection control environment, or I.C.E. The I.C.E. is entered through full-length, non-touch, sliding-glass doors, which open and close automatically by an infrared eye. This also affords patients and practitioners privacy for discussions and minimizes sound bleed-through to other treatment rooms. Even disposal of sharps is handled in a high-tech manner. Specialized equipment is used to melt down all sharps into a plug form, which is then compacted and disposed of in an ecologically appropriate way. The sterilization, rotation, and management of instruments is processed in a highly engineered manner, resulting in increasing both productivity and patient safety.

Most importantly, within this twenty-first century office is an awareness of, and attention to the heart of the practice, people. The team recognizes that along with increased attention to patient protection comes additional responsibility to build and maintain patient relationships. So it is within this unique environment that patients receive exceptional care, both as patients and as people.

TOP TIPS:

1. Initiate discussions on patient protection with patients. Most patients will not feel comfortable bringing up the conversation, but will appreciate your doing so.
2. Take new patients on a tour of the office. Show and discuss the sterilization area.
3. If you send out a welcoming packet to new patients, include printed information on patient protection and steps taken in your office.
4. Display signage about infection control in the office.
5. Have available for patients in reception, brochures and flyers about the infection control procedures followed. Don't wait for the new patient to see or take one, offer the information and explain it.
6. When a patient asks questions about sterilization or infection control, acknowledge and reinforce their appropriateness in doing so. Encourage questions and offer responses that help the patient feel confidence in the practice.
7. Don't make changes in your infection control procedures unless you are truly committed to the change. Recanting what you earlier had presented as an important means of patient protection may concern patients.

REFERENCES

[1] Numerous organizations offer patient education pamphlets on the subject of patient protection. One that patients in focus groups liked very much is "Talking Infection Control" (item W113 available from the ADA Catalog Department).

[2] Lemonick, Michael E. "Killers All Around," *Time*, New York, NY, September 12, 1994.

14

The Power of Positive Self-Presentation

"I expect to pass through this world but once. Any good therefore that I can do, or any kindness that I can show to any fellow creature, let me do it now. Let me not defer or neglect it, for I shall not pass this way again."

—A N O N Y M O U S

I was visiting the office of a highly respected specialist. He was known for providing top quality care in a physically beautiful environment. The office was decorated so that it looked like a very elegant, yet comfortable reading room. When patients arrived, they were offered herbal tea or coffee and it was brought to them in a china cup. This was not your ordinary office.

In interviewing the staff members, I learned that each of them had been with this practice for a minimum of fifteen years. They knew their patients very well and had developed real friendships with many of them. During our conversation, Gail, the office manager, suddenly jumped up and said, "I'm feeling just a bit chilly. I'm going to get 'our' sweater." I thought that was an odd turn of phrase but I understood it better when I saw her don the sweater. You may have one of these in your office too. It's the one that everybody wears, it's a communal piece of clothing. This one once was white; it was now gray. It had little woolen pills over the arms and front of it. It had been worn, so many times, by so many people who had put their hands in the pockets that the front of the sweater was now about three inches longer than the back. Some might say it had "character", others would say it was incongruent with the office.

No sooner had Gail put on the sweater, than a patient entered the office. This was a patient she had known for many years. Gail proceeded to make the patient a cup of herbal tea and take it out to the reception area.

I marveled at the lack of consistency in this scenario. Somehow, "our" sweater looked out of place. This team had worked together so long and they were so comfortable with each other in the office that they no longer noticed these idiosyncrasies. After all, they were all sharing the sweater! But what about the new patients who visited this office? How might they have viewed this? How might this reflect on other aspects of this practice?

How you self-present will have a significant impact on patients of the practice. Because of this, it is important that team members become more aware of the elements of self-presentation and manage the impression they are making on patients and office visitors. Whether it is visual, vocal, or verbal, you will be sending messages about yourself to those around you. Naomi Rhode, RDH, CPAE, puts it this way, "You cannot *not* communicate."

APPAREL AND APPEARANCE: HUMAN PACKAGING AND PATIENT PERCEPTIONS

When it comes to appearance, particularly in the areas of clothing and grooming, patients are very critical. Because they do not know how to judge the clinical, they use criteria more familiar to qualify the practice—clothing is one of those items. It's something they understand, something they can judge fairly accurately.

In focus groups the issue of appearance is frequently raised by patients. They will make connections between the appearance of the staff and the cleanliness of the office. If the staff looks crisp, clean, and well put together, then the office is probably sterile and safe as well. If the entire team is well groomed then it's likely that the patient will expect positive clinical results from this practice. Obviously, these judgments can be wrong. The clinical skills by the practitioner and the team could be borderline even if the team looks terrific. The doctor who looks a bit disheveled could produce beautiful aesthetic results. The challenge in this latter example is that patients may never give this doctor a chance.

An attorney, who is also a dentist, related an incident that occurred at the close of a malpractice trial. The dentist on trial in the case was found to be at fault and judged guilty. The jury noted, "If he can come to court with spots on his suit and he can't even get it to the dry cleaners for something as important as his trial, then how hygienic was he during the treatment? If he can't get his shoes shined for court, then how clean was the equipment?" These are the parallels patients make in relation to appearance.

THREE CATEGORIES OF OFFICE APPAREL

Patients have indicated in focus groups the benefit of seeing three distinctly different levels of apparel in the office. When they observe the following three categories, they understand the responsibilities of each and patients are then more likely to be appropriate in directing their questions and communication. The three categories are:

• Business staff should wear mainstream business apparel that is appropriate in the community. Be careful of being too informal. Patients may feel, "If they're informal about how they look, what else are they informal about?" This carries special significance as related to infection control and sterilization. It is better to err on the side of formality rather than informality.

• Hygienists and clinical staff are well received in clinical apparel such as scrubs and lab coats.

• Dentists' style options vary depending upon office location, patient demographics, and whether the dentist is male or female.

When it comes to determining the appropriate apparel for the dentist there is no hard and fast rule relating to style. There is a range of acceptability for both male dentists and female dentists in the viewpoints of patients. Regionality does come into play as well as the demographics of your patient base. For example, if your office is located in a downtown metropolitan area and you work primarily with business executives, then take your cues from the business executive as to what he or she might perceive as professional for a dentist. The attire may be more formal than one might find in a suburban or rural practice.

At the same time, apparel needs to be in sync with the image of the practice and with the personality of the practitioner. The male dentist who is very informal and whose practice image is very relaxed may find a high degree of patient acceptance to wearing a knit shirt and khaki pants. A look for men which is acceptable in many different environments and for many different patients is the long sleeve shirt with dress pants or crisply creased casual pants. When a man wears a crisp, starched, long sleeve shirt, it can be dressed up or dressed down based on how it's worn. If a spread collar is preferred, it will call for a tie and will appear more formal. If he wears a buttoned down, oxford cloth shirt, open at the neck, he's saying he has more relaxed attitudes.[1] The more formal practitioner may feel most comfortable in a lab coat over street wear.

The female dentist is presented with a special challenge in that she must differentiate her role from that of the clinical staff. If the staff is primarily female and the dentist is female, the patient needs to be able to immediately recognize who the dentist is by way of the difference in apparel. This may mean that if the staff wears scrubs, then the dentist wears a different color scrub or chooses to wear a dress or tailored pants with a lab coat over it. The lab coat for the female doctor is particularly effective in that it can be made more formal or more relaxed by buttoning or unbuttoning and it will look appropriate with almost any style of apparel worn underneath. In addition, a name tag or name embroidered on the lab coat can be helpful in reinforcing the doctor's role.

Scrubs are also an effective choice for either male or female dentists. Patients from all demographic groups responded to the doctors' wearing of scrubs. Ideally, the female dentist would wear a different color scrub than that of other clinical team members. If desired, the nonverbal message can be made more authoritative or formal by addition of a lab coat over the scrubs. However, lab coats are not recommended wear when treating children. The starched, white formality can look forbidding to a child.

We've also queried patients about disposable gowns. These are typically well received by patients and send a message of sterility and safety.

Most important to patients is the cleanliness and the crispness in all three categories of apparel. There is little room for error when it comes to attention to detail and perceptions of cleanliness. Patients frequently view shoes as a means of determining the attention to detail paid by the wearer. Men appear to be even more cognizant of this factor than women. Shoes that are well shined and in good condition tend to speak well of the wearer. This applies just as much to the individuals working at the front desk. That old pair of white heels that is run down and has the black scuff marks on the right shoe from driving is a real turn-off. A patient may look at this and say, "How well is she going to take care of my records?"

Clinical apparel is available in a great range of styles, colors, and patterns today. The important point in relation to the clinical team is that they provide a cohesive and unified message to the patient. This means wearing a similar look. Within a team it's difficult to narrow down a particular style or cut that pleases every member of the team. I have seen a few clinical apparel wear lines where different styles are available in the same color and pattern. Team members even could choose two styles that suit them best. This still presents a cohesive team appearance because the colors, fabric, and pattern unify them. This must be done with great care or it could confuse patients.

In focus groups, patients have indicated their preference of scrub colors. Scrubs in the blue family were favored by all demographic groups. "Blue" could mean anything from a pastel blue to navy to turquoise and teal. The entire blue family was favored with a slight preference towards the pastels and the aqua to teal shades. Also, many focus group members liked scrubs in the pink to fuchsia family. There was a decided dislike for olive drab scrubs. Many focus group members remarked that it reminded them either of the hospital or the military.

In discussing patient preferences of appearance and apparel, focus group participants consistently remarked about their appreciation of the team that wears name tags. It matters not whether it's a name tag or a garment embroidered with the team member's name, although tags *are* more noticeable. Patients find this very helpful. On behalf of dental patients across the United States I will pose this request to readers: Please get name tags, and if you already have them, *wear them*! Patients feel a lot more comfortable speaking to you when they can use your name, and that certainly helps in building a relationship as well.

PERSONAL PROTECTIVE EQUIPMENT FROM THE PATIENT'S POINT OF VIEW

The barriers that exist to protect can also create a barrier to communicate. Patients are reassured by the personal protective equipment they see worn by staff, yet responses to this apparel and equipment can vary depending upon how it's worn and when it's worn.

Masks should only be worn during the actual clinical exam or treatment. Ideally, the mask would not be placed around the practitioner's neck prior to or following clinical examination of the patient. This is not always feasible, however. Masks, visors and protective eye gear are the most distinctive barriers worn by the team. Because they so clearly separate you from the patient it becomes more challenging for the patient to feel at ease and able to connect with the practitioner when you are wearing these. People feel more comfortable communicating person-to-person instead of patient-to-practitioner.

The type of mask that you wear can influence patients as well. Approximately half of the patients in focus groups indicated that it didn't matter to them what type of mask was worn by the team. The other half indicated a style preference when presented with options. Approximately one-third of this last group liked the pre-molded style mask, the balance preferred a flat, pleated style mask. When presented with the option of seeing the team member in a printed or tinted mask, approximately two-thirds of the mask preference group responded favorably, particularly when staff members were wearing these. A significant number of patients did prefer that the dentist, whether male or female, wear a plain white mask. "It just looks more 'doctor-like', as one patient put it.[2]

Patients voice appreciation for the wearing of gloves during exams and treatments. They are very aware of the need for gloves and are far more observant than the dental team may be aware in relation to the subject matter. (See also chapter 13). There were no negative comments in any focus groups in relation to the wearing of gloves. Patient concerns do revolve around the cleanliness of the gloves however. Questions patients may ask themselves include: "Is this a new pair of gloves?" (Make sure the patient sees you take them out of the box), "What else are they touching in the room that could be contaminated?" (Be aware of what else you touch when you are wearing the gloves during treatment or exam).

Patients are typically not aware of the OSHA regulations regarding personal protective equipment. They are not likely to recognize the need for long sleeves or a closed neckline during an invasive procedure. Their awareness and knowledge related to this issue depends in large part on the amount of education provided them by previous practitioners. In many cases, you will not know if you are treating a patient who had discussed this issue with a prior clinician. However, when patients do see and recognize a disposable garment, similar to a paper surgical gown, they respond positively. It does heighten their awareness to the sterilization and safety measures maintained in this practice.

PERSONAL GROOMING AND THE IMPACT ON THE PATIENT

I had been hired as an undercover patient by a general dentist. All of the details in this practice were in place—the office was physically beautiful and all of the collateral materials were congruent with the facility. I was seated in the reception area when the assistant asked me to join her in the treatment room. Her demeanor was very pleasant and she helped me feel comfortable in the office. As I was being seated, she offered to take my purse and place it on the counter. In doing so, I noticed that her fingernails had been professionally manicured. It was in October and almost Halloween. She'd had her nails done specifically for the season. They were painted black with an orange-colored decal on each fingertip. I was floored! The rest of her grooming was very positive, but her nails were in questionable taste for a dental practice.

The subject of personal grooming can be a sensitive one. It is one that patients also discuss in focus groups. They look at the grooming of the staff members and the doctors as an indication of the cleanliness in the office, i.e., sterilization and infection control. They also use this as a gauge of what the practitioner considers acceptable.

Worst case scenario for the patient is to be in a dental practice where any member of the team has bad breath or bad teeth. This can, and does happen. It is perceived by patients as, "do what I say, not what I do." Patients consider it particularly unpardonable for a practitioner to discuss aesthetics with a patient as the patient peers into a clinician's unaesthetic mouth!

The following list addresses specific elements of grooming and patient responses:

• **Hair:** Patients expect the doctor and staff members' hair to be neat and orderly. Consider what you see when you go into a cafeteria. The servers typically wear hair nets to prevent "hairy mishaps"! This is not to suggest that the dental team wear nets, but that they be aware that the same sensitivities occur in the dental practice. Keeping the hair back and off of the face is going to help patients feel more comfortable with the grooming of the individual. Those women who have long hair might consider using headbands, barrettes, or pulling the hair back into a ponytail during working hours.

Many mainstream patients today have some difficulty in relating to the male healthcare professional with long hair. It's possible that this will change, but currently there is a segment of the population which either will be confused or have some difficulty with this issue. Much depends on the practitioner, the clientele, and the image of the practice. This is a very personal matter and one which must be judged objectively by the dental professional.

The most important aspect of hair in relation to patient perceptions is that it be neat and orderly. In the words of one focus group patient, "The doctor had her hair pulled back in a pony tail, but it was so disheveled and straggly that it looked really bad. If she can't keep her hair orderly, what is she going to do in taking care of my mouth?"

• **Facial hair:** Patients are more accepting of mustaches than beards. Again, the most important aspect of this is neatness. Patients indicate that a mustache is acceptable as long as it's trimmed and neat. Patients do find questionable those unusual mustaches such as the handlebar or the "Fu Manchu" style. Either of these looks idiosyncratic and most patients find them in questionable taste.

• **Nails:** The way you take care of your fingernails is interpreted in much the same manner as the way you take care of your shoes. It's a matter of attention to detail. Nails that look ragged and bitten may be interpreted as a lack of care. Some patients are concerned that if you bite your nails, you may be high-strung or nervous. Nail polish makes a statement to both male and female patients. Patients communicate that they would prefer to see members of the dental team without colored nail polish. They find clear nail polish or a French manicure to be more acceptable and they prefer shorter nails on all team members.

I recall being seated next to a female dentist at a luncheon. She had a habit of gesturing expressively with her hands as she spoke. I couldn't help but notice that her nails had been manicured with brightly colored polish. However, the polish had chipped on almost every fingernail. I was shocked that she appeared before her peers in such disarray, but what must patients think? It was a statement about the doctor and a possible lack of attention to detail.

• **Fragrance:** Patient response to this one is simple. So long as you bathe daily you don't need to wear fragrance in the work environment. Throughout the day you're working with so many different kinds of patients. Some of them may be allergic to certain fragrances, some may have an aversion to the scent you wear. Some patients may say to themselves, "That's the same perfume my ex-mother-in-law used to wear!" You are working in such close proximity to your patients, you are in their comfort zone. You won't go wrong if you don't wear fragrance, you could go wrong if you do. If you have strong feelings about wearing fragrance, go lightly with it. Better to underdo it than overdo it.

• **Makeup:** Patients are very much turned off by excessive makeup in the office of a healthcare provider. This is particularly offensive with those who come in direct contact with the patient during clinical exams or procedures. As with fragrance, makeup can be overdone very easily. It's important for the team member to look good and well groomed, but not look like she is going out for the evening. In this case, less is more.

I was out of town and was dropping a car off at the rental agency. Next door there was a dental office, so I dropped in to ask a few questions. The young lady at the front desk had on so much makeup that it looked like a mask. She was not a healthy looking front line person for a healthcare provider. I then became aware of my surroundings which were questionable in decor with a pervasive medicinal smell hanging in the air.

• **Body piercing/tattoos:** Some readers may be saying to themselves, "Is this *really* necessary to address?" The reality is it is a changing world and although I have not experienced seeing this myself in a dental practice, it is an issue that has been discussed among healthcare providers in news groups on the Internet. Practitioner/owners communicated concerns about staff members who opted for such decorations. These decorations are clearly not mainstream at this point.

A significant portion of the practice clientele would be confused, concerned, or put off by viewing such. The purpose of including this issue is not to be judgmental but to consider the reality of what patient responses might be. Some patients would be concerned about cleanliness and sterility in viewing either of these elements in a healthcare setting. One might argue, that's a matter of ignorance, however the practice is still forced to deal with the reality of patients' perceptions.

• **Jewelry:** Jewelry is a form of adornment that ties personal grooming to style and apparel. It's a very personalized form of expression and in some cases, may say more to patients than they want to know! Bear in mind that it is your hands and neck-to-face that patients notice the most. A simple watch and basic rings are acceptable to most demographics. Women should avoid wearing dangling earrings in the dental practice; the movement can be distracting. A clip-on or pierced earring that sits close to the ear is going to look the best.

Avoid anything that's too flashy. One patient in a focus group noted, "The doctor wore one of those big, jeweled Rolex watches, and I thought to myself, 'I can forget the veneers, this guy's going to be too expensive.'" Jewelry can be fun and a highly individualized way to express yourself. Just don't overdo this during office hours. Again, less is more.

BODY LANGUAGE: PATIENT PERCEPTIONS OF THE "REAL YOU"

Patients quickly gain an understanding, right or wrong, of who you are based on your actions, demeanor, and body language in the office. Because patients are in your office typically for a very short period of time, they are making judgments about you based on that same small window of time.

Let's say you've just come back from lunch where you had an argument with a friend. It affected your mood and on return to the office you moved in an abrupt and quick manner. Internally you were still focused on the heated discussion that had just occurred. However, your patient doesn't know this. If it's the first time that the patient has met you, the impression is that this is the way that you are all the time. A lack of eye contact and a lack of patient awareness can lead to patient discomfort.

Patient perceptions of the entire practice are influenced by each member of the team. Some issues relate to specific patient demographics and responses may vary based on the group.

We conducted a focus group with African-American patients and discussed their feelings about and interpretations of staff demeanor in various dental offices. Although they expressed some preference for being a patient of an African-American practitioner, their concerns were more for how they were treated by any member of the team regardless of ethnic origin. Regardless of gender or age, and we had patients from age 22 through 50 in this group, the consensus was that staff needs to communicate in a consistent manner with any non-white patient. Several participants expressed an awareness of being treated differently in the office of an Anglo dental practitioner. One young women put it this way, "It was my first time in this office and there were two white patients at the counter. I waited for the receptionist to help me. When it was my turn, she acted differently than she had towards the whites. She acted *normal* with them, but seemed *self-conscious* with me. It was as if she felt she needed to be *Miss Perky* for my benefit."

The patient was indicating that the staff member was trying too hard to be ingratiating. As she described the scenario, some of the other group participants nodded their heads and smiled. They were indicating that the demeanor of the Anglo team member communicated a discomfort with the situation. These patients would have felt more comfortable if they had been communicated with in a "no different than anybody else" manner.

ON ENTERING THE OFFICE

Your office is like a second home to you. You're so accustomed to being there that you see things as you expect them to be. But the first time the patient walks in to your office can be a very uncomfortable feeling. We are on unknown turf and the one thing that can help us feel the most comfortable immediately is a welcoming person at the front desk. As soon as patients walk in the door, they should receive eye contact and a smile from the individual at the front desk. Some readers may be saying, "Oh, you don't know our front desk. We are so busy all the time we don't have time to notice every patient who walks in." My response is, "You must find a way to manage this. Patients today will not forgive being ignored. You cannot risk this in today's challenging marketplace."

Let's say that you have two patients at the counter, you're on the phone with a third patient and a new patient enters the office. You can turn and look at this patient, make eye contact, smile and lift the index finger indicating, "One moment". It is *acknowledgment* that is the *most* important aspect of communication with patients when they first come in the office.

The appropriate greeting for a new patient is to orient yourself towards that patient, shake hands and introduce yourself. It is amazing to me, as many times as I have been a new patient in offices, the number of staff members who never introduce themselves to me, never tell me their names.

Introducing yourself and giving the patient your name is the very first, most elementary step upon which a relationship can start to build. If we don't know who you are, it is pretty hard to really communicate with you. Give the patient a warm, full handshake, not just fingertips. And verbally add a gracious welcoming such as, "Oh, Mrs. Smith, I'm Nancy and I spoke with you on the phone. I've been looking forward to meeting you and we're so pleased that you're here."

If you really want to communicate a very gracious and warm welcoming, stand when you meet this new patient. When you rise from the chair and shake hands with the new patient, you are indicating a level of respect and "specialness" of this patient, as if you were greeting a guest in your home.

Once patients are seated they are able to observe any members of the team who are within view of the reception area. If you have a very open office area, they are also able to observe how you interact with each other and how cohesive you may appear as a team. This influences patients' sense of ease and comfort by being in a stable office.

How you sit and how you stand regardless of your role in the office is communicating not just about you but about the practice as well. Patients like to feel they are in an office where there is positive energy and that partly can be seen in your posture and how you move. When you were a child, your mother may have slapped you on the back and said, "Stand up straight!" As simplistic as this may sound, its importance still holds true. People look more confident and more credible with good posture.

In one office I visited, the young lady at the front desk lazed back in her chair as she talked to other staff members. The young doctor approached the counter from the clinical side of the office, extended her arms across the counter and stretched her back like a cat. Obviously the staff member's demeanor was acceptable to this practitioner who communicated nonverbally in a very similar manner. This was an office that was lacking in credibility in many areas and the nonverbal elements were consistent with the rest of the weaknesses there.

MEETING THE PRACTITIONER

When the dentist enters the treatment room, this is what frequently happens: he or she shakes hands, offers a brief self introduction and then focuses on the file. Sometimes the doctor remains standing, sometimes the doctor sits.(Fig. 14-1 and 14-2.)

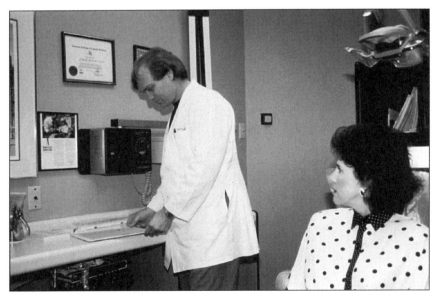

Fig. 14-1 When the doctor enters the treatment room and focuses on the file, the patient can feel ignored and unimportant.

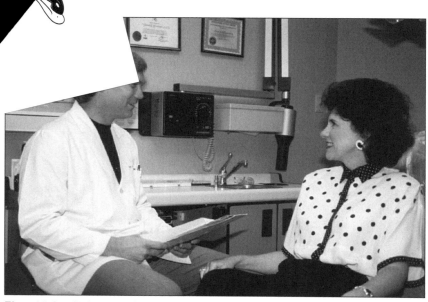

Fig. 14-2 Patients prefer the practitioner sitting at eye level, facing them, communicating their importance.

Here's what patients want and what they prefer:

• Doctor enters the room and approaches the chair.

• Doctor greets patient while standing at a one o'clock to two o'clock position in relation to the patient's chair.

• Doctor shakes hands, offering a full hand shake with males and females offering direct eye contact and a smile at the same time.

• Doctor introduces self with first name and last name, or just first name; avoid use of "Doctor X". You are positioning yourself in a manner that is off-putting to many patients. For example, "I'm Susan Jones" or "I'm Dr. Susan Jones," not "I'm Dr. Jones."

• Use the patient's preferred name. This should be determined by the front desk staff or from information requested on the patient information form.

• Doctor seats self in the one o'clock to two o'clock position in relation to the patient. This allows for full eye contact between both parties and allows the patient to gain a greater sense of the practitioner. The file should be placed on the counter or should be closed and in the doctor's lap.

The first moments with the patient are to develop some level of rapport and to allow the patient to get a sense of the doctor. The doctor needs to verbally and nonverbally communicate to the patient at this point that he or she is a person as well as a practitioner! This means engage in some form of small talk that will help put the patient at ease. It is best if the topic is centered around the patient or what may be of interest to the patient. It should not be of such a personal nature that would cause the patient discomfort. This should also be an opportunity for the doctor to observe the patient's behavioral style to know how to communicate best with this individual. (Fig. 14-3 and 14-4.)

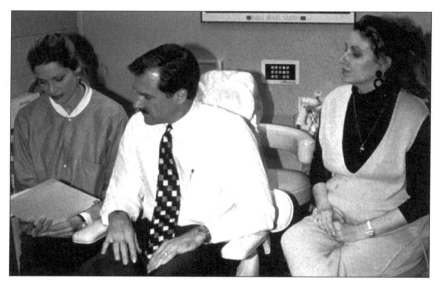

Fig. 14-3 The patient's spouse has been left out of the conversation by a doctor placing primary focus on the file, rather than the patient.

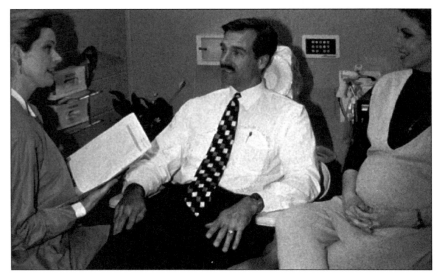

Fig. 14-4 The focus is the patient and spouse and the doctor presents as a caring practitioner.

What occurs in these moments can be crucial to the balance of the appointment and the relationship. It's as much an opportunity for the doctor as it is for the patient. Research has shown that the "tone of the relationships [with patients] rests primarily with the dentist rather than with the patient."[3] Gaining treatment acceptance, patient compliance, and patient referrals frequently can be traced back to interpersonal issues. It is clear that a large part of the responsibility for the interpersonal relationship falls on the shoulders of the practitioner.

The clinical team works closely with the patients. As a patient sits in the chair, you move into his/her comfort zone. This can be a very unsettling feeling for some patients. In a focus group I asked participants, "Tell me something you really like and something you really dislike about your dentist." One patient made an interesting observation. She said, "I don't like that he gets right up in my face." I kept my amusement to myself thinking, "Well, yes, he's a dentist. That's what he does." But I understood what she meant. What she was expressing was that this doctor entered her comfort zone before she was ready, before she had given him permission to do so. The entire team must ensure that patients are given time and opportunity to gain a comfort level with them prior to the exam or treatment.

There must be a level of trust developed before the practitioner moves into the patient's comfort zone. How do you know when that is established? It would be wonderful to say, "Exactly seven minutes after you enter the treatment room, it's acceptable to start the clinical exam." There is no such time frame. In order to determine what is appropriate, one must look at issues of the behavioral style of the patient and the many ways that one develops trust. Both of these areas are discussed at length in chapters 15, 16, and 17 of this book. The important point here is, be careful how you position yourself in relation to your patients and the time frames within which you initiate the clinical exam or the procedure. Take your cues from your patients.

As we sit in the chair and look up at you, we have two views. One where your face is covered with a mask and the other where we can see your expression more readily. In either case, your eyes are communicating to us. Even with the mask on we can guess at the hidden expression, whether that's a smile, a frown, whether we see eyes darting at a staff member who also might hide a frown underneath the mask.

Your face is truly your primary expression source, not your words. Your face communicates your feelings to us, not what you are thinking. Sometimes we look at your face and we may guess, right or wrong, what you are thinking.

Picture a patient with a mouth full of cotton and instruments. The patient can't talk, other than garbled mumbling. Patients detest this situation and they talk about it in our groups. "I've got all this stuff in my mouth, and then she asks me a question!" Patients cannot ask questions much of the time because the mouth is numb or stuffed with cotton! So please, help us out, explain what your expression means. Tell us what you're seeing but don't ask us questions if we're not able to respond. This is a very common complaint and request from patients in our groups.

Much in the way that we may look in your eyes and at your face and try to read you, patients also want you to recognize verbally when we give you "clues" through our own facial expression. For example, eyes which suddenly make eye contact with you, a sudden furrowing of the brow, etc. Patients may not be able to, or want to tell you verbally that they're in stress, but they want you to recognize it and "get it".

GETTING IN TOUCH WITH YOUR PATIENTS

The great anthropologist, Ashley Montagu, wrote in his seminal book, *Touching; The Human Significance of Skin* of the power of touch to heal and connect human beings.[4] Patients do respond to caring touch by practitioners and team members. The gentle touch is most appreciated in the treatment room before, during, and immediately after the procedure or exam. It is interesting to note that what some people perceive as patronizing may be responded to positively in a clinical environment. Many men and women, old and young, respond well to touch on the shoulder and on the arm area.

This form of communication is frequently addressed in focus groups by patients. One woman did note however, "One doctor would give me a little pat on the shoulder and say, 'You're not even going to feel this' right before he was going to give me a shot. That little pat, along with his words, made me feel like he was talking to a little girl. I didn't like his manner." The touch that is given to a patient in order to communicate a caring attitude and to reduce patient anxiety must be extended in a genuine, heartfelt manner. Otherwise, it can come across as insincere and contradict what the doctor means to say.

I conducted role playing sessions with team members in a general dentist's office. Fran, one of the hygienists, was a formal and highly analytical individual. Her focus was typically on the treatment that she was providing and she had excellent clinical skills. However, she did not feel at ease when addressing interpersonal issues that influenced patient relationships. It was clear that Fran understood the impact of a reassuring touch on the shoulder prior to treatment. But the way that it was done, she came across as contrived and practiced instead of sincere and spontaneous. In a case like this, if *you* don't feel comfortable doing it, don't do it.

I had been seated in an airport waiting for a flight that had already been delayed for an hour. The gentleman sitting next to me was awaiting the same plane. We got into a most interesting conversation. He was an oncologist from New York. He daily faced the issues of cancer patients, as well as the stresses placed on family members. We discussed the impact of touch in relation to his communications. He said, "I touch the patient within the first 15 minutes of meeting him or her. I want to make that connection very quickly. Also, I use touch in communicating with relatives of the patients; I want them to know that I care about them also."

Social psychologists note that appropriateness of touch varies dependent on gender of both parties, relationship between them, and the part of body being touched.[5] What is deemed appropriate also varies widely by culture. In America it is generally considered acceptable for a patient to be touched on the arm or shoulder. Obviously, practitioners "are licensed to touch in ways we would not tolerate from anyone else with whom we were not emotionally involved." [6]

Today there are numerous societal issues that can influence this. Therefore, some degree of care needs to be taken. With the number of sexual harassment suits being filed, practitioners are wise to be sensitive to how touch may be interpreted. Touch is seldom acted in isolation. That is, its meaning is often interpreted based on other verbal or nonverbal indicators accompanying it, such as words spoken, eye contact, body positioning, etc. Be aware of your entire message. This matter is also crucial in interacting with children today.

Helen Keller, a most remarkable woman, had neither the benefit of sight nor hearing. It was touch that initially enabled her to connect with those around her. Touch became an all-important language for her and she learned more about the people she met through their touch. In her own articulate way she said,

> *The hands of those I meet are dumbly eloquent to me. I have met people so empty of joy that when I clasped their frosty fingertips it seemed as if I were shaking hands with a northeast storm. There are others whose hands have sunbeams in them, so that their grasp warms my heart. It may be only the clinging touch of a child's hand, but there is as much potential sunshine in it for me as there is in a loving glance for others.*

THE TOPIC OF THE TALK

What you talk about and *how much* you talk is a subject that patients have strong views on. When this is addressed in focus groups, I can almost count on a discussion of what one patient called, "stuffed mouth syndrome." This occurs when the patient's mouth is stuffed with cotton, there's a suction tube in place, and the doctor asks questions of the patient or chooses to chat, requiring patient response. Patients joke about this, but they also intensely dislike it! If you must carry on two-way communication with patients, prepare them for it. Let patients know you may need to ask some questions during treatment and let them know how they can best respond to you.

Two other discussion issues for focus group patients seem to be diametrically opposed. They are:

- the "chatty" team member
- the cold, uncommunicative team member

The Chatty Team Member: The "chatterer" talks more than the patient likes. Sometimes it's a matter of *what* this team member talks about. Patients say that it is most offensive when a chatterer focuses totally on himself or herself.

The Uncommunicative Team Member: The "non-talker" may be focused on tasks or concerned about staying on schedule, and does not engage the patient in *any* discussion. The result may be that the patient feels uncomfortable. The discomfort intensifies for a highly expressive patient who feels ignored.

Here are tips to increase likelihood of patient-friendly communications.

- Recognize the behavioral style of the patient (See chapter 15). This alone can help to ensure an appropriate amount and style of patient/practitioner communication. Take your cues from the patient.

• Focus on the patient more than on yourself. Start the discussion focusing on the patient. It's fine to respond to patient questions about yourself, or to interject comments about yourself, but the overall focus should be on the patient.

• At least half of the discussion with patients should be related to clinical matters, with a healthy portion of this being patient education. This increases patient perception of value.

Vocal Quality: Packaging of Your Words

The way you use your voice has an enormous impact on the way the words are perceived. Vocal quality is like the packaging that wraps up the words you say. You can make that appealing or you could push people away just by your vocal tone.

Patients frequently talk about vocal tone in relation to how messages are conveyed either with the patient or between team members. Here are some comments patients have made that relate to vocal tone:

• "The assistant yelled down the hall at the hygienist that I [the patient] was ready."

• "I felt like a naughty little girl, her [hygienist's] words and tone were scolding me for not doing a better job. It was her tone that really bothered me the most!"

• "I could hear the doctor in the hallway reprimanding the assistant. He talked down to her and his voice was grating. I felt terrible for her."

- "His voice was so soothing and reassuring. I don't remember what he said, but I felt like I was in good hands by the softness and caring tone of his voice."

- "She sounded so hurried on the phone, I figured that's the way they'd be in the office."

- "They were laughing behind me and it made me feel uncomfortable. I couldn't see them and I felt like they were laughing at me."

Patients often refer to voice in describing circumstances of their contact with your office. Your voice is truly a marvelous instrument, one which we often take for granted. Yet it is voice that has such an enormous impact on patient perceptions of the verbal.

Tone and Timing

Your vocal tone and the speed with which you speak influence patient perceptions of you as well as influences their interpretation of the verbal. In order to connect most effectively with your patients, in order for them to feel most comfortable with you, it will be important that you first listen actively to the way that the patient is communicating. If you hear anger or anxiety in the patient's voice then slow down and soften your tone. This action can frequently help patients feel calmer and more settled. However, this should not be done in such a manner that it is perceived as an adult patronizing a child. It must be communicated in a caring way.

Every one of us has a range of vocal tone and vocal timing. There are times when you speak faster than other times, and there are times when you speak more strongly or more softly than other times. People feel most comfortable when they are communicating with those who speak in a similar manner.[7] By adjusting your tone and timing to that which is natural to you but closest to the patient's, you will be helping the patient feel more comfortable with you. As the patient becomes more comfortable with you he/she is more likely to hear the verbal message.

Therefore, if you speak very quickly and the patient you're talking with speaks much more slowly, then slow down! I'm not suggesting that you imitate the patient, but that you adjust to the pattern that is still natural to you and closest to that of the patient.

If you are enthusiastic about something, if you feel strongly about the subject matter at hand, the patient needs to hear this in your voice. Once again, it's a matter of congruence. This is particularly important when addressing issues of a serious nature, such as finances, insurance, patient no-shows, and cancellations.

For example, if a patient misses an appointment and you call the patient but reach a recorder, your voice needs to convey concern. If you use a lilting, soft, or ethereal vocal tone, then you will cast doubt on the words that you have just said. Your words and your vocal tone must convey the same message. Likewise, you will be taken more seriously in discussing finances and insurance when the words that you say are communicated in a definite and self confident manner.

Even our pets respond to voice and know the difference between an angry, sharp tone versus a friendly tone. A world champion hog caller, in citing his unique abilities noted, "You've got to have appeal as well as power in your voice. You've got to convince the hogs you've got something for them!" Here was a man who truly understood the power of voice!

If a patient comes into your office and he/she is very enthusiastic about something, perhaps a trip he has recently taken, he would like to hear a responsiveness from you as well. If you hear enthusiasm in patients' voices, they also would like to see and preferably hear your responsiveness.

An important note here relates to the behavioral style of your patients. Understanding your patients is crucial to developing a rapport and building a long-term relationship. This means listening closely, not only to their words but to their vocal patterns as well. The way an individual uses his voice is an indication to his mood and behavioral style. (See chapter 15 on behavioral styles) If you are a highly enthusiastic, outgoing individual and your patient is perhaps more introverted or analytical, this individual may not be responsive to an overly expressive vocal pattern in communication. Take your cues from the patients and help them feel comfortable within your environment.

The power of voice is particularly influential on the telephone. Because visual elements have been removed, the words and the way that you say the words are all important. Also see chapter 11 for more extensive information about vocal tone in telephone use.

A poem appeared in a "Dear Abby" column that sums up the topics addressed in this segment. The author of the poem was unknown.[8] What is particularly significant about this is that a patient found the poem framed and on the wall of her physician's office. It certainly sums up the concept of voice as the "packaging" of our words.

THE TONE OF VOICE

It's not so much what you say
As the manner in which you say it;
It's not so much the language you use
As the tone in which you convey it.
"Come here!" I sharply said
And the child cowered and wept.

"Come here," I said

He looked and smiled

And straight to my lap he crept.

Words may be mild and fair

But the tone may pierce like a dart;

Words may be soft as the summer air

But the tone may break my heart;

For words come from the mind

Grow by study and art

But tone leaps from the inner self,

Revealing the state of the heart.

Whether you know it or not,

Whether you mean or care,

Gentleness, kindness, love and hate,

Envy, anger are there.

Then, would you quarrels avoid

And peace and love rejoice?

Keep anger not only out of your words

Keep it out of your voice.

— AUTHOR UNKNOWN

TOP TIPS:

1. Help the patient understand the different roles in the office via the apparel worn. Have three distinct categories of apparel: business staff, clinical team, doctors.
2. Be particularly sensitive to patient perceptions of personal protective equipment. Remove personal barriers when not needed and recognize that patients

observe what you touch in the treatment room while
you are wearing gloves.

3. In personal grooming, neatness is of prime
    importance. Hair must be neat; wear minimal jewelry,
    make-up, and fragrance.

4. Keep fingernails, short, well-trimmed. Dark or brightly
    colored fingernail polish is best avoided for clinical
    team members.

5. Introduce yourself to new patients and use the
    patient's preferred name.

6. At the front desk: stand and shake hands with the new
    patient.

7. In the treatment areas, during discussions sit at the
    patient's eye level. Face the patient and focus on the
    patient, not on the file.

8. Match the patient's vocal tone and timing except when
    you hear anger or anxiety. At those times slow down
    and soften your voice.

REFERENCES

[1] Boswell, Suzanne. *Menswear: Suiting the Customer*, Regents/Prentice Hall, Englewood Cliffs, NJ, 1993.

[2] Some focus group patients commented that pre-molded styles looked like those available to consumers for painting or for allergy sufferers. These patients perceived the flat, pleated masks to look more "professional."

[3] Rankin, MA, Jane; Harris, Ph.D., Mary B. "Patients Preferences for Dentists' Behaviors," *Journal of the American Dental Association*, Vol. 110, March, 1985.

[4] Montagu, Ashley, *Touching: The Human Significance of Skin*, New York, NY, Harper & Row, 1978.

[5] Morris, Desmond. *Body Watching*, Crown Publishers, Inc., New York, NY, 1985.

[6] Marsh, Dr. Peter. *Eye to Eye; How People Interact*, Salem House, Topsfield, MA, 1988.

[7] Cialdini, Ph.D., Robert B. *Influence: How and Why People Agree to Things*, William Morrow and Co., Inc., New York, NY, 1984.

[8] _____, "Dear Abby" column, *Dallas Morning News*, Dallas, TX, May 19, 1996.

15

Behavioral Styles of Staff and Patients

"You can make more friends in two months by becoming interested in other people than you can in two years by trying to get other people interested in you."

— D A L E   C A R N E G I E

I feel so uncomfortable, said the hygienist, Sally, in reference to her next patient. Bill Britton is so difficult to work with. He's always in a hurry and he never seems to pay attention to what I'm suggesting in terms of periodontal treatment. He keeps saying that he wants his condition to improve, but he wants it to happen overnight without any work on his part.

I was working with the entire staff of a practice and we were preparing to do some role playing. Sally was discussing the types of patients she had the most difficulty working with; she was seeking answers about how to deal with them. She is a very people-oriented individual and likes to build positive, warm relationships with her clients. She is interested in them as people—not just as patients, but as she put it, "there are just some people I can't seem to get through to." What Sally was experiencing was a contrast in styles. As an Amiable behavioral style, Sally found great satisfaction in building friendly relationships with her patients. Because she preferred to work at a steady and measured pace, she presumed that her patients would also appreciate, and find soothing, a very calm and steady appointment time. However, Sally was not taking into account the fact that in her role as hygienist, she deals with many different people every day. Their needs and their behavioral styles vary.

Because Sally operated out of her own comfort zone, there were numerous times when she was not meeting the needs of her patients. As a result, some of her patients were calling the office and requesting a different hygienist, one whom they were able to relate to more effectively. In the case of her upcoming patient, Sally was feeling stress because the behavioral style of this patient was in such great contrast with hers. She didn't know specifically why she was feeling this tension, but she knew that the relationship with the patient was not moving in the right direction.

The patient, Bill Britton, was a classic Driving style. He was a salesman and an entrepreneur. He frequently had numerous projects he was working on simultaneously. Bill had great concerns about time constraints for his dental appointments and always seemed to be rushed. He was very goal oriented and he wanted the end result of healthy teeth and gums, but he was frustrated with the lengthy explanations, the chat about family and personal topics. He just wanted to get to the bottom line, "take care of my mouth, do it quickly and give me the quickest steps to get the results that I want."

In order to help Sally and the rest of the team become more comfortable in treating all behavioral styles of patients, we conducted an in-depth behavioral profile on each team member. Our next step was to discuss at length the ways that each behavioral style within the team could best interact with each other. This process includes learning how to listen effectively and how to obtain feedback that increases human understanding and rapport. The next logical step was applying these same concepts to patients and thereby knowing how to communicate and relate well with all styles of patients.

The results? Sally not only felt more comfortable in treating Bill Britton, but she gained self-confidence with other team members and patients. A long-term outcome was a more cohesive team and patients who exhibited increased confidence in the practice.

THE STUDY OF BEHAVIOR AND ITS IMPACT ON HUMAN INTERACTION

Every day the entire dental team is dealing with four basic behavioral styles. This model, developed by David Merrill, Ph.D. and Roger Reid, MA is one that aids in understanding others through increased awareness of their behavior; it is behavior that the team is dealing with during the day.[1] Once the behavioral style of the patient is determined, likely response to circumstances within the appointment time frame can be predicted fairly well. The exception is, of course, outside influences that affect the patient prior to entering the office. However, understanding the style of the patient means that the attending staff members can more confidently know how to respond to the patient's behavior.

BEHAVIOR VERSUS PERSONALITY

Behavior is what's on the outside. It's what the world sees, it's how you interact with others. To simplify this, it's what you say, it's what you do; it's observable behavior.

On the other hand, personality encompasses much more. It includes behavior but it also incorporates all of those elements that we hold inside and we may not exhibit or we may not share with others. This can include, for example, your deepest hopes, dreams, fears, and desires. Your personality is like a whole ear of corn whereas your behavior is what appears on the outside. It's the husk!

The significance is that *behavior* is what the team must deal with during the patient's appointment. The inner being exists in the patient, but the staff members must deal only with the reality of the patient's behavior during the appointment. For example, a patient arrives at the office after the stress of rush hour traffic. The same patient arrives at the next appointment after a leisurely and pleasurable luncheon with friends. Here we have seen in the same patient, two very different circumstances and it is the resultant behavior the team must handle.

SOCIAL STYLE™₂

In using the concept of SOCIAL STYLE™ to increase effective communication with your patients, you must fine-tune your powers of observation. In recognizing a behavioral style, or SOCIAL STYLE™ first you must be able to observe the patient accurately and recognize the

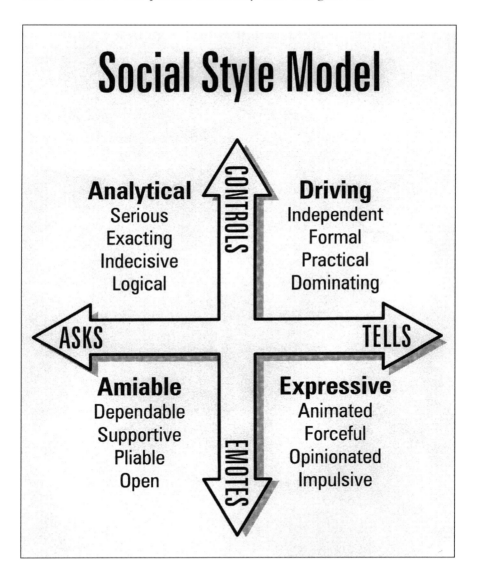

Social Style Model

Analytical
Serious
Exacting
Indecisive
Logical

CONTROLS

Driving
Independent
Formal
Practical
Dominating

ASKS

TELLS

Amiable
Dependable
Supportive
Pliable
Open

EMOTES

Expressive
Animated
Forceful
Opinionated
Impulsive

Fig. 15-1 By putting the dimensions of Assertiveness and Responsiveness together, you identify the four patterns of behaviors, or styles, of the Social Change Model. (Courtesy the TRACOM Corporation, Denver, CO)

clues that will help you determine that patient's style. In order to do this, you need to back off and allow the patient room to exhibit enough of his behavioral clues to be identified.

There are two dimensions of human behavior which are key elements in understanding the SOCIAL STYLE MODEL™[3] (Fig. 15-1.) The first is *assertiveness*. People are assertive in two different ways. They may be *ask assertive* or *tell assertive*. Ask assertive people are the ones who tend to pose questions more often than to make statements or offer information. Sometimes they make statements in an asking manner. These are the people who seek information and often avoid taking a position on a subject matter until they have gotten enough answers. The tell assertive individuals are the ones who more readily verbalize a position on an issue. They are more willing to voice their opinions and make statements more readily.

The ask assertive individual frequently speaks more slowly, makes fewer statements, and may be quieter in volume. They also may be recognized by some other nonverbal clues; they may make less eye contact during conversation, and hand movement and body posture may be more reserved.

The tell assertive individual may be recognized by a quicker speech pattern, by making more statements and using louder volume in speaking. In addition, their gestures may be more directive. They also tend to make more eye contact during conversation.

The second dimension of behavior is called *responsiveness*. Responsiveness is an indication of how much emotion a person may be willing to display to others. The individual seen as controlling his/her emotions may be perceived to be less responsive, and the individual who exhibits emotions more freely is seen to be more responsive. The behavioral clues indicative of emotionally controlling people are that they may have a more monotone voice and focus on tasks rather than people; they frequently use data and facts in conversation. Their body posturing, use of hands and facial expressions may also be more controlled, closer to the body, and sometimes seem to be rigid.

The person who is seen as more emotionally responsive, frequently uses a wider range of voice inflection; his focus is on people and relationships, and he will frequently use stories and personal opinion in conversation. These individuals may be more animated than the controlling behavioral styles. Their attitude is more casual and their gesturing may be more open. It is the degree of responsiveness and assertiveness that combines to determine an individual's style.

RECOGNIZING THE FOUR TYPES

Sally, the hygienist mentioned earlier, is very people oriented and tends to ask a lot of questions about interpersonal issues. She is slower, more measured, and softer in tone. She exhibits Amiable behavior in numerous ways, making identification of her style quite easy. Her patient, Bill Britton, exhibits his Driving behavior through faster speech patterns, more controlled motions, focus on results, and speed in conversation. (Fig. 15-2)

People of the Expressive behavioral type make more statements. They speak faster, use more variety in their vocal tone and they're frequently very animated in conversation. The Expressive style tends to focus on issues with people, relationships, and they often use stories in making their points.

In contrast, the Analytical style is one which is more restrained in communication. The voice is more subdued, frequently monotone. The focus is on tasks.

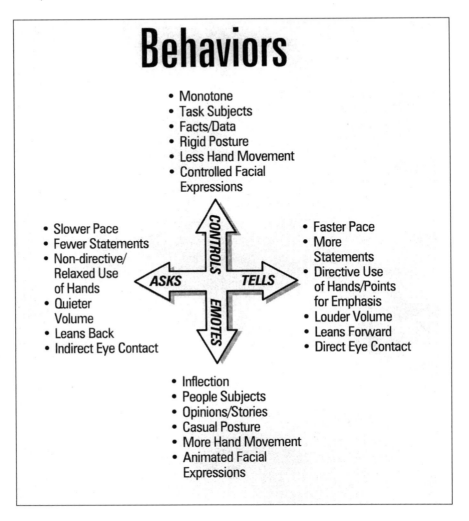

Fig. 15-2 This illustration helps identify behavior typical of the four behavioral styles. (Courtesy the TRACOM Corporation, Denver, CO)

They have great interest for, and appreciation of, fact and data in making points. The Analytical style is reserved in the pace of speech, speaking more slowly, and offering fewer statements. Their tone is quieter and their body language is more controlled and reserved.

YOUR OWN STYLE

It is extremely difficult to make accurate determination of one's own style. This requires real objectivity and an outsider's perspective on the self. Research has shown that given difficult circumstances, we frequently find or make, excuses to cover our own shortcomings. Researchers refer to this as *Self-Handicapping Strategy*.[4]

Self awareness is an important key to understanding behavior and helping to relate to others more effectively. Attention to how we're communicating and behaving does not mean that one "gets carried away by emotions, overacting and amplifying what is perceived."[5] True self awareness is a neutral mode that allows the individual to look at himself in an objective manner. In the same way that it's easiest to recognize the styles of other individuals by "stepping back", it is also easier to recognize one's own behavior and style by objectively moving away from the emotional connect "rather than being immersed and lost in it."[6] Consequently, self determination of behavioral styles is a challenge but it can be addressed through application of the Social Style Model™. (Fig. 15-1) Recognizing behavioral cues can aid in understanding yourself and others. (Fig. 15-2)

Understanding that comes with self knowledge is key in helping you to communicate most effectively with your patients and with your peers. So what style are you? The ideal method for determining your behavioral style is through objective feedback from others. This process can be effected through completion of a questionnaire by individuals who observe your behavior in the professional arena. These questionnaires are then submitted to an organization which processes them by computer and the profile that results from the compilation offers a perspective of how others may view the individual in question.[7]

BEHAVIORAL STYLE AND TEAM COHESION

The more cohesive the team is, the more likely that productivity will rise and members of the team will gain greater satisfaction on the job. The concept of a cohesive team is a crucial one in the patient's eyes. Patients want to be part of a dental practice "family" that is functioning well. A team that is not operating cohesively can cause patient anxiety. There is no question that patients feel tension that exists within the team.

As an undercover dental patient, I've experienced this myself and it doesn't take expressed words for patients to recognize team stress. The team may think that they're hiding it, but patients can sense it. They often bring this up in focus groups we conduct with patients. One patient commented, "I saw the looks that flashed between the doctor and the assistant as they worked together. But more than that I felt the tension in the air, and it made me feel very uncomfortable. Maybe they were thinking more about the stress between them, than my periodontal problem!"

The more you can learn about your team members and recognize the predictable pattern of communication, the more likely that you can learn how to communicate to gain positive and productive results.[8]

CASE PRESENTATION, TREATMENT ACCEPTANCE, AND COMPLIANCE

When you start communicating with your patients in a manner that earns endorsement, you are more likely to see a positive response to case presentation, and treatment acceptance should rise. For example, if you are presenting a case to an Analytical style patient, your approach would be very different from presenting the very same treatment plan to a patient of the Expressive style.

The Analytical patient will respond to in-depth data that provides a solid foundation for your suggestions. This patient will appreciate and value your offering some history of how the treatment has been successful with other patients. Information should be offered in a logical and orderly manner, perhaps prioritizing a treatment schedule and presenting it in steps.

Your Analytical patients will not be as responsive to a "warm, fuzzy" approach. They will be making judgments based on your ability to offer sufficient details, pros and cons of a treatment, and research supporting your perspectives.[9] The Analytical patients particularly, will take note of your attention to details when it comes to issues of informed consent. Make sure you dot the "i's" and cross the "t's" when informing about risks, benefits, and options to this patient.

If you are an Expressive style, you will need to adjust your speed to a slower, more methodical pace that the Analytical will feel comfortable with. In addition, be extremely careful not to put any pressure on this patient. Analytical patients will resist and respond negatively; they need time to evaluate all you've told them.

If you were presenting the same treatment plan to an Expressive style patient, your approach would need to be quite different. The Expressive patient will respond to a faster, more high energy style of presentation. They will be interested in how others will feel about the treatment, particularly if it is aesthetic in nature. Give them personal approval and credit for their decision to consider the treatment. These individuals will respond to a personal approach with acknowledgment of their decision-making.

The Expressives will accept and appreciate a more broad-based presentation of information. Start communicating with this patient in terms of the "big picture" and based on feedback and questions from this patient, provide additional details that may be appreciated. Relate success stories of your other patients who have had similar treatments and take an informal approach in communicating with this patient. They will also respond to a stimulating verbal and visual approach to the subject, using inflection in your voice and more open, animated facial expressions and gestures.

If your style is quite different from your patient's it is crucial to recognize that in the case presentation, you will be meeting your patient's needs by modifying your approach to be in sync with the patient. "It is naive, at best, to assume that the same verbal communication will work equally well" with all style patients. Instead, an awareness of, and sensitivity to, the different styles of your patients will best be exemplified through your versatility and adjusting to each individual patient. It is key to understand that one doesn't *change* one's style, but rather one adapts and manages one's behavior to aid in communication's effectiveness. You are far more likely to gain patient endorsement and certainly increase patient compliance when the patient feels you understand his needs. As George Bernard Shaw put it, "It is unwise to do unto others as you would have them do unto you. Their tastes may not be the same!"

PATIENT RETENTION

One of the factors that influences whether a patient stays with a particular dental practice is how comfortable they feel there. That comfort is in large part due to the relationships built with the dental team. Patients in focus groups frequently talk about their feelings about the team. They value the team that communicates a genuine caring attitude.

The perception of "caring attitude" can vary dependent on the style of the patient. In one focus group we conducted, there was a very reserved, thoughtful gentleman. He was methodical and organized in his thoughts and focused on details and data as he spoke on each issue. He was clearly an Analytical style. When we discussed team communication, he talked about a staff member in his dental office who caused him great concern. He put it this way, "When I come into the office and I'm led to the hygiene room, she gives me a hug. Then the whole time I'm in the chair she's talking incessantly about her family and asking me personal questions. I feel it's inappropriate behavior and I've gotten where I hate to go in for my cleaning." A conflict in style, indeed—and one that could cause the patient to leave the practice. The staff member was doing what was comfortable for her instead of adjusting to the style of the patient.

The Amiable patient will have greater need for a personal approach by staff. This is the person who will value the staff that remembers details about the patient's family, interests, and history. This patient will respond to personalized nurturing by the practitioners. Be aware however, that this is also the patient who can engage in chatting that may result in getting behind schedule. There's a delicate balance where the staff needs to communicate with personal interest toward this patient and at the same time, maintain some degree of control over time.

In a similar vein, issues of time can be a very serious matter when it comes to both the team and the patient. It is the Driving and Analytical patients who can become the most disturbed if you start very late for the appointment, and/or you run overtime. A verbal acknowledgment of the patient's time concerns or challenges in relation to time will tell this patient that you are aware and sensitive to his issues.

With all patients, issues of confidentiality and privacy are important. As a mystery patient in numerous dental offices, I've experienced the challenges that are presented to patients of different styles when there is a lack of privacy. For example, the Expressive and Driving patients may be more likely to openly verbalize in the reception or business areas, their discontent with fees or insurance coverage. Some of these patients will not be at all intimidated by the presence of other patients who can overhear the conversation. This can present awkward situations for the staff.

On the other hand, patients who may be more reticent to state their concerns, perhaps the Amiables and Analyticals, may not verbalize their thoughts at all. They may feel uncomfortable doing so in such public areas. However, this is a distinct disadvantage for the dental team. Until you know the objections of the patient, it will be difficult for you to deal with him. Privacy for communications on financial matters or insurance issues is extremely important for all styles of patients.[9]

Patient retention can certainly be affected by the communication styles of the staff. In order to help the patient feel most comfortable in the office, the team must be versatile enough to recognize the patient's style and modify behavior to increase patient ease and to gain patient endorsement.

Understanding and responding to your patients' behavioral styles can go a long way toward helping to retain those same patients. Once you understand the behavioral style of the individual it is frequently possible to predict behavior.[10] The accuracy with which you can predict a patient's likely behavior may be based on how well you have observed and understood his past behaviors. Future behavior by patients may be situational; that is, the situation in which the patient is placed will have an impact on the behavior. But the patient's responses will still fall within the behavioral realm of that patient's social style. Therefore, it is of great benefit to the practice to recognize and respond appropriately to each patient's style. The patient will feel more at ease, can feel more understood by the team, and will be less likely to "graze" away from the practice because of this very basic connect.

TAKING THE FIRST STEPS

In starting to apply the concepts of SOCIAL STYLE™, it's key to avoid trying to determine the style of a patient or peer too quickly. Observe the individual closely, in as many different situations as is possible. Most importantly, get out of the way! That is, you can't begin to recognize a behavioral pattern or observe style clues if your feelings get in the way of being objective. Pay less attention to how you are feeling about the person, and pay more attention to the behavior of the individual. It's through observing what they say and what they do that you'll be able to start to clarify the style of the person you're interacting with!

The dental offices that most successfully incorporate this system, make it a part of their everyday process with patients. From the moment of the first phone call from a prospective patient, the receptionist listens actively to the communication style of the caller. Notes are made as to initial perception of style. If the caller schedules an appointment, the initial perception of style is noted in the records. When the patient visits the office, the attending team members use this information in evaluating the patient. They add their observations to those already accumulated and ultimately the determined style is noted in the patient's permanent records. Reference to this style prior to the patient's appointments can aid appreciably in increasing patient endorsement, compliance, and treatment acceptance.

This concept is particularly effective when patients are discussed in the morning huddle. In this way, the entire team is communicating in a manner that is cohesive and meets the patients' needs in the most comprehensive manner.

When it comes to gaining endorsement of all the different individuals you come in contact with daily, remember the power of being versatile. We can't expect patients to adjust to the team, the team must adjust to the patients. In the words of Mae West, "It's not what you do, it's how you do it. It's not what you say, it's how you say it. And it's how you look as you do it and you say it!"

TOP TIPS:

1. Separate your subjective feelings about an individual from your objective observations of the individual.
2. Recognize the important clues to an individual's style that come by way of what the person says and what the person does.
3. When meeting a new patient, restrain exhibiting your own style until you have been able to

observe and more closely identify the patient's style.

4. Give and receive feedback in a manner which will be most comfortable for your patient. Be open and versatile and recognize that each person is a unique individual.

5. Recognize the strengths of all styles. The most effective teams are frequently made up of all four behavioral styles.

REFERENCES

[1] Merrill, David, Ph.D. and Reid, Roger, MA . *Personal Styles and Effective Performance,* Chilton Book Company, Radnor, PA, 1981.

[2] SOCIAL STYLE is a service mark of The TRACOM Corporation.

[3] The SOCIAL STYLE MODEL is a trademark of The TRACOM Corporation.

[4] Forgas, Joseph. Interpersonal Behaviour: *The Psychology of Social Interaction,* Pergamon Press, Oxford, England, 1985. Goleman, Daniel.. Emotional Intelligence, Bantam Books, New York, NY, 1995.

[5] Goleman, Daniel.. *Emotional Intelligence,* Bantam Books, New York, NY, 1995.

[6] Goleman, Daniel.. *Emotional Intelligence*, Bantam Books, New York, NY, 1995.

[7] Self Perception instruments also are available. When implemented by the entire team in a staff meeting, the team is better equipped to understand each other and patients. Instrument packets and Staff Meeting Outline are available from Boswell Presentations; (972) 243-2086.

[8] Moine, Donald and Heard, John. *Modern Persuasion Strategies: The Hidden Advantage in Selling*, Prentice Hall, Inc., Englewood Cliffs, NJ, 1984.

[9] Goffman, Erving. *Behavior in Public Places*, The Free Press, Division of Macmillan Publishing Co., Inc., New York, NY, 1963.

[10] Kleinke, Chris. *Meeting and Understanding People*, W. H. Freeman and Company, New York, NY, 1986 .

16

Encouraging Patient Ease in the Dental Office

"To him who is in fear, everything rustles."
— S O P H O C L E S

There's no way I'd change dentists. I finally found an office where I feel okay." Deborah was not only a member of this focus group but was also one of the leaders of the non-profit organization where the focus group was being held. When I had spoken to her in the process of organizing this group, Deborah had told me how strongly she felt about her dentist and the whole team at that office. Here was a patient who was a true ambassador for this practice. She explained to me her family history of dental problems. Both her mother and grandmother had periodontal disease and had lost most of their teeth. Deborah had seen these severe problems and she had vicariously experienced the pain and embarrassment that both of them had felt.

Now in her forties, Deborah was experiencing some of these same problems. However, she made a decision that she would do whatever was necessary to avoid losing her teeth. In our focus group, she talked about having gone from dentist to dentist to find the office where she would feel most at ease. She had an extremely high anxiety level about the dental office experience.

But Deborah was also very fortunate. She had found a practitioner and a team that understood and helped her through her fears. Because she was on a three-month recall with her periodontist, she had come to know the team well. "I still do get nervous when I go in there," she said. "I can't even sit down, I have to stand, or walk or talk to staff until I go to the treatment room."

Her comfort level with the office was primarily based on the interpersonal skills and the understanding that was exhibited by all members of the team. Of all the focus group participants we have interviewed, Deborah stood out as having the highest expressed fear level. She was also one of the patients who was happiest with her dental practice.

FACTORS THAT CAN CAUSE PATIENT ANXIETY

It is no surprise to the dental team that a high percentage of patients experience tension in relation to a dental appointment. The subject matter of patient fear and anxiety is a huge one and far more complicated than the goals for this book. Patient fear and anxiety may be rooted deeply in the history of the patient, early experiences, or attitudes of relatives or friends that have influenced patient behavior. My goal is not to investigate these matters but rather to look specifically at what is likely to increase patient anxiety in the office and, regardless of the source, how it can be reduced.

DEFINING THE TERMS: FEAR VERSUS ANXIETY

Often the concepts of fear and anxiety are interchanged and used in a synonymous manner. In actuality, they are quite different. Fear is the appraisal of danger. "It is a cognitive process as opposed to an emotional reaction."[1] "Fear can be learned vicariously by hearing about or witnessing other individuals' traumatic experiences."[2] Anxiety is an emotional state, frequently an emotional response to fear.

The following are items that patients frequently indicate cause tension or increase patient anxiety. It is possible that some of your patients experience fear and anxiety in relation to these items and, as we have learned in focus groups, your patients might not be communicating these concerns to you.

FEAR OR ANXIETY IN RELATION TO:

- Painful injections
- Pain during treatment
- The unknown, not knowing what will happen during the treatment.
- Insensitive practitioner who doesn't relate to the patient.

- Practitioner who has a rough or hard touch.
- Uncommunicative doctor or team member.
- Appointment not starting on time or extended wait prior to treatment starting.
- Lack of privacy.
- Fees
- Clinical conditions and proposed treatments.
- Sounds of equipment or sounds of other patients who are experiencing discomfort.

In focus groups, patients have indicated that the following concepts help to reduce tension or anxiety while in the dental office:

- **Give a Painless Injection.** Learn how to give a painless injection. It is possible to do so and I know from responses in my seminars that the majority of doctors recognize this. Whether they have learned to do this or not is another matter. This is always one of the top items that patients bring up in relation to anxiety or fear in the dental office. The dentist needs to learn how to give a painless injection, and the entire team needs to recognize the importance of verbalizing this learned skill to patients. In effect, this is a marketing concept that patients respond to very positively.

- **Have a Sense Of Humor.** Patients truly appreciate when the practitioner is able to "loosen up." This helps the patient feel more relaxed and breathe a little easier. Voltaire said, "The art of medicine consists of amusing the patient while nature cures the disease." Although the reality of this may not be completely true, it is certainly true that the attitude of the practitioner will influence that of the patient. Humor is typically appreciated—appropriate humor, that is. We have heard stories from patients about inappropriate jokes and "humorous" stories being related in the treatment room and within patient earshot.

Inappropriate subject matter includes anything related to religion, politics, sexual in nature, or anything which is demeaning or derogatory to others. I have experienced forms of humor I feel are very inappropriate in the dental office. On more than one occasion, doctors have joked to the patient about the patient's dental experience with statements like, "Well, I'm glad it's *you* sitting in the chair and not me!" A statement like this might be intended as a moment of levity to loosen up the patient and communicate that the doctor is poking fun at himself or herself. However, this is actually affirming to the patient that there may be cause for some concern! Doctors who are using this form of humor need to make a 180° about-face and reevaluate the kind of message being sent to the patient. Goethe said, "Men show their characters in nothing more clearly than in what they think laughable."

- **Explain the Treatment Before You Begin It.** This is a major complaint by patients, not just in relation to reducing patient tension but in discussing complaints about the office as a whole. Patients want to know what is going to happen in a treatment before the treatment begins. Patients also want to know how to act, what they may need to do, and they want to know it before the procedure starts. The more information that the patient can be provided prior to treatment, the more likely that anxiety will be reduced during treatment. Consequently, you will probably find an informed patient is a more cooperative one.

- **Offer Attention Distractions.** Use headsets, TV's, and virtual reality glasses that involve the patient and over which the patient has control. When the practitioner has been particularly effective in preparing the patient psychologically for treatment and when the patient has some control over communication and environment, patient fear and resultant anxiety can lessen. In focus groups, patients talk about the benefits of putting on a headset and listening to music or watching a TV in the ceiling.

Patients remarked that these are highly effective in helping to decrease patient tension. The act of the patient using a remote control means that to some extent the patient is managing his or her own environment. Virtual reality glasses take this a step farther in that the patient has the option to view the electronic image or look through the glasses and communicate directly with the team.

The most common form of positive distractions that I have experienced as a patient are art work, posters, and photographs on the ceiling as well as view out a window. (This issue is discussed in greater depth in chapter 12 on decor.)

• **Ensure That the Entire Dental Team Is Well-Groomed.** For patients with high concerns about infection control, clinical team members who are not well-groomed can be source of fear and anxiety. The patient may question his or her own personal safety in the office. Poor grooming will reflect on the doctor's judgment and the doctor's acceptance of this type of appearance.

• **Communicate as a Cohesive Team.** This is a fundamentally important concept. When a patient is placed in an environment where the team communicates well with each other the patient is reassured. When the team likes and respects each other, the patient feels more at ease.

Patients talk about this in focus groups and I have experienced it myself on several occasions when there is a high tension level among the team. Patients do feel this. The tension may be perceived in the way the team members move, how quickly and/or sharply they speak, the words that are used, eye contact with each other, etc. If a patient is in such an environment and the doctor says, "just relax," it means very little to the patient. No amount of electronic or decor distractions can eliminate awareness of this type of tension around the patient.

- **Exhibit Sincere Caring for the Patient.** "Sincere" is the operative word here. If the patient perceives team members are insincere or patronizing in any way, the opposite of the desired result can occur. One patient in a focus group noted, "I overheard the doctor and assistant exchanging heated words outside the room. He sounded really angry at her, then he came back into the room and said to me, 'I know you're a little nervous about this treatment. Just sit back, you're in good hands, just relax now.' But he said it like he'd memorized it and it didn't mean anything. I was really bothered because I knew that he was upset from the argument with the assistant; so his words didn't mean a thing to me.

In reality, the dentist who says, "just relax" is communicating to the patient that he/she does not know how to manage the situation; making a statement like this is equivalent to saying, "I really don't understand what you are feeling, so try to relax by your own will because I don't know what to do to help you." This is far from a comforting thought for a patient!

- **Establish a Relationship With the Individual as a Person First, Then as a Patient.** Many patients remark on the importance of the doctor knowing something about the patient, his interests, her work, their hobbies. For the patient, this is an indication that the practitioner or the team member sees the individual as a person not just as a patient. In addition, there is a sense of greater "belongingness." The patient's thinking is, "You know me and I know something about you, we are a part of the same family. I 'belong' here and feel at ease here."

One doctor I spoke with said, "I don't do 'chit-chat' with patients. I don't have time for it and most patients don't have time for it. They are in the office for treatment, not for friendship." He said this in a quick, abrupt vocal pattern probably very similar to the way in which he communicated with his patients. Interestingly, his staff was very warm and friendly. He had surrounded himself with people who counterbalanced his strident manner. Perhaps his patients remained with him due to his staff and his clinical skills rather than any interpersonal skills he had.

In focus groups, patients comment that they prefer the doctor to have some level of people skills that will help them feel more at ease in the office. But they quickly add a disclaimer of, "I don't expect him/her to be my best friend. Clinical skills are more important in the long run but if I could find someone with both the clinical skills and the interpersonal skills, that's what I'd prefer."

Many issues can influence patients' anxiety or tension in the dental practice. Those patients who do not have a high fear level also can be influenced by these elements. The more that tension can be reduced within the patient, the more effective and efficient the entire appointment time for the patient will be. Consider this a type of "universal precaution" wherein steps are taken to create the most tension free environment possible for all patients whether there is a high expressed level of fear or not. The following material will aid in developing this tension free environment and can result in patients who are more receptive to treatment in your office.

ON THE PHONE

Each time the phone rings, regardless of what else may be occurring in your surroundings, recognize that the caller is not aware of your circumstances. The vocal tone you use, your manner in communicating with this patient is going to define for the patient the type of practice your have. A welcoming tone, caring words and a sincere interest in the patient will help the caller recognize that yours is an office where patients will be treated with kindness and respect. The receptionist needs to listen closely to the vocal pattern, timing, and verbal message of the caller. If there is any hint of anxiety, then the caller should be reassured with specifics that address the patient's issues. For example, if a new patient is calling about his/her appointment, and if this new patient expresses fear of dental treatment, the receptionist should pose questions to seek out the source of the patient's discomfort. Then that specific cause for concern can be addressed.

When a receptionist makes a comment like, "Oh, don't worry about a thing, you'll be fine here!" This is not really addressing patient concerns since there was no specific response as to *why* the patient should feel comfortable in the office. Therefore, the patient has not really been given reassurance. A response like, "I understand you've had some bad experiences with injections in the past. Our patients repeatedly comment that Dr. Smith really *does* give Novocain so they can't feel it." Now the patient's specific concern has been addressed in a manner and using the words that are familiar to the patient and that the patient understands.

Ideally, the receptionist can make a note about this patient's concern in his/her records. When the patient arrives at the office the patient can be reassured once more about this issue. This is a message that the patient is important and that the practice recognizes the patient's concerns.

In Reception

Ensure that the reception area is comfortable. As much as possible, create a living room type environment that will help to put the patient at ease. (Fig. 16-1) Be aware of the sounds that can be heard in the reception area. Patients should not hear conversations or equipment sounds coming from the clinical areas. The reception area should be devoid of any type of medicinal smell and there should be aesthetically pleasing visual elements which help to create a comfortable environment.

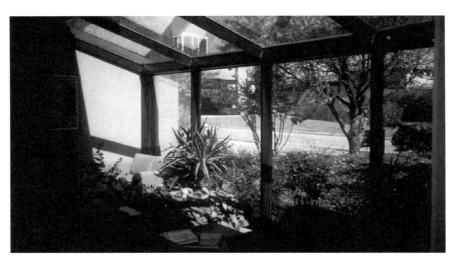

Fig. 16-1 The central patient seating area of Dr. McDougal's office is very much like an atrium, to develop a soothing environment.

Immediately upon a patient's entering the reception area, he/she should receive eye contact and a welcoming smile from the greeting staff member. If this staff member is assisting a patient at the counter, acknowledgment of the incoming patient is still crucial. If a patient, particularly one who is experiencing tension, is ignored it can result in increased anxiety on the part of the patient.

In Clinical Areas

Sit in the treatment chair and see the treatment room in the same way that the patient does. Do this during regular office hours so that you can become more aware of the sounds in the room as well. If you are highly aware of what is occurring in the adjacent treatment areas, recognize that this can be a cause for concern with high anxiety patients. A fearful patient can have his or her fears confirmed by the sound of another patient experiencing discomfort. Also, equipment sounds can be a trigger for some fearful patients. The less sound from adjacent rooms, the better.

What do you see sitting in the chair? If there are electronic diversions or distractions, can they be controlled by the patient? For example, TV's, headsets, and virtual reality glasses need to be controllable by the patient. These elements can be extremely helpful in overcoming any sound leakage from other treatment areas.

Patients do like to see clinician degrees and certificates. However, they are best placed on the side walls rather than on the wall directly in front of the patient. A window that looks out on a pleasant scene, or a print or photograph which is visually pleasing will aid in reducing tension. Place art work in the direct line of vision of the patient. Prints and posters on the ceiling directly above the treatment chair are helpful in providing distraction during treatment. Amusing and whimsical prints are appreciated by patients.

Dr. Terry Dickinson of Houston, TX offers his patients a unique view of the dental team. He takes photographs at staff retreats and meetings, has them blown up to poster size and positioned on the ceiling above the patient.(Fig. 16-2) This offers the patient an "insiders view" of the team and helps the patient feel more a part of the practice family. This is an excellent way to build additional rapport between the patient and the team and to increase patient awareness of ongoing team continuing education as well. As patients sit in the chair they can look up and see the team smiling back at them! Dr. Dickinson periodically changes these posters, and patients gain an unusual perspective of a cohesive and enlightened group!

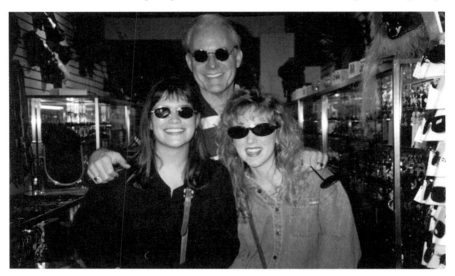

Fig. 16-2 Dr. Terry Dickinson puts light-hearted posters of the team on the treatment room ceiling to relax the patient and to demonstrate a cohesive and educated team. (Courtesy Terry Dickinson, D.D.S., F.A.G.D.)

Dr. Mark Friedman of Encino, CA puts television monitors in treatment rooms to enable patients to view a travelogue that includes aerial views of strikingly beautiful land and sea images. A music soundtrack aids in making this a very soothing, pleasant sensory experience for the patient. With a headset in place, the patient can separate himself or herself from the clinical experience by controlling the sound level of the music to block out equipment sounds.

In another office I visited, the doctor had a neck massage unit available.[3] Dr. Jan Balsiger of Richardson, TX offers this device to patients who are experiencing longer treatments and may find that the massage unit helps them feel more comfortable. Perhaps even more important, however, is the message that it sends to the patient, "You are important and valued. We want to help you feel at ease here."

TEAM INTERACTIONS AND PATIENTS

A most significant element in reducing patient anxiety is the interaction and communication between the patient and the team. When the patient is surrounded by a team who like and respect each other, the patient feels that he or she is in a stable place. If there is any sense of discord among the team members, patient tension can rise.

In the clinical areas a caring touch on the shoulder or arm while preparing the patient for treatment or during treatment can be very settling. (Fig. 16-3) Patients talk about this in focus groups and a caring, gentle touch can be very significant to patients. When it is accompanied by a warm smile and eye contact, it is a significant nonverbal message of, "you're in good hands, we care about you as a person."

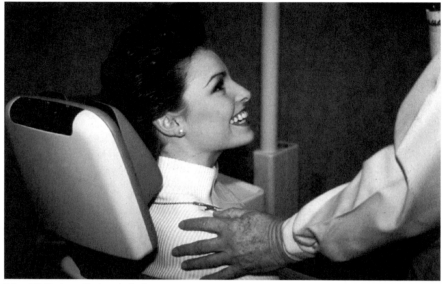

Fig. 16-3 A gentle touch during a treatment can communicate a practitioner's caring and sensitivity towards the patient. (Courtesy Ronald Goldstein. D.D.S.)

The Touch of Human Hands

The touch of human hands

Not vain, unthinking words,

Not that cold charity

Which shuns our misery;

We seek a loyal friend

Who understands,

And the warmth, the pulsing warmth,

Of human hands.

Thomas Curtis Clark

The patient should be left alone as little as possible once in the clinical area. In the ideal situation, the patient would always have a staff member in the room. This is particularly significant with the patient who is experiencing high anxiety. However, the attitude and demeanor of the staff member is important. This needs to be a person who can help to reduce the patient's anxiety through verbal or nonverbal communication.

On conclusion of the treatment or the exam, the patient should be walked to the counter by a team member. If staff members at the front desk are busy assisting other patients, the staff member should remain with this patient until "handed over" to the business staff person. A patient who has a high stress level in the dental office will be reassured by the presence of a caring staff member.

On conclusion of the business transactions, this patient should receive closing comments from the staff member at the front desk indicating appreciation for the patient. If the patient in question is one who is known to have a very high level of fear or anxiety in relation to the dental appointment, this individual will appreciate recognition of accomplishment in completing treatment. One patient in a focus group commented,

> *The whole staff knows I'm terrified to come in for my appointments, but they make me feel so good about it when I'm through. Inevitably, I get a few pats on the back and one of the assistants always gives me a hug. It makes me feel good about coming to the office and proud when I've made it through an appointment. It helps me feel a little less scared about my next appointment.*

PATIENT COMMENTARY ON "WE CATER TO COWARDS"

I see this phrase in promotional pieces, in advertising, and in collateral materials. We have asked fearful patients how they feel about the term, "coward" in relation to their self perceptions and their perceptions of the dental offices that used the term. Interestingly their responses were very similar regardless of demographics. On the whole, patients do not like the term and don't like someone else referring to them as a coward. However, many patients accepted the "title" somewhat begrudgingly. Tom, a patient with a very high anxiety level, expressed it like this,

> *"Yeah, I guess I am a coward, and I admit it. People laugh about being scared of the dentist, but underneath I don't think it's funny. It's very real to me. Some of my friends kid me about being afraid. It's like, because I'm a physically big man, I shouldn't be scared. I think it's similar to some jokes. It's okay for me to joke about being a coward, but I don't really like hearing it from someone else and it's certainly something I'm not proud of."*

A female patient noted,

> *Well, a phrase like that might get my attention in the phone book, but it doesn't mean I'd go. It sounds a little cheesy! I'd rather go to an office that says it offers 'gentle and understanding care'. Since I don't really like to call myself a 'coward' I'd rather not go to an office that calls me one!*

During this discussion, we showed patients display ads from the yellow pages. Those ads that had cartoons, like a cowardly lion, were often perceived to be offices of inferior clinical skills more so than those offices that did not use such cartoon-like devices.

Here's another view of this reality: the truly fearful patient is taking a very brave step in making and keeping the dental appointment. He or she is facing a great fear head on; this is far from cowardly. If a deeply fearful patient says to you, "I'm terrified of being here. I've had some awful experiences in dental offices and I'm a real coward." This is an opportunity to build a very meaningful practitioner-patient relationship. A response like, "I think you're very brave to face what has been so frightening for you—together we can work on making this a more positive experience for you. Tell me about what happened in the past so we can be sure that doesn't happen to you here." This information-seeking conversation can be the foundation for a long-term mutually beneficial patient relationship.

REASSURANCE VIA NONVERBAL COMMUNICATION

Joan was a fearful patient. In our focus group she explained that she had moved and had found a new dentist,

> *I'm terrified of going to the dentist. I told the staff that I was a real chicken and that I needed a lot of 'hand-holding' just to get through a cleaning. The hygienist was gentle, kind, and caring. She told me that the dentist was very understanding and that he'd be gentle too. But he wasn't! He seemed in a hurry and left the room several times to check on another patient.*

*I got the feeling that I was sort of an after-
thought and an inconvenience. I couldn't
talk to him—I guess it didn't matter—I
don't think he would've listened anyway. I
won't go back there. I haven't been to a
dentist in a year and a half.*

Joan added that even after telling the group that,
she felt ashamed and embarrassed about it.

Effective nonverbal communication is exceptionally
important in reducing anxiety for your patients and in
helping you understand your patients. The moment that
you walk into the treatment room, you are speaking
nonverbally, as well as verbally, to the patient. You tell that
patient how you feel about him/her and how you feel
about yourself. Warm and caring body language can go a
long way in helping to reduce stress that patients may feel
about the dental appointment and the treatment.

PATIENT PREFERENCES IN PRACTITIONER NONVERBAL COMMUNICATION

Here are some of the most important elements of
nonverbal communication that patients say can aid in
reducing patient stress:

• Sit at the patient's eye level when in discussion.
Face the patient and allow some space between you.
Ideally, the practitioner is seated at the patient's one
o'clock position. The patient must be able to see you and
gain a comfort level before you initiate any type of exam
or treatment. These moments can be used by you to gain
greater understanding of the patient as well. Do not start
an exam or treatment prior to patient's readiness.

• A most important aspect of body language is
facial expression. Facial expression is not an accurate

indicator of what people think, but rather what they feel. Patients want to see that you can be empathic in addressing patient anxieties and fears. I've been a patient in numerous practices where practitioners exhibit a lack of facial expression and I've presumed that in some cases this represents a goal of communicating objectivity toward the patient. A practitioner's face that is totally nonexpressive can cause patient stress.

Patients don't know how you are feeling about them. They will be less likely to express their real feelings to you if you appear unfeeling toward them. A facial expression that appears at all inflexible or rigid is off-putting to a fearful or anxious patient. Instead, he/she will respond to an expression of kindness, caring, and openness. Most particularly, the fearful patient will seek the practitioner who appears understanding and nonjudgmental.

• When the patient is talking, be aware of your own eye contact. Ensure that you acknowledge the patient's message through an eye pattern that indicates interest and concern. Patients frequently judge how much you are listening by your eye contact. This does not mean that constant eye contact will be appreciated, it may well be interpreted as intrusive and unsettling, like the "staring" game so many children play. Instead most patients will respond to eye contact that is maintained approximately 75% of the time the patient is talking. Patients do understand when you look away to think about what the patient just said or to reflect on the condition or treatment.

• Listen to the patient's vocal tone and timing to gain a perspective on the patient's mood. If you detect anxiety expressed vocally, use a softer, slightly slower vocal pattern than usual to aid in reducing patient anxiety.

• Most importantly, when the patient is talking, make sure that your body orientation, facial expression, words and voice communicate a consistent message.

ALTERNATIVE FORMS OF PAIN MANAGEMENT

Because of the high incidence of patient fear of injections, alternative forms of sedating the patient may be considered. We have discussed the following concepts in focus groups and though there is a low patient awareness of these options, there is high responsiveness to the concepts. However, focus groups are decidedly not held in clinical settings and our participants do not experience these treatments. Therefore, it is important to note that actual applicability and effectiveness is not tested in a scientific manner. Inclusion here is solely to offer patient viewpoints.

We have shown patients promotional materials about electronic anesthesia units.[4] Though there are technical differences among available products and there may be efficiency variations, patients viewed these technologies favorably in relation to the concept of managing pain. Those patients who were most fearful of injections were also most responsive to the concepts. Some of our participants expressed concern about gaining complete blocking of uncomfortable sensations. The patients who had concerns about infection control issues liked the fact that needles were not used and the process was non-invasive. Many patients said they liked the fact that the patient was able to control the amount of signal, and resultant blocking, of the targeted area.

It became clear that use of these new technologies would require excellent communication skills on the part of the practitioners. They would need to be skilled in discussing with the patient the technical aspects of the devices while instilling patient trust and reassurance that their fears would not be realized. Certainly effectiveness of any such technology can be positively affected by the ability of the practitioner to build a strong bond of trust with the patient.

As with so many issues relating to patient trust, when team members can speak from experience about this technology, the patient's likelihood of acceptance and compliance can rise. A team member talking about what to expect and the type of sensations to be experienced also can be very powerful to the patient.

Use of hypnosis also was discussed as an alternative or adjunct to injection. Patients were very receptive to the *concept* of hypnosis. The majority were aware and responsive to the mind-body connect and could understand that it would be possible to use either hypnosis or acupuncture in dental/medical procedures. However, and this is a big however, a significant 50% of the responsive participants changed their minds when the word *hypnosis* was used in conjunction with description of the process. Though this process of deep relaxation has been recognized by the American Dental Association, the American Medical Association, and the American Psychology Association, there is still a significant holdover in thinking from the days of the parlor game hocus-pocus so long associated with it.

In conducting seminars from coast to coast, I invariably meet practitioners who successfully use the principles of hypnosis to aid in reduction of patient pain and anxiety. I find it interesting that many of these doctors also have mentioned the resistance of some patients to the word itself, although they readily accept and value the principles. Most of these same doctors no longer use the term, *hypnosis* for that very reason. It is likely that as society continues to be receptive to the mind-body connect (See chapter 7) we will find hypnosis used with greater frequency in the dental office.

TRUST

Much of this book addresses the issues that can aid in building a trusting patient-practitioner relationship. This is a particularly important matter when it comes to reducing tension and earning patient endorsement. The word "trust" is used frequently by patients in focus groups when discussing their feelings about anxiety and tension in relation to the dental practice. In looking at the definition of the word one can understand the power that it holds for patients. It is derived from a medieval word, "traust" which meant covenant, protection, safety. Today trust signifies "an assured reliance on another person for help and protection in a risky situation."[5] You may not feel that dental treatment is risky, but to the patient it is often considered to be. Trust is powerful. Simply stated, "fear is soluable in trust".[6] Take, for example, how much trust affected this focus group patient.

> *I start getting nervous the day before my appointment. My last dentist didn't let me know what was going to happen. He'd tell me how he wanted me to feel and just go on with it [the treatment]. I lost trust in him. That nervousness carried over to this new dentist. I trust him, but I'm still apprehensive from my past experiences.*

Harold was a highly expressive member of one focus group we conducted. He was a principal of a public high school, stood 6'3" and looked like he could handle anything. It was normal for him to manage challenges and stress every day. But when it came to dental appointments, it was a different matter. Harold related in a focus group his experiences in a military clinic. He said,

> *I had a lot of work done by the dentist over the years I was in the military. But a few years after I got out, I started having*

*problems with that work. There was a lot
of pain and I had to do something about
it, but I couldn't afford a lot. So I found a
'cut-rate' dentist who did 'cut rate' work. I
think the treatments were worse than the
condition. He gave me nothing for pain—
said I was a big guy and I could handle
it. When I finally could afford a good
dentist, I needed everything done over, but
I was terrified of dentists at this point!*

Given Harold's history, I was curious how he
found a dentist he could trust and he related a very
detailed process he went through. He explained that he
was determined not to go through another terrible
experience and that he wasn't going to even make an
appointment with dental office without first "investigating"
the office. He got referrals from friends and family, then he
called each office and asked what the office does for the
fearful patient and what they offered in pain reduction. He
then visited the offices and asked if it was possible to meet
the doctor. He said, "I wanted to find an office that looked
clean, where the staff was kind, and where the doctor
really seemed to care about patients." Once he located
that office, and developed a trusting relationship with the
dentist and staff, he said, "If I lived in another state, I'd still
come here to this doctor. I trust him. He is very sensitive
to my past experiences and he takes his time to make sure
that I'm okay throughout any treatment."

Trust and strong communication skills go hand in
hand. We hear this from patients consistently. When
patients talk about the dental teams they trust, they
typically tie this in with the way that the doctor and all
team members interact with the patient.

Control as a Matter of Trust

There is another identifying factor that is frequently seen in the trusting relationship between patient and practitioner, and that is control. Numerous patients in our focus groups have cited the importance of patient control, although most often they don't use the word, "control." Lynn, a patient with a very high fear level due to experiences as a child noted,

> *I get the most nervous when I feel like the dentist isn't paying attention or doesn't care about how I'm feeling. I've tried to give him nonverbal clues during treatment. Since I can't talk because of all the 'stuff' in my mouth, I try to communicate with my eyes that I'm getting nervous or feeling pain, but he doesn't respond. What I'd like is if we could have a signal—I could raise my hand and he'd stop—then I could catch my breath then we could go on. But I feel dumb suggesting this.*

Lynn was really addressing the issue of some patient control during the treatment.

Patients sincerely value team members who address this situation openly. Similar to your initiating a discussion on infection control in your office, patients appreciate it when *you* raise the subject of patient control. Before starting a procedure, offer a couple of signals that patients can use to talk to the doctor or to catch their breath. This indicates that you recognize that the patient may have this need and that it is permissible to do so. You're offering valuable information to the patient in the manner of a caring practitioner.

Nathan Friedman, DDS, Clinical Professor and Founder of the Department of Behavioral Dentistry at University of Southern California School of Dentistry in Los

Angeles, CA affirms how important effective communication is in helping the fearful patient. Dr. Friedman has developed the Iatrosedative Process wherein the practitioner, through a very specific dialogue with fearful patients, is able to eliminate patient fear or markedly reduce the fear. This minimizes the anxiety to a level that allows the patient to face the dental experience with feelings of security. Through a process of getting and giving information, the practitioner is able to help the patient reach a place where treatment is possible. One element of this process relates to offering the patient some type of control so that the treatment will be stopped if the patient feels threatened. [7]

Focus group participants have communicated that trust of the practitioner increases as the doctor talks to them, explains what is going to happen prior to proceeding, and offers the patient some form of control during the proceedings. Dr. Friedman's extensive research on managing the dental experience for the fearful patient validates the importance of effective communication with the fearful patient. He states "in order to help people with their fears, you have to know what they are fearful of and how they reached that point. Then you must promise to protect the patient from what caused the fear and ensure that it won't happen again." He suggests that the dentist must be both a "danger control authority" and a "protective authority" for the patient. In an interview with Dr. Friedman, he offered these suggestions to the practitioner:[8]

• Recognize the verbal and nonverbal cues from patients that may indicate you are about to treat a fearful patient. These cues may range from an outright statement like, "I'm terrified of coming to the dentist" to body language typical of anxiety or nervousness.

• Initiate dialogue that will encourage the patient to express and acknowledge concerns and problems.

Verbalize empathy and understanding with statements like, "I understand that this must be difficult for you. Let's look at this first [before starting treatment] because we *can* do something about it."

- Ask "what" and "tell me" questions that get the patient talking like, "Can you tell me what happened?", "What is it that you are afraid of?"

- Offer protective assurance that the things that happened to the patient before are not going to happen in this relationship and that you will work together to ensure this. A statement like, "We will work together so that what happened before is not going to happen between you and me."

- Inform the patient of what to expect in terms of pressure, noise, and all things that will happen to him/her during the treatment. If the practitioner makes a statement like, "I'm going to share my control and my knowledge and I'm not going to do anything without your knowing what I'm about to do," the patient feels more in control and part of the process.

Dr. Friedman notes that "when patients know exactly what will be taking place, patient anxiety is lessened." This does not imply that the practitioner explain each clinical step, rather prepare the patient by telling the patient what to expect before it occurs. This approach can be used by any team member who communicates face to face with the patient. Hygienists can use the same concepts in easing patient anxiety and increasing patient compliance. A practitioner benefit of implementing these steps is the opportunity to treat a patient who is now more relaxed and easier to work with.

The focus group patients we have interviewed who are highly fearful have verbalized a dread of the dental appointment, in large part due to past experiences. Some of these patients admitted having "missed" appointments because of overwhelming fears. These same patients have affirmed the validity of the concepts addressed by Dr. Friedman above. Had these same patients experienced the kind of protective promise from the practitioner that is described above, certainly they would be less fearful. There is no doubt that they would also be loyal and long term patients of the practice. The kind of patient bond that grows from this relationship can weather challenging outside influences and will certainly result in loyalty and enthusiastic referrals.

On a personal note, I have a history of very high fear of the dental experience. That fear has dissipated through being a patient of many practitioners who recognize the power of communicating care and compassion for the patient both verbally and nonverbally. I only wish that, as a child, I'd had the good fortune of being a patient of a practitioner who practiced Dr. Friedman's philosophy. I wish for all fearful patients that they find this caring environment and team in your office.

TOP TIPS:

1. Most meaningful to patients is a genuinely caring practitioner, one who communicates well and listens actively to patients.
2. Offer the patient preparatory information about the procedure prior to starting it and solicit questions from patients. Actively listen and respond to patient concerns by offering information that will aid in reducing anxiety.
3. Encourage the patient to verbalize his/her feelings about dental treatment and/or dental history.
4. Learn to give a painless injection. Not only will patients appreciate this, they will tell others about it.

5. Offer patient distractions. Patients appreciate headsets to aid in tension reduction. These can be an inexpensive "high tech" patient distraction in each treatment room.

6. Be aware of body language, both yours and the patient's.

7. Create an environment that is soothing and comfortable.

8. Ask the patient, "What else can we do to help you feel more comfortable?"

REFERENCES

[1] Nathan Friedman, DDS, "Fear Reduction with the Iatrosedative Process," *Journal of the California Dental Association*, March, 1993.

[2] Beck, A.T. *Anxiety Disorders and Phobias: A Cognitive Perspective*, Basic Books, New York, NY, 1985.

[3] This is a "shiatsu" style electric massager that is widely available at retail outlets for public purchase.

[4] The two devices for which promotional materials were shown in focus groups were the Cedeta Mk2 Electronic Anesthesia unit and the 3-M Electronic Anesthesia unit. Additional information on these devices may be obtained by contacting Cedeta Dental International, Inc., Westport, CT, (800) 350-8232 and 3-M, Minneapolis, MN, (800) 362-3455.

[5] Nathan Friedman, DDS, "Fear Reduction with the Iatrosedative Process," *Journal of the California Dental Association,* March, 1993.

[6] Nathan Friedman, DDS, "Fear Reduction with the Iatrosedative Process," *Journal of the California Dental Association,* March, 1993.

[7] Nathan Friedman, DDS, "Fear Reduction with the Iatrosedative Process," *Journal of the California Dental Association,* March, 1993.

[8] Information related to the Iatrosedative Process was taken from a phone interview conducted with Nathan Friedman, DDS, Clinical Professor and Founder of the Department of Behavioral Dentistry at University of Southern California School of Dentistry in Los Angeles by Suzanne Boswell on September 21, 1996.

17

The Patient's View of the Service-Oriented Practice

"Service is just a day-in, day-out, ongoing, never-ending, unremitting, persevering, compassionate type of activity."

—LEON GORMAN, OF L.L. BEAN

Prior to being a Mystery Patient, I was a Mystery Guest for hotels. I stayed at properties undercover and rated the facility as to quality, service, impression management, self presentation of staff, etc. I continue to work with the hospitality industry on these same issues and find many similarities in comparing the challenges of the hospitality industry to the challenges of the dental profession. Two obvious and significant similarities are the importance of service and guest/patient loyalty.

THE LITTLE THINGS MAKE THE BIGGEST DIFFERENCE

As in dentistry, the smallest things can make the biggest differences in perceptions of service for hotels. This was beautifully illustrated in a conversation I had with a couple of hotel valets. I'd visited a five-star plus facility that repeatedly traded places for #1 or #2 hotel in the country. Their international and celebrity clientele demanded the very best and they provided it. I asked one valet, "So are you #1 or #2 this year?" He responded, "Oh we lost #1 slot and we're #2 this year." "So what happened that you dropped a slot?" I asked. "Well we had a 'spotter' stay undercover to rate the hotel. We were tied for the #1 spot nationally until he came out to get his car. He was given change in dirty, wrinkled, torn dollar bills. That's when we became #2." The second valet laughed as he pulled his wallet from his pocket and fanned out the dollars. "So that's why I've been getting only brand new, crisp dollar bills in the morning when I go in to get my change for guests!" It was a dramatic story that shows just how much the little things can make a difference.

GETTING RID OF THE DIRTY DOLLAR BILLS

Following this incident, I stayed at a Ritz Carlton and was curious how widespread this issue was. Of course Ritz Carlton is known for superb service in all areas so on departure from the hotel, I said to the valet, "Say I'm just curious, can I see the change you give to guests?" With some degree of amusement, he pulled out his wallet, and yes, he had all clean, crisp dollar bills!

What does this have to do with dentistry? It's simple. For the hotels that strive to maintain top levels of service, that strive to earn and maintain guest loyalty, they do everything they can to differentiate themselves from others. They pay attention to the smallest details, even the condition of the dollar bills that are given to departing guests. That same challenge holds true for dentistry. If you want to differentiate yourself, if you want to stand out as superior, you've got to attend to the small details. You've got to get rid of the dirty dollar bills! And you've got to have departing patients thinking, "Wow! This office is really special!" When that occurs the experience is burned into the patient's brain. If patients leave your practice for a managed care plan or for another office on their lists, they'll make comparisons and you want the comparisons to be dramatic. You want the void between your office and the patient's next office to be so great that they want to return to your practice, where they received exceptional service. That's your challenge, and in that challenge are innumerable opportunities to provide your patients with remarkable "Wows".

OFFERING DISTINCTIVE DENTISTRY FOR THE DISCERNING PATIENT

Many offices today seek to develop an office that meets the needs and wants of the discerning patient. What's happening in dentistry is very similar to the evolution that's been occurring in the retail industry. Stores like Nordstrom's and Neiman Marcus have risen to the top due, in large part, to spectacular service. There is also an increase in discount stores. WalMart is a significant retail force and mainstay in cities and small towns across the country. You can see the growing divide in the middle.

There is a proliferation of dental plans today that offer patients low fees with a mixed range of services and quality. Although there is a growing market for these practices, there is also a growing market for the practice that offers cutting edge treatments and exceptional service.

Some of these offices are being referred to as "boutique dental practices." I have mixed feelings about use of this term in patient communication. My mixed reactions are to the term, not the concept. I believe that the highly individualized practices offering specialized treatment are a real and significant wave of the future. However, I question applying the term, "boutique" to it. A boutique is a small shop that usually offers specialized and unique service. So far so good. However, it is most often associated with women's apparel or accessories. Women may well respond to the term, and a large percentage of your client base is women. However, this is *not* a term that most men will relate to.

My background includes 13 years in the menswear business, a significant portion of which was spent as a designer and consumer relations manager for an international menswear firm. An important part of my work required understanding the attitudes and decision-making processes of male customers. What I'm about to say is based on experience and access to extensive research by national advertising and marketing firms.

Most men currently will not respond to this type of terminology. Try suggesting to some of your male business colleagues that they consider "going to a *boutique* practice for some *cosmetic* treatment." Put these two terms together and you're dead in the water with a high percentage of men. The point is this, if you're marketing this type of service, use the concept, not the term when talking with patients.

MOMENTS OF TRUTH

Webster defines service as "an act of helpful activity." That's a pretty broad statement with which I'm sure you'd agree. Nearly every interaction with a patient could be said to be a service according to this definition, or it would be if the team member recognized the opportunities that exist in the interaction. Bearing this in mind, everything you do with or for a patient is a part of your service to that patient.

Every point of contact with a patient offers opportunities to the practice and moments of truth for the patient. That means the way the phone is answered, how questions are answered, the attentive body language while in conversation with a patient, your awareness of patient confidentiality issues, your concern to patient sensitivities, how you say good-bye to a patient. All of these "speak" to the patient about your service attitude, and each of these interactions actually offers you the opportunities to cement relationships.

Early in this book we addressed the concept of three phases of patient perceptions, all three phases offer opportune "moments of truth" for the patient: Pre-Appointment, Appointment and Post-Appointment. Each phase must be consciously managed in order to anticipate patient needs and to provide *WOW* moments of truth for the patient.

The following points of contact very commonly hold powerful moments of truth for patients and must be carefully managed by all involved:

- The first phone call
- First visit to the office
- Prompt responses to inquiries and patient requests
- Appearance of anything sent through the mail to patients
- Management of patient complaints

- Patient requests that demand some degree of flexibility by the office
- Emergency treatment situations
- Management of patient fear or pain
- Ability to be empathetic during challenges for the patient
- Attentiveness to patient during conversation
- Manner of dismissing the patient at the close of the appointment
- Follow up with patients after difficult or painful treatment

There are wonderful seeds for a brainstorming staff session in the items above. Investigate as a group the many ways that you can take each item on the list and fine tune the service provided to patients. How can you develop little jewel-like "moments of truth" for your patients in each point of contact? Every staff member can have an impact on the patient. *Create* your opportunities to make *WOW* moments for your patients, don't expect them to just happen!

THE IMPORTANCE OF GIVING FAIR WARNING

If you are making changes or anticipate "glitches" that could result in raising patient blood pressure, it is advisable to prepare patients for what to expect. Patients don't like surprises—at least not those of the unpleasant sort. When patients know what to expect, they are more likely to prepare for it and, hopefully adjust.

An Illinois dentist sent me the following letter that he'd received from his paperboy. It is a superb example of the paperboy preparing his customers for an upcoming temporary change. This young man was aware that by communicating openly about this from the beginning, he'd be less likely to deal with complaint calls. In addition, he was paving the way for his young protege!

To my customers,

This is your paper boy, Jake Harvidson. The papers will be delivered a little late starting Wednesday because I am on the track team at Shepherd Junior High School. You will have a different paper boy on the days that I have track meets. Your papers will be delivered between 5 and 7 p.m. on the days I have practice. On Tuesdays your papers will be delivered at the regular time because we have no practices on Tuesdays. Your paper boy, when I have meets, is only 7 years old so just try to work with him.

Sincerely,

Jake Harvidson

If you have temporary changes that may affect your patients, give them fair warning. They'll find you more service-minded and sensitive to patient concerns.

A Confidence-Shaking Moment of Truth

I had an unforgettable experience as a patient in the office of a dentist who was known for having very high rates of patient retention and treatment acceptance. I had heard a great deal about this doctor. I'd heard about the professionalism of his team, the quality of his clinical skills and the attention to detail provided in his new patient process. I wanted to experience it myself, so I made an appointment as a new patient in his office.

On arrival at the office I realized this was not the ordinary day; the tension was so thick among the team members that I could feel it as I approached the counter. It was evidenced in the way team members spoke and interacted with each other. It felt a little like being around a married couple who were trying to hide that they'd just had a fight! You know it, you can see it, you can feel it, even though they're doing a valiant job of trying to hide it. It became clear very quickly that an emergency patient had just left the office. I overheard team members discussing that a hygienist and an assistant were both out sick that day, and that the schedule was booked full. The office was going to have a real challenge throughout this entire day. By the time I got into the treatment room my appointment was already starting 25 minutes late.

This doctor about whom I'd heard so many wonderful things, who was supposed to be so friendly and warm, came across as tense and focused on data. Following the clinical exam he invited me to join him in the consultation room to discuss proposed treatment. This was the part of the exam that I had heard that he handled so beautifully. He directed his attention to my file and the front desk. He positioned himself where he could see the front desk through the consultation room door.

He sat on the front half of his chair and he was practically hyperventilating as he spoke. Throughout the consult his eyes darted from me, to the file, to the door. I had a hard time concentrating on what he was saying because of his obvious distraction from the moment. On conclusion he mumbled a "pleased to meet you", gave me a half-hearted handshake as he checked his watch and slipped out of the room. At the front desk my paperwork was processed in an efficient, though rushed manner. I felt like the entire team was racing through the steps without any heart in it.

THE PATIENT'S WINDOW OF TIME

This was truly a moment of truth for me. Here was an office known for high clinical skills and service for whom the morning had definitely *not* started off right. Yet, that was my reality. What if I had been a "real" patient and had been referred to the office by a friend or by another dentist? I'd have entered the practice with high expectations and would have left wondering about the judgment of my referral source! It was a *WHOA!* experience not a *WOW!* experience.

Patients and dental teams have very different views of the office. The dental team may view the office in a much larger "window of time" than that of the patient. The patient is only able to view the office from the brief interactions or appointments experienced. That is the patient's reality of what your office is like. But the dental team may view their performance over the span of a day, or a week, a month or even a year. So the patient's view is vastly skewed from the view of the dental practice. It's very difficult, if not impossible, for any member of the team to be aware of what the patient's view really is. There's just too much going on within the practice environment to separate the experiences of one person.

WHATEVER IT TAKES—MMFI

A valued patient should *never* leave your office feeling unimportant or ignored. Whatever it takes for the team to do so, ensure that patients feel valued and important. An acronym used often by service-oriented businesses today is MMFI, which stands for Make Me Feel

Important. This is what patients will respond to—help them feel important in your office. When patients leave your practice with this feeling, they are far more likely to refer you to others and to remain a part of your practice family. However, the message of patient importance must come from the heart or it means nothing. Worse, offering platitudes that supposedly represent service attitude can backfire and work against you.

Three Levels of Patient Friendly Service

There are three levels of service that fall in the patient-friendly category. They are listed here in order of positive impact on the patient and one level builds on the previous level. Level III is the most highly evolved and includes all elements of levels I and II:

I. Meeting Patient Basic Needs and Expectations

II. Anticipating Patient Needs

III. Offering Patients the Unexpected WOWS

Each of these levels is defined below and accompanied by patient comments that relate to it. The concepts listed are just a few that are possible to move the practice to each consecutive level. However, there are many, many more that you and your team can develop.

Carpe Diem. I suggest that the following sections be used as a basis for a staff meeting wherein you determine the service levels within your own practice and enumerate the steps you can take to move to the next level.

I. MEETING PATIENT BASIC NEEDS AND EXPECTATIONS

At this level, patients find congruence among the three phases of the patient process: Pre-Appointment, Appointment, and Post Appointment. Typically the practice has communicated well on the phone, and patient questions are answered competently. The patient experiences a smoothly flowing appointment with no untoward surprises. They get what they expected and are not let down. However, there is nothing stellar that occurs. The patient feels good about the experience and will return, but may not be as likely to refer others, as the patients that experience levels II and III.

• **Appointments run on schedule:** If patients consistently must wait more than 15 minutes it will have an impact on perceptions of your service attitude. Patients have said that they would be able to accept this situation more readily if the team members would be open about it. If it's going to be more than 15 minutes for the patient to wait, can you notify the patient in a pleasant manner when the patent arrives? Some patients have said, "If they're really running late, could the office just call and let me know? If they're running 45 minutes behind, then I won't break my neck getting there for an earlier time." One man noted, "I was racing to my appointment and got a ticket that cost me $210 dollars. Then, when I got to the office, I ended up waiting an hour. I was fuming by the time I sat in the chair, and the doctor really heard about it!"

• **Team has finely-tuned communication skills:** This comes as no surprise but it is becoming of increasing importance as patients become more critical. An office that cuts the amount of communication time with patients will be perceived to offer inferior service and many patients associate that with clinical skills as well. It is here where the team must be extremely conscious of what they do and say with the patient during appointment time. Patients have said, "He really listened to me!", "I felt important because of the questions they asked me". "She wasn't running from office to office, but sat down and really talked with me."

Other patient comments that relate to this level include:

- "As long as the doctor is nice and does an adequate job, I'm fine. Plus I like to get free stuff." [Toothbrush, ad specialties, etc.]
- "Doctor's caring attitude, I don't have to wait a long time."
- "They have a nice waiting room and good magazines. They have coffee for patients."
- "I like the staff, they're friendly and helpful when I make an appointment."

II. ANTICIPATING NEEDS

The level above is acceptable for a large percentage of patients, but it doesn't really separate you from other offices as much as levels II or III do. It is in level II where the team starts to go beyond what is expected. The team anticipates patient needs that the patient may not have even expressed. When those needs are met, the patient finds it exceptionally caring. This can often require a deep sensitivity to patients.

When it comes to anticipating needs, it means being empathetic. If it appears that the patient might be cold, before the patient asks for a blanket, ask the patient if he/she might like one. Help the patient with it. If the music is loud and the patient seems not to be able to hear you, indicate you'll lower the sound so it's easier to communicate. There are so many ways that one can anticipate needs of the patient, but it means extending outside yourself and into your patient's moment. Try to experience what the patient is experiencing and finding a solution before the patient might even have thought about it. This is exceptionally meaningful for patients.

The areas below address issues patients bring up in focus groups that also fall in this category.

• **Appointment availability:** The practice is "accessible" to patients within a reasonable time frame and hours are varied. Patients find it "unfriendly" if a practice is only open Monday to Thursday from 7 to 4. The point patients make is, "We want to get an appointment within a three-week time frame maximum. We want the office to be open some nights after 5 p.m. and on Saturdays." The office that offers varied hours is perceived as anticipating patient needs and is as a result more accommodating.

• **The team establishes positive feedback loops:** They ensure patient comprehension and indicate an interest in the patient via asking the right questions and listening actively. This is truly rare today. If you develop this skill, you will go a long way in increasing patient retention, treatment acceptance, and referrals. Questions like, "Tell me how you feel about—(whatever is the subject of discussion)" will aid in communicating sincere interest in the patient.

• **The office is "up-to-date" in continuing education and technology:** Up-to-date is a term consistently used by patients in focus groups. They want to know that the team, particularly the dentist(s), are staying current on clinical issues, infection control, and technology. This may be reality in your office, but it's crucial that you let your patients know, and that may be via your answering machine, or on hold tape, newsletter, office discussion, etc.

• **Strong emphasis on patient education:** When we ask patients to describe the "ideal dentist" they typically use the word "teacher", and that holds true for all members of the dental team. Teaching the patient is one of the ways that the patient perceives value. Make sure that patients leave your office understanding more about their oral health and oral hygiene than when they entered.

• **Rapid emergency contact and response:** This type office is highly accessible to patients, in many cases making the doctor's home phone number available for emergencies. The office responds rapidly to patient calls. How you handle patient emergencies will have an enormous impact on your patient retention and referral rates. Here is where you truly can earn a reputation for being service minded for patients. In numerous focus groups we have heard patients offer rave reviews of their dental offices because of the service they were provided in an emergency. A patient who has experienced attentive service in this situation typically will not forget this. Here is where a strong bond of relationship can be forged that won't be broken.

• **The team is cohesive:** Patients often tie the concept of a cohesive team with that of service. When patients view team members communicating seamlessly with each other there is a perception that the office is operating in an efficient and effective manner. Although this may not be the case, much of the time it is a reality. Patients also remark consistently about the importance to them of staff continuity and what it means to them. When the team members know the patient, they feel more important and more a part of the practice family.

• **Complaints are handled well:** How the office handles a problem or a complaint is a major predictor of how satisfied and how long a patient will remain with the practice. Problems arise. You'll always have them. However, they might also be looked upon as opportunities to build stronger bonds with patients. Frequently the patient who experiences a problem and finds it handled well by the team, becomes a more loyal patient than if he had not experienced the problem in the first place.

III. OFFERING THE UNEXPECTED: WOW SERVICE

It's here where the practice self-actualizes and reaches the highest levels of service for the patient. There is a focus on the patient and the team thinks more about the patient needs than their own needs. However, they go beyond level II in this area. They now offer unique and special benefits that aid in helping the patient feel comfortable in the office and increase the patient awareness of being special and valued to the practice.

Here are some comments we've heard in patient focus groups that relate to this level:

• "I couldn't believe it, the doctor actually came out to the reception area to greet me. It was my first time in the office and I've *never* had a dentist or physician do that. It blew me away!"

• "My car had broken down and I couldn't get to the appointment. I was floored, the office sent one of the staff members to pick me up and drive me home. I thought that was remarkable!"

• "Talk about service, I was in the office for an all-morning treatment and had to rush to a business appointment in the afternoon. When the treatment was over, the assistant gave me a warm facecloth that smelled of lemon. Then they had a fruit plate delivered from a restaurant nearby for me so I could go straight to my business appointment. That's service! I told the clients I was meeting and they'd never heard anything like it! That made me feel really good."

- "There's always something great going in my office. Last visit I was there around Mother's Day and they had long stemmed roses on the counter. At the end of the appointments, they gave one to every patient—including the men!"

- "I stop by my dentist's office about once a week on the way to work. They always have unusual coffees brewing and the office manager brings freshly baked muffins from a bakery every morning. It's okay with them—I drop in; they have paper cups for coffee "on the go" and I grab a muffin. They're great!"

- "I had an appointment on my birthday and the whole team came into the treatment room and sang happy birthday to me and gave me a birthday favor and funny paper hat. I hadn't even said anything about it being my birthday. I went back to the office and kept the hat on my desk all day!"

- "The doctor not only called me the night of my surgery, but he called my home every day after until I could report that I was feeling back to normal. I really felt that he cared for me. I thought that was a rare thing to do and I've never had another doctor do this. I trust him tremendously, and I've told a lot of other people about this."

- "The office sent me a gift certificate to a great restaurant in town because I'd referred two patients to the office. They didn't need to do that, but I really appreciated it and we had a great time there. It's a place I couldn't have afforded to go on my own!"

It's being different that raises you to this level. It's a matter of going beyond the extra mile into the exceptional. These are truly *WOW* experiences. It's at this level that you are likely to increase referrals from proud patients! The concepts above are examples only, what are the ways that you can create wonderful experiences for your patients?

IMPORTANCE OF PATIENT EDUCATION

This topic is especially important in relation to perceptions of service today and it offers special opportunities in the dental practice. The practice that actively educates the patient not only is perceived to be service-oriented, but there is an additional benefit to both patient and practitioner. As the patient becomes more educated, the dental IQ rises. When this occurs and the patient has increased appreciation for and value of dentistry, the likelihood is that treatment acceptance and referrals will increase as well. It's a win-win investment, and that's exactly what it is, an investment. For it may take some time and some effort, but this typically pays off in the long run in more satisfied patients.

Here are some of the ways that patients in focus groups have indicated responsiveness to patient education:

• If you have the patient watch a video or read a pamphlet regarding a proposed treatment, give the patient a pad and pen first. Ask the patient to write down questions so that you can make sure that you don't miss answering any of them. This is also helpful relating to informed consent (see chapter 8).

• Patients like the laminated clipboards with illustrations that can be annotated.[1] When you use these to illustrate a condition or treatment, the patient perceives that you care. You are taking the time and effort to provide information to the patient and you are perceived more positively. Also, the patient perceives that you value the patient more.

• Use of models or books in demonstrating or illustrating conditions or treatments. Any time you use a visual to educate the patient you are perceived positively by the patient.

• If you take a patient into a consult room and conduct a "show and tell" with slides or x rays this is impressive and aids in building trust.[2]

• Intraoral camera: I have mentioned in several other areas in this book the power of this educational tool and patient perceptions. Acceptance crosses all demographics and skilled use of this tool will position you well in relation to patient education and service.

MARKETING AND SERVICE: HOW DO THEY RELATE?

Where does marketing end and service begin? Or, can these concepts be reversed? In dentistry, I propose that these concepts are inextricably entwined. To patients, excellent service is the best possible marketing that you can do. (Fig. 17-1) For the most part it is low cost and has the biggest impact on patient retention, treatment acceptance, and referrals. We know this from feedback in our focus groups.

However, it's exceedingly important that the practice not confuse these two concepts, though they are related. A practice can put so much meaning and money into marketing that service suffers. Be sure that you are able to deliver what you promise! If you talk "quality service" in your collateral materials or in your marketing efforts, you better be able to live up to your words, or patients will be let down. Incongruence can lead to

---

OUR PROMISE

Our promise to you, our patient, is that you will always be treated as if you were the most important person in the world to us - OUR FRIEND.

- *To be kind, gentle and caring at all times.*
- *To keep our time appointment agreement as a sign of our respect.*
- *To always discuss fees, expectations, schedules and issues as often and in as much detail as **you** wish.*
- *To become aware and always mindful of your overall and long term vision of your dental health and appearance.*
- *To make suggestions and recommendations from time to time to aid you in achieving your dental health goals.*

Steve Carstensen, D.D.S.
General and Restorative Dentistry

Fig. 17-1 This simple card says the dental team is aware and sensitive to the patients' major concerns. (Courtesy Steve Carstensen, D.D.S.)

weakened trust and that is something no practice can afford. Efforts of marketing become wheelspin when the practice does not meet, anticipate, or exceed the patient's expectations

HOW'RE WE DOIN?

Past Mayor of New York City, Ed Koch, had a line he frequently used that won him favor by the public. With a lot of style and enthusiasm he'd call out to crowds, "How am I doin'?" He was asking for feedback from his constituents and these New Yorkers were well known for telling him! By making this statement to voters, he was saying, "Your opinions are important. I care what you think." Of course, the bottom line was what he did with that information.

The same concept can be taken into the dental office to understand patients better and increase levels of service. Retailers and hoteliers have successfully employed this type of feedback for years. These are businesses that can only survive on the loyalty of their customers and guests. There is much to be learned from this!

I am a big proponent of the patient survey. Obviously, I believe that objective input is crucial; I initiated the dental patient focus group concept because I wanted to get real-world information from patients to take to dental teams. I know how powerful this information can be and how surprising the outcomes can be also! My company conducts extensive, in-depth patient surveys for clients. The questions are customized for the specific needs of the practice and, because they are processed totally by us, we gain more objective responses from patients than if they responded directly to the dental practice. Other groups offer survey compilation as well. [3]

You can also create your own survey either to be given at patient point of departure or to be mailed. Here's a way you can conduct a survey that is very low cost and can be implemented in the office with a high rate of patient response. This concept is not a new one, but I believe it has been fine tuned most effectively in the hospitality industry. If you want to see the hotel survey that I've found to be the most "guest-friendly" take a look at Hilton's "15-second Quality Quiz" available in their lobbies. Here's how to implement this concept in an efficient and cost effective manner:

1. Create a brief survey, no more than six questions and include a place for comments at the bottom. Print it on a small sheet of paper (8.5" x 5.5" or smaller). Avoid "yes/no" questions and instead ask questions that can be checked off according to a scale of agreement. Ask

questions that relate directly to your practice or address concerns you have about patient preferences or feelings. The survey can be created and duplicated in house. Don't spend a lot of money on production, because you may find it beneficial to update it or change the survey quarterly.

2. Get a box with an insertion slot on the top and a highly visible padlock on it. The lock is significant, be sure it is visible to patients and looks like it cannot be easily opened. A combination style padlock is effective for this purpose.

3. When a patient approaches the counter, and before the statement is prepared, hand the patient one of the survey forms and say, "We want to be sure that we continue to meet and exceed the needs of our patients, so we're conducting a brief survey and would truly value your feedback and suggestions. While I'm preparing your paperwork, would you take just a few moments to check off these questions? If you have any comments that you think we should know about your treatment today, please write those in. Please don't sign the survey! When you're through slip it in the locked box over there. We open the box and compile the responses _____(whatever frequency you expect to do this, once a week, twice a month). By the time you're through I'll have your statement ready for you!"

4. You are telling the patient:
• We care about you as a patient and want to be responsive to your needs.
• You will remain anonymous.
• This won't take any more time than you're already going to be here while I prepare your paperwork.

When this is handled in a caring manner with a warm vocal tone and a sincere expression, you will find a very high rate of response. It is crucial that patients put the form in the box themselves and that they know they will remain anonymous and that the feedback is sincerely appreciated by the office. If you ask the patient to mail the form back to you, even if you give a stamped, self-addressed envelope, you can bet that your response rate will be much lower.

Reviewing the compiled responses is an important process for the entire team. This can form the basis for a highly productive staff meeting. Identify the weak areas of service and consider this an opportunity to get rid of the dirty dollar bills so you may fine tune the image of your practice in your community.

SAMPLE SURVEY QUESTIONS

The ideal survey is customized to the needs and interests of both the patients and the practice. Offices that create their own surveys should change them every three to six months, or even annually, as the practice evolves. I know that many offices can use a jumpstart in developing an in-house survey, so here are some very basic, starting-point questions to consider in developing your own. These questions would offer responses in a scale of agreement ranging from strongly agree to strongly disagree.

1. Staff was friendly on the phone.
2. Appointment time was convenient.
3. Reception area is comfortable and well-maintained.
4. Appointment started on time.
5. Hygienist was gentle and caring.
6. Assistant was accommodating and helpful.
7. Dentist was caring and communicated well.

8. Billing was explained well and efficiently handled.

These statements are extremely general and should be rephrased for your office. They are included here as a *starting point only*. Ideally, each question would address only one concept. For example, you might rephrase question number three to address either *comfortable* or *well-maintained*. After all, a patient might think the reception area was comfortable but not well-maintained, and therefore have a difficult time accurately answering the question. Determine what criteria *you* think are most important in *your* office and phrase your questions accordingly. The shorter the survey is, the better. The fewer questions, the higher the rate of responses you'll get. At the bottom of your survey include an area for additional comments. These comments can often be the most valuable information gathered from a survey.

COMMUNICATION OF PATIENT APPRECIATION

A most important element of service is the skill with which you communicate to the patient your appreciation of the patient and the value of the patient to the practice. This is crucial today. If your patient doesn't know this, you have a weak relationship that can result in patient grazing from the practice. If you are sincere in communicating patient appreciation, the likelihood of patient perceptions of service will rise. When it comes to this issue, however, the verbalization of appreciation must be genuine, it must be sincere. Patients must see it, hear it, feel it, in order to know it and believe it. Service is most appreciated when it comes from the heart, not when it is practiced and perceived as unfeeling.

For the bottom line here is, patients don't care how much you know until they know how much you care! Help make your patients feel valued and important in your practice through finely tuned service.

TOP TIPS:

1. When with the patient, be in the moment!

2. Address the patient by the patient's preferred name.

3. Anticipate the needs of the patient as much as possible; this communicates that you are empathic and thinking of the patient more than yourself.

4. Offer the patient options whenever possible. Patients like this and perceive the practice to be service-oriented.

5. Avoid talking "office policy" to the patient. It makes you sound inflexible and not patient-friendly.

6. Choose positive words to address challenging issues, instead of negative words. Patients want to know that you see the glass as "half full" instead of "half empty."

7. Show the patient that you try to find answers to challenges as a team. If you don't have the answer, ask a team member to assist you in finding a patient-friendly solution to a problem. Patents like to see more than one person working on their behalf!

8. Make sure that the front line people are empowered to handle problems, or don't put them on the front line! This is a major irritation for patients, and unfortunately a common one!

REFERENCES

[1] Clipboards like this are available from numerous companies like Smart Practice in Phoenix, AZ.

[2] Not all patients will respond to movement to another room. Much depends on the demographic. See chapters 12 and 19.

[3] The ADA offers a survey service called ADA-Checkup. Information may be obtained by contacting, (800) 849-0869. Also, the ADA offers a booklet, *Measuring Patient Satisfaction in the Dental Practice* (item M027). This booklet can be helpful in determining the direction of questions to ask and includes a sample survey. In addition, Hancock Management Services (800-214-7576) offers a unique service called "The Boxx" wherein they structure and manage patient, in-house surveys.

18

The Significance of Team to the Patient

"They said you have to use your first-best player, but I found out you win with the five that fit together best."

— RED AUERBACH, COACH, BOSTON CELTICS

W e were opening the meeting of a new focus group. As I often do, I posed the first question to the entire group, "Tell me one thing that you really like about your dentist and one thing that you don't like." Brian offered a response that is not an uncommon one in these groups. Although I asked specifically about "the dentist", Brian responded, "What I really like is, the staff." He described the dental team and his feelings of comfort in the office because of the highly developed interpersonal skills of the dental office group.

What was interesting, was that although I'd asked about the *dentist*, his response was about what he liked in the *team*. This is significant, though not unusual. An office that has done an excellent job of pulling itself together as a cohesive, well-functioning team has accomplished a great deal, not only for the practice itself, but also for the patients. I can say without a doubt, that the most powerful "marketing tool" a practice can have is an upbeat, well-functioning team especially when the members of the group have long tenure with the practice.

TEAM VS. STAFF

Let's first investigate what a "team" really is. A team can be defined as a "group of people working together towards a common purpose or goal."[1] This commonly accepted definition of team does not specify any levels of responsibility or hierarchy within the group. One can infer that all members working in the dental office are a part of the team, including the dentists, hygienists, clinical and business staff members. This is an extremely important point, because it signifies the responsibility and importance of every single member of the group to aid in reaching goals. Consider this: TEAM is the acronym for: Together Everybody Achieves More!

When patients remark, "The reason I like my dentist's office is because it feels like family," it's actually a statement that reflects on every single member of the team. We certainly hope that any patient making that statement is reminded of a healthy, functioning family, not a dysfunctional one!

Patients often view team compatibility as a barometer of how satisfied they will be with the practice. Obviously, this has nothing to do with the clinical skills of the practitioners, but until given a history with the practice, patients have nothing else to go on. Patients do not know how to judge the clinical so they use other criteria.

In continuing education programs and in books and articles, the term "team" is frequently used. Interestingly, this is not a term that patients use very often. More often, patients differentiate between the staff and dentist with one exception. When patients are very happy with the practice, when they like their dentist and the staff, when the staff has long tenure and there is rapport between staff and patient, patients refer to the group as "like family." Those patients in focus groups who are most likely to remain with the practice and accept treatment can be spotted because they say, "It's not like a dentist's office, it's more like 'family.'" The feeling of warmth and comfort that comes through in their discussion clearly communicates that the office has done an excellent job in building relationships with these patients.

TEAM CONTINUITY

This issue of team continuity is more important to patients than practitioners may realize. Patients make many judgments based on the longevity of the staff and the rate of turnover. Staff continuity is a significant indicator in predicting the likelihood of patient retention and treatment acceptance. Patients talk about how they feel in the dental practice. When they relate a feeling of comfort with the team, frequently these same patients may mention how long they have been a patient of the practice and/or how long they have known the team members in the practice. There is a sense of comfort that comes via familiarity, as long as the patient is treated well and with respect. Many patients in our groups comment that they would not want to change dentists because of their comfort with team members in the office.

Patients also have made observations about the likelihood of their own happiness in the practice based on the longevity of staff members. When we've asked patients, "Specifically, what is it that you like about being a patient in a practice where the staff has long tenure?" Patients frequently respond with the following answers:

- "The staff members have stayed with this practice for a long time. If the doctor treats *them* well, then the doctor will probably treat *me* well."
- "The staff members have been in this office for a long time so they're probably more efficient and knowledgeable than newer staff members might be."
- "If they like working together in this office, I will probably like being a patient here also."

The most frequent conclusion by patients is that if the staff is happy with *this* doctor and *this* office, this is a good indicator that the patient may be happy there also. Conversely, patients do not like numerous staff changes. This is unsettling for patients in many ways, some of which are listed below:

- "If the doctor can't keep staff members, what is the problem in the office?"
- "If team members are leaving the practice because they're unhappy, maybe I'll be unhappy too."
- "I don't like being a part of a training process with a new staff member."
- "I just got used to the last [staff member], and now they change again."

Patients are looking for comfort, a sense of "belonging", and familiarity in the dental office. Finding these elements in the practice is likely to encourage the patient to stay. These are factors that also help reduce patient anxiety.

One of the biggest challenges a practitioner has is developing a strong team and maintaining equilibrium within the team. This doesn't happen by itself. It takes conscious effort. That effort must originate with the dentist or primary leader of the group. Ensuring open lines of communication and keeping one's sights set on goals are very important for every member of the team.

THE PRACTICE MISSION STATEMENT AND ITS IMPACT ON PATIENTS

The dental teams which seem to have the greatest sense of purpose also have developed a mission statement or vision for the practice. I've been in many offices where I have seen mission statements beautifully framed on walls and yet the behavior exhibited is not congruent with the message of the statement. In order for your mission statement to have any value it must be the foundation upon which the practice is built. Every team member needs to know the statement, what it really means, and needs to live this and exhibit it for patients. Otherwise, a beautifully framed statement is only a wall decoration at best. At worst it is an anathema to the practice, causing the patient to be confused and resulting in lack of credibility for the practice.

I was discussing the matter of mission statements at a major dental meeting. I was conducting a round table session and asked the practitioners present, "How many of you have a mission statement?" Half of the doctors raised their hands. I asked them, "How many of you can state with assurance that your team members really know the statement?" At that point, a Canadian doctor pulled his business card out of his pocket, he slid the card across the table to me and suggested that I turn it over. On the flip side of his business card was written his mission statement and as I read it, he quoted it to me word for word from memory. I'd never seen anyone do that before and haven't experienced it since.

He commented that every member of the team was able to do that. The team had written the mission statement together and so each member of the team had a vested interest in it.

The mission statement that you write should not be static. Just as our society evolves and issues change for the public, (See Part 1, Sociotrends) your mission statement needs to be updated periodically as well.

From the patients' perspective, a well-written mission statement viewed in the reception area is patient-centered. That all-important message guides the team in such a way that their behavior and decisions in relation to patient issues are congruent with the message.

PATIENT "IMMERSION" INTO THE PRACTICE

Patients have made their feelings known strongly and clearly in our focus groups: Staff is extremely powerful in influencing patient perceptions of the practice. Patients see the team as human indicators of how satisfied they will be with their experiences in the dental office. They may sit in the reception area and view the way the team interacts with each other and with other patients. They notice the way staff communicates with the dentist and how effectively they appear to work with each other.

In focus groups we noticed a repeated pattern among patients that appeared to be very pleased as patients in a new practice. There was a similarity in feelings from different offices that these patients communicated in relation to the team. There were even similarities in what occurred in their first appointments.

Frequently, these pleased patients would describe a dental practice team that appeared to be highly supportive of each other. Team members spoke well of each other, staff spoke well of the dentist and vice versa. Patients often talked about a combined feeling of warmth and confidence that emanated from these teams.

In my own experiences as a mystery patient, I started to look for the same specifics that I kept hearing about from patients. Those offices that were the most finely tuned did, in fact, follow a similar pattern to what was described by our focus group participants. I interviewed some dentists who were known for having high rates of patient retention and treatment acceptance. Once again, the same pattern of communication was evident in these offices.

We now refer to this process as, "Immersion". The new patient who visits a dental office for the first time and finds a highly cohesive and productive team is frequently "immersed" into the practice using the following process. From my own experiences in the most successful offices, I don't believe that this is a technique, but rather a method of communicating that emanates naturally from a highly evolved group.

The following represents the similar elements that are manifested to new patients in an office that effectively immerses patients into the practice:

• Phone call(s) instill confidence in the patient via supportive words spoken about the team members, hygienists, assistants and doctor(s). Some offices use third-person credibility to instill additional confidence in the patient. That is, they tell patients how *other* patients feel about the doctor and the staff.

• On the phone, callers gain the feeling of patient appreciation by the office. They are thanked for calling the office and welcomed into the office and/or community.

• On arrival at the office, the patient is promptly greeted and warmly welcomed as a new patient. Patients frequently relate feeling "special" in this office. They also experience consistency in approach in comparing the phone call to the actual office visit.

• Team members introduce themselves and/or their colleagues to the patient.

• The dentist sits and faces the patient in the first minutes prior to the clinical exam. The doctor communicates with the patient as a person first, allowing the patient the opportunity to feel at ease with the practitioner.

• The patient views team members interacting positively, efficiently and supportively with each other. Patients remark that among team members, verbal words of support and respect are communicated in a genuine and natural manner. This behavior does not appear contrived or practiced.

• Team members are proud of the practice. They verbalize it and the patient sees this exhibited nonverbally as well.

• When the patient is in the treatment chair, focus by team members is on the patient. There is little in the way of practitioner distraction. If the dentist is in the treatment room, he/she is not interrupted with phone calls and is not continually leaving the room to check on other patients.

• On closure of the exam or treatment, the patient is walked to the appointment counter by an assistant.

• Acknowledgment of the patient's value to the practice is communicated as the patient prepares to depart, with a message like, "We're really pleased you're part of our practice and we look forward to seeing you in _____."

The most important thing I can tell you regarding this entire process is that patients consistently remark that the feelings conveyed throughout are those of sincerity and recognition of the patient's value to the practice. If a patient perceives that any of these elements is being used as technique to gain favor or manipulate the patient, it is perceived as extremely negative. In other words, if a team member talks about the quality of service provided by the practice or addresses how much the practice cares about patients, it better be communicated genuinely and from the heart or not said at all.

There is no "quick-fix" that will achieve this same end result without the risk of team members coming across as being insincere or using technique. Instead, immersion seems to occur most naturally when a team has worked together for a significant period of time, respects each other genuinely, has a common goal and sense of purpose, and then exhibits strong ethical characteristics. With these concepts in place, immersing the patient into the practice occurs naturally. Also, when patients experience this, they recognize it as a rarity, and choose to remain part of a practice where they feel nurtured, safe, and know they will be treated fairly.

STAFF BEHAVIOR REPRESENTS DOCTOR'S STANDARDS

In our focus groups, patients say they find the credibility and confidence of staff members to be extremely important in influencing their perceptions of the doctor. The patient's thinking is this, "The doctor has chosen this staff member to represent his/her office. The behavior of each staff member represents what is acceptable to the doctor. Therefore I know more about the doctor by observing the staff member." With this kind of thinking there is a need for the doctor to hire staff that will represent the office well, and to offer training on the procedures and service values of the practice. As a result of doing this well, the patient can feel confidence in the practice, and the doctor can feel confidence that staff represents the practice in a friendly and professional manner.

Most important in this concept is the fact that the communication with patients must be genuine—sincere. Anything, any behavior, that smacks of manipulation, can result in the opposite outcome from that which is desired. Given these circumstances, patients will avoid the practice that appears to be disingenuous.

SEGUE TO THE CLINICAL STAFF

Patients welcome the kind of statements that support the abilities and skills of other staff members when they are verbalized in a genuine manner. This can begin the moment the patient is called to move into the clinical area. The front desk person can introduce the patient to the assistant or hygienist with a few statements of salutation. In the ideal situation, the patient is given brief words of introduction about the staff member. For example, the receptionist might say,

Ms. Boswell, this is Shelly, she's our dental assistant who'll be with you today. Shelly has been with us for seven years and patients say that 'Shelly never meets a stranger'. So you're in really good

hands—Shelly will make sure that you're comfortable.

The receptionist can jump-start the conversation for Shelly with an introductory statement like, "Shelly, Ms. Boswell moved here last month from Dallas, and she's just had her braces removed after two years!"

This is not meant to sound like party introductions! This brief personal connect in interactions can help patients to feel more at ease. It also helps them to understand that they are placing themselves in confident hands. This is indeed reassuring! It's a solid foundation on which to initiate a clinical exam. Patients want to believe they've made the right decision in choosing your office, and staff affirmation of this is comforting.

The *nonverbal* approach to clinical communication that patients like includes:[2]

- Focus on the patient, not on the file.
- Sit at eye level, rather than standing or sitting at a level higher than the patient.
- Sit facing, not beside the patient, in the first moments. It's friendlier and the patient can observe you more readily.

The *verbal* approach to clinical communication that patients like includes:

- A personal connect before jumping into the clinical topics—i.e., "small talk."
- Use of lay terms. Terms basic to dental professionals, like "prophy," may be foreign to patients.
- Supportive talk of other members of the dental team.
- Introductions to other members of the team.

- Use of a communication style that is in sync with that of the patient.
- Use of active listening with the patient and responding before changing the subject.

AN EXAMPLE OF COMPLETE IMMERSION

I personally experienced a most dramatic and effective example of immersion. I had been hired as an undercover mystery patient for a cutting-edge office. The doctor had neither seen me, nor had he talked with me prior to my "appointment." He'd gotten my name as a referral from another client of mine and he had an intermediary make all the necessary arrangements. He did not even know when I'd schedule the new-patient appointment. It was the ideal situation for this type of visit—I had complete anonymity.

My pre-appointment impression was one of a well-orchestrated office, smoothly run. The receptionist was knowledgeable, professional, and friendly on the phone. I had received a welcoming packet in the mail that included information about the staff as well as the doctor. Also included were patient forms and a stamped, self-addressed envelope for forms return. A strong, cohesive picture of the office was presented before the appointment.

The day of my appointment arrived. Sandra, the person I'd talked to on the phone, greeted me by name as I entered the door. She stood, shook hands, and introduced me to the office manager who had been working with her at the counter. I waited less than five minutes before Betsy entered the reception area and introduced herself. She explained that she was the assistant and would be working with me today. As she walked me to the treatment room she said, "We're really proud that you chose our office, and I feel sure you're going to feel at home here." She had incredible people skills—she was predisposing me to feeling good about the practice. She knew what to do and say to instill confidence in the practice and to alleviate my "new patient" jitters.

After seating me she sat at eye level in front of me. She placed my file on the counter and focused on me instead of on the file. She sought out areas of commonality. It was obvious that she'd studied my file before seating me, because she proceeded to ask me how I was making the transition from Massachusetts to Texas. Her body language was relaxed and her manner communicated genuine interest. She listened to me and responded to my comments before changing the direction of the conversation. It was obvious that, although she was a very young woman, she had the kind of people-skills savvy that usually comes from experience and maturity. Also it was obvious that she really liked working with people.

I'd observed her earlier with another patient and she had been very low key. She'd been interacting with a patient who was rather introverted and Betsy's behavior mirrored that of the patient.[3] In the first moments of our discussion, I felt that she was evaluating me as to behavioral style; she listened more than she talked. It wasn't long before she started to loosen up and she seemed to be adjusting to the style I was exhibiting— behavior quite different than I'd seen in her earlier!

She wanted to take my photograph for the office files and I objected. I said I really didn't want to have my picture taken that day and asked if we could do it next time. There was no problem with that on her part. Although I was to realize later that she already knew how she was going to handle that challenge! Betsy proceeded to take the patient history, then offered to take me on a tour of the practice before the doctor conducted the clinical exam.

Here is where Betsy really outdid herself. We visited each treatment and hygiene room in the office. She introduced me to each staff member and told them something about me, and told me something about them. This procedure communicated belief in the clinical skills and caring attitude of the practice. By the time we reached the last treatment room, she was talking about the doctor. I had written on the new patient form that I'd had a history of fear of the dental experience. I explained that I had some terrible memories from childhood and I was hesitant to have clinical treatments performed due to that history as well as fear of injections.

Betsy chose to talk about the gentleness of the doctor and his skill in giving an injection that I wouldn't even feel. She told me what other patients said about his abilities, and about how much the staff enjoyed working with him. I was sold! To hear a staff member speak so strongly, with such conviction about the doctor and each staff member was a rarity! But most importantly, I felt she was genuine. I was not having smoke blown at me!

On the way back to the treatment room, she stopped at the sterilization area and briefly addressed issues related to infection control. She talked about the standards of protection for patients and all members of the dental team. She invited me to ask questions about this important subject. Then she segued to a supportive mention of the practice philosophy. The mission statement of the practice was written in calligraphy and was in a beautiful frame on the wall. With some pride, she noted that the mission statement was written by the entire team at a staff retreat three months earlier. Then she seated me prior to the clinical exam with the doctor. She mentioned that the staff members all had been a part of the practice a minimum of nine years and that one person had been with the doctor for 21 years!

This was a lot of information in a very short office tour. However, Betsy was finely attuned to people and she was confident in her communication skills, so she did not appear as contrived or patronizing. If she'd handled this in a "practiced" manner she might be perceived as insincere. She came across as an individual proud of her work, her peers, and the practice—and she wanted me to feel confident in my decision to choose this office.

Then, with a playful smile, she asked if I wouldn't please reconsider having the photo taken now. She had done a great job of building rapport with me and I think she knew that the likelihood of compliance was greater now than earlier. I was so amused by her handling of this that I laughed and let her take my picture. She was not "Pollyanna" but a genuinely enthusiastic ambassador for the practice! In the over 500 undercover mystery visits I've made to dental offices, I've never experienced a staff member who so seamlessly integrated me into the office with such confidence, credibility, and finesse.

Consistency, Congruence and the Doctor

At this point the doctor joined us in the treatment room. Like Betsy, he chose to sit at eye level facing me. He was just as she had described, sincere, warm and he seemed to be genuinely interested in me as a patient. Had he been anything other than what was described to me, I'd have been terribly let down. The entire process to this point had built up my expectations. A lack of consistency and/or congruence on the part of the doctor would have led to patient confusion and decreasing credibility. I then might have questioned Betsy's sincerity and her truthfulness. Doubt would have been cast on her, the doctor, and the practice as a whole.

The doctor spoke well of Betsy and told me that she'd been on the team for 10 years. As he talked he looked at her as well, and his words were congruent with his demeanor. He exhibited a real respect for Betsy as a person and as an assistant. My confidence in her also rose as a result of seeing and hearing him. This kind of affirmation is extremely powerful for the patient. Also it helps the patient to understand the heart of the practice. The earlier that the patient can be immersed into the heart, and understand the heart, of the practice, the more likely that the patient will become a long-term member of the dental family!

IMMERSION AND BEHAVIOR MODIFICATION

As in effective communication with anyone, the team member needs to be acutely sensitive to the communication style of patients. Staff members must modify behavior and adjust to the style of communication that will help the patient feel comfortable. This means closely observing the patient as well as listening to the pattern of verbal and vocal communication.[4] Once the patient's style is recognized, then the immersion process can be modified to "fit" that individual. For example, an introverted, analytical type would need to be immersed into the practice in a different manner from an animated extrovert. The modification would not affect the process itself, but how the information was presented to the patient. The patient who is very people-oriented and appears to be a socializer will respond positively to an emphasis on the humanistic elements. The detail-oriented introvert may prefer to hear specifics about the education of the staff members and their clinical skills.

The tour of the office would be conducted similarly with both types, but would be altered to emphasize different perspectives of the staff members and of the practice itself. This behavior modification and customization of the immersion process is a way to provide information in the manner that patients would most like to receive it.

In order for a long-term patient-practice relationship to thrive, the entire team must earn the endorsement of the patient. The process of earning endorsement is not the responsibility of any one person, not that of the doctor alone, and not that of any individual team member alone. Instead it takes a concerted effort as a team to communicate with confidence to the patient, to exhibit pride in self and in each other. Most importantly success depends on the ability to maintain a fine-tuned awareness to the changing needs of the patient, whether the patient has been with the practice for one week or for 10 years.

SELECTION OF STAFF MEMBERS

For the practice owner and/or office administrator, selection of staff members and the hiring process is certainly a challenging one. It is a process that cannot be taken lightly because it so strongly influences patients' perceptions of every aspect of your office. Also, the choices you make are ones which you, patients, and every other team member must live with.

SELECTING TEAM MEMBERS

In one of the offices where I found an extremely cohesive team I asked the doctor what method he used to select and hire staff. He responded that that responsibility was not his alone, that the balance of the team all played a part in the decision making process. He then described a creative process that involved team participation from the very beginning. His office manager initially collected the applications, made cuts, and narrowed down the number of likely candidates prior to the interview process.

Business team members who would be speaking with patients on the phone were initially interviewed over the telephone in order to hear vocal quality and evaluate their self presentation since this would be the primary form of direct communication with patients.

The first interviews with key candidates were conducted by the office manager. As the process continued, additional team members were involved in order to further narrow the field, and the final selection was made by the dentist himself. What was so powerful about this process is that the team members became invested in selection and consequently they would have a greater interest in ensuring the success of this new team member. The doctor commented, "Once the new staff member comes on board, a very basic level of rapport has already been built and the team wants this person to succeed." This process also helps to explain how a team can form a very tightly knit family and feel some level of responsibility toward each other.

Caveat: Staff members at the front desk are your ambassadors to the world. Select them carefully! No matter how sharp the person is, *do not* risk putting someone on the front lines who would be most effective working alone on the books in a back room. This person is probably not going to be happy dealing with people all day, and patients probably won't be as happy either! This is *not* the staff slot to "try out" someone! You need to know that this person can manage two patients at the counter and three ringing phone lines with a smile on her face!

Team members are truly the heart of your practice and their relationships with patients can have very serious bottom-line impact on the success of your practice. I was meeting with a dentist client at her office when one of her long-term patients arrived. This is a person who had just driven 30 miles for the dental appointment. She lived in a small town on the outskirts of a metropolitan area and had fought heavy freeway traffic to get to her appointment on time.

It was interesting to observe her interactions with the team members. She was greeted warmly by two of the business staff members. The hygienist walked out into the reception area, gave this patient a hug and said, "I've missed you. It seems like more than six months since we've seen you!" It was obvious that there was a genuine fondness from the team for this patient. From what I saw in those few moments, it was clear to me why this patient would continue to come to this practice even though she had to drive so far.

TOP TIPS:

1.   Develop or update your mission statement as a team. Then walk your talk!
2.   Let patients see *genuine*, mutual team liking and respect for each other. This builds patient confidence.
3.   Have staff meetings at least once a month to build team understanding and ensure focus on common goals. A *short* team meeting once a week is more

effective in the development of a truly cohesive team. Encourage different team members to be responsible for topics to be covered.

4. Encourage discussions of each other's strengths. Make sure all members of the team understand the importance of everyone's roles in the office. Take a tour of the office as a group and have each team member explain what he/she does so that all understand each other's responsibilities. When the team is more knowledgeable about each other and the office, both the team and the patients benefit. This process can be a real eye opener!

5. Offer a weekly or monthly award to the team member who exhibited exemplary service to patients. Make this a team decision that involves discussion of all the exceptional patient interactions that have occurred. This helps to build appreciation for each other and heightened awareness to patient responses to excellent customer service.

6. Engage the entire team in periodic group functions *away* from the office that are *not* work related. Give the team options to choose from, and/or ask for their ideas. Positive and enjoyable experiences as a group aid in developing greater team spirit, mutual appreciation, and understanding. Renewed enthusiasm for each other and the practice are important outcomes. This influences patient perceptions of the practice.

7. Have a suggestion box for employees and give incentive for participation. Let the team see that their ideas have value and are taken seriously.

8. Have team members participate in the recruiting and interviewing process of new team members. You're more likely to have a team that works well together and the members of the team have a

vested interest in seeing the new team member succeed.

9.   Interview prospective office staff members on the phone to evaluate the effectiveness of their "phone personalities".

10.   Include an office tour for new patients. Introduce team members to new patients throughout the tour.

REFERENCES

[1] Lewis, Ralph. *Team-Building Skills*, McGraw-Hill, Inc., New York, NY, 1994.

[2] Boswell, S. "Practice Made Perfect/Managing Patient Perceptions," J*ournal of Esthetic Dentistry*, Volume 6, Number 6, 1994.

[3] Brooks, Michael. *Instant Rapport*, Warner Books, New York, NY 1989.

[4] Brooks, Michael. *Instant Rapport*, Warner Books, New York, NY 1989.

19

Financial Matters: The Patient's Perspective

"They wanted to discuss payment plans while I was at the front counter. There were two other patients standing there and I felt like I was 'on display!'"

— F O C U S   G R O U P   P A R T I C I P A N T

The subject of the focus group was financial matters and we were addressing the issues of primary concern to patients. One of the participants brought up an incident that had occurred during his most recent dental appointment. He described an office where treatment areas were separated by six-foot "privacy dividers." There were plants on top of the dividers, but there was actually little privacy. "I could hear quite clearly the conversation going on in the next room where the staff member was explaining the fee to that patient. The patient was saying that he couldn't afford the crown and was asking if he could make payments on it." This focus group member stated that he wanted to get out of the chair at that point. "There was no privacy, and I knew that I was going to have a similar discussion about fees for my bridge. I didn't relish the idea of everyone else in the office hearing it!"

Another focus group participant, Joan, related an incident that shook her confidence in the office. She had been a patient in a sole practitioner's office for more than seven years. Sitting in the reception area, she overheard a conversation between two staff members. They were out of sight, but not out of earshot. One team member questioned the other, "Is Nancy Bruner on a plan or do we charge full fee for her prophy?"

That one sentence was enough to leave Joan wondering about her relationship with the office and whether it should continue or not. Joan was an assertive individual. She presented herself with confidence and seemed the type of person who would openly express her concerns to the doctor. I asked her, "Did you talk with the dentist about your concerns?"

> *No, she said, it wouldn't have made any difference anyway. But I don't like the idea that someone else is getting the same treatment that I pay a lot more for. If that's they way this office operates then, well, I'm still thinking about it. I might change dentists.*

THE PATIENT'S "BIG THREE"

The big three issues frequently addressed in continuing education programs are of major concern to patients. These factors that influence likelihood of patient treatment acceptance are:

1. **Money:** The patient thinks, "How much is this going to cost and how am I going to pay for it?"
2. **Pain:** The patient thinks: "Is it going to hurt? How will I manage the pain?"
3. **Time:** The patient thinks: "How long is it going to take and when can I get it taken care of?"

The typical patient wants these questions answered and appreciates the team helping to facilitate each issue. Eliminating objections to each of these issues is critical for treatment acceptance. The doctor may opt for a knowledgeable team member to manage the financial discussion. (This is addressed later in this chapter.)

Pain issues must be addressed directly by the clinical team with assurances and specifics to the patient of how pain will be managed. If there are options in this regard, the options should be explained to the patient. The more the patient knows about this, the more receptive the patient will be. In mainstream business this process is referred to as consultative selling. You are offering information and gaining patient input into the process. This "partnering" with the patient gains high acceptance by patients. One focus group patient rebelled against the dogmatic tone by his dentist. This patient said, "I wanted to tell the doctor, 'Doc, don't dictate to me what I have to do. Give me some options and let me choose!'" For example, let your patients choose from what options there are in relation to pain management; they'll be more responsive to you in other areas when they can take some part in the process.

Help the patient understand and manage the time issues—not just the phasing of the treatment, although this can be crucial to gaining treatment acceptance in relation to ease of monthly payments. But an important element of time that is becoming increasingly evident in our focus groups is the time required away from the office or job for the patient. Patients are expressing their concerns more about the hours the dental practice is open and how much time the patient has to take off from work to receive treatment. Those offices that meet the patients' needs by being open a few extended hours a week will find less hesitancy to book appointments due to missing work. Help patients by discussing their schedules and evaluating how you can treat them without their losing valuable time from their work.

When it comes to issues of money, pain, and time, patients value you more when you indicate a sincere interest in patients and a genuine desire to meet their needs. When you verbalize a desire to work with the patient in these areas, the patient is more likely to want to work with you.

COMMUNICATION ISSUES FROM THE PATIENT'S PERSPECTIVE

The entire team must be acutely aware of patient concerns in relation to financial and insurance issues. Inappropriate attitude or approach can drive a patient away from the practice. Sensitivity also must be maintained with the discussion of any financial or insurance matters in earshot of other patients.

Another patient said, "I thought their fees were exorbitant. I paid my bill but I never went back to them." We've heard this kind of statement many times in focus groups and the scenario is almost always the same. I asked this patient the question I pose to every patient who makes that statement, "Did you talk to the dentist or any member of the team about your dissatisfaction?" She responded, "Well, no I didn't. I would have felt uncomfortable doing that. Besides, they wouldn't do anything about it." Patient dissatisfaction or distress over fees is often not communicated to the dental team.

Frequently these patients leave the practice and seek another office where they believe the fees are more reasonable.

Those patients who do speak with you openly and directly about fees are in the minority and are actually doing you a service. Each patient who voices mainstream opinions about any issue in the office probably represents at least 10 other patients who are not talking to you about it. Listen to what the outspoken ones say. I'm not suggesting that they are right, I am just proposing that they may have an important perspective to be heard.

Whenever I hear patients talk about fees, insurance, or managed care issues, I always wonder about the communication skills of the practitioners in their offices. Assuming that the practitioner has good to excellent clinical skills, my feeling is that many members of the dental team have not learned how to address their patients about what can be an awkward subject matter.

The following are issues that patients have raised in focus groups:

• "I got a notification from the insurance company that the doctor's fees were more than what is considered usual, customary, and reasonable (UCR). The insurance company did not cover as much of the fee as I had hoped they would. This makes me feel really uncomfortable and it makes me question the ethics of the doctor."

Patients don't like surprises. It is much better for them to have been educated about UCR prior to receiving a notification like this from the insurance company. Explaining what UCR means, how the insurance companies evaluates fees, and delineating the quality of care that would be provided under the umbrella of UCR is all crucial in practice-patient relationships. Most importantly, this communication must occur prior to the patient receiving any such notification from the insurance company. When the office must explain this after the fact, it is awkward. To the patient, it appears that you are scrambling for excuses. When you explain it early, the information can be provided in the form of patient education and in the form of helping to raise the patient's dental IQ.

• "When I got to the counter to pay, the bill was more than the fee that had been quoted to me!"

We do hear this in focus groups and invariably, the patient did not receive a written treatment plan prior to the procedure itself. It is very easy for patients to misunderstand or not even hear information that is being provided to them in the discussion of treatment plans and fees. Sometimes this occurs because of a fee or fee range that is quoted over the phone. *You* may be very aware of giving the patient all of the information in discussion. However, your patient's attention may not even be in the room during the discussion. At a key point in your explanation, your patient may have "gone away" to think about what the balance was in the checkbook or to worry about a child who needed to be picked up at school. A written treatment plan provides three benefits:

1. Clear cut communication with patients in black and white.

2. A record for your files and for the patient.

3. Higher perceived value of the treatment by the patient.

• "The doctor proposed an expensive treatment that I don't think I really need. I've got great insurance and I think that's the reason he's suggesting this; he thinks I'll accept the treatment because of the insurance plan I have."

Unfortunately, this is not uncommon to hear. Patients probably are not verbalizing this to you in the same way they tell us. If there is pain, they understand the need for treatment. If there are aesthetic considerations, the patient is more likely to understand because these are considerations that can be seen. However, if they can't feel it, if they can't see it, it is more likely that patients are going to have questions. This is the place where an intraoral camera can aid immeasurably in communicating with both the patient and the insurance company.

Putting the intraoral camera aside, there is a basic issue here of effectively educating the patient. If the patient cannot see the condition, then the practitioner must educate the patient as to the problem and what the consequences may be without treatment.

One doctor noted that he does not address money or the time span of treatment until the patient indicates that the treatment is desired. Initial discussions revolve around (1) the condition (2) the treatment needed to improve the condition and to maintain good health. This keeps the focus off of insurance issues and on the value of treatment for the patient.

- "Don't assume I can't afford the treatment—let me judge whether I can afford it or not."

This statement is most typically made by the low income patient or elderly patient. Implying that a patient cannot afford a treatment is a very sensitive issue and a matter of pride for many. Without full information provided by the patient, you really *don't* know if the patient can afford it. Perhaps a family member wants to assist the patient. Patients do not appreciate the team member who says something like, "Well, this is not an inexpensive procedure." This will be interpreted by some patients as "Well, you're really not able to afford this." Be careful about qualifying your patients without all the information, and avoid making judgments about what is "best" for the patient in relation to highly elective treatments, most particularly aesthetic treatments.

I was an undercover patient and talking with the doctor about replacement of a front filling that bothered me. It looked discolored to me and I thought it should be replaced. I was surprised when the doctor said, "No, I wouldn't do that; it doesn't look that bad. Why don't you wait a while." It was important to me yet he was applying his own standards to the quality of care I was requesting.

There are many points-of-view on this issue, I recognize. But the important point here is, don't let patients feel that their perspectives are without value or that you perceive the patients to be incapable of paying for treatments. Either one of these attitudes can be perceived as demeaning or insensitive to patients.

• "Don't quote fees or discuss payment plans with me in front of other patients."

This is discussed at length in this chapter as well as in other areas of this book. This is a crucial issue and serious attention must be paid to maintaining patient privacy and confidentiality. Ensuring patient privacy for these discussions is critical for patient trust. Every practice *must* ensure confidentiality of patient discussions on financial matters. A cavalier attitude here is enough to encourage a patient to look for a more "professional" caregiver.

• "Give me a written statement on financial arrangements. I don't like having to ask for one."

There is a perception of decreased value when they can't see the treatment plan and fee on paper. It becomes more tangible when patients read this. Always give a statement, even if you provide a treatment for free. What a great feeling for a patient to receive a printed statement with the actual fee shown and then *no charge* written over it. This is a significant message to the patient.

• "Why won't you accept assignment of benefits? I think that should be part of your service!"

This is a touchy issue for some patients and practices. If the office has been doing such and considers stopping, the practice can expect to lose patients as a result. In our focus groups we have had patients indicate a resentment when a practitioner halts this "patient benefit". Patients do appreciate those offices that handle this matter by accepting assignments of benefits. If the office doesn't accept assignment and never has, that's another matter. If patients know this from the beginning, then they can accept it far more readily than if the office decides to stop the process.

- "Even though it's not covered in my insurance plan, can't you just list a couple of treatments so that I can get the cost of the full procedure covered?"

This is an ethical issue that deserves direct response by the office. How you address ethical issues will communicate to patients how they can expect you to act when you are managing their clinical and financial matters. An honest and direct answer will gain the respect of most patients, even if it is not financially in their favor. At the same time, your response must not infer that the patient is wanting to be unethical. Instead ensure that the patient understands the options that are available in payment plans. It should be clear to the patient that any type of hedging is not an option.

- "Why are you charging me an "infection control fee? You didn't used to do this; were you not sterilizing equipment before?"

This is certainly another touchy issue for the dental practice. I've been a patient in offices that include separate infection control fees on the statement, as well as offices that include the fee as a part of the treatment fee. How do patients feel about it? As in so many other areas, it is a change that bothers them. Some ask the question above, and some are more understanding (even though they may not *like* the response.) Yet others state that this should be a part of doing business and should not be passed on to the patient at all. This last perspective is typically from one who has not managed or owned a business!

There is no single solution to this issue that will blanketly cover all the patient objections and questions.

Although, if the infection control costs are a part of the treatment fee, then this is typically not an issue

Throughout this book there is an underlying message of, "The responsibility is on your shoulders to communicate to the patients about your skills, your proficiency, the benefits of your office, and the value of your treatments." Patients only know what you tell them, what they may gather from friends, and their own personal experiences. When a patient comments, "I can get the same work done by another office for a lot less," my feeling is that the practitioner has not effectively educated the patient or instilled in the patient belief in the value provided by the office. Dr. Robert Frazer Jr., of Austin, TX speaks nationwide on the subject of values based, fee-for-service dentistry. He states, "Never quote a fee until you are certain that the patient's perceived value has been raised to an appropriate level."[1] This places the responsibility squarely on the shoulders of the dentist and the finance person to ensure that there is accurate comprehension of the treatment to be provided and the respective fees. This requires excellent communication skills and the ability to develop a feedback loop that will verify practitioner's communication and patient comprehension.

STAFF ATTITUDES ABOUT FEE DISCLOSURE

As a patient, I often detect discomfort by both the dentist and team members when approaching the subject matter of fees. Many times dentists act as if they are avoiding the subject, evidenced by way of non-verbal communication: eye contact avoidance, a sudden shifting of weight, and movement toward the door! This usually occurs when they're discussing higher fee treatments.

I recognize the reasoning behind having a staff member who has been trained to discuss finances with patients. However, the doctor must present the concept of staff fee presentation to the patient in a manner that builds confidence in the office, and the team member. Unfortunately, many doctors feel great discomfort at this point and that discomfort can manifest itself nonverbally.

An issue that must be addressed here is the position that staff members take in discussing fees with patients. I have experienced the discomfort that can be heard vocally and verbally by staff members when talking about fees with patients. In some cases, it's almost apologetic. It's clear that the staff member feels uncomfortable about quoting a fee or charging a patient a dollar amount that the staff person might not be able to afford. This is a very critical matter because if the patient perceives any semblance of doubt in the staff as to the value of treatment, those same doubts are then placed in the patient's mind.

Because staff attitudes influence patients greatly, anything that might look or sound like an apologetic tone will be received negatively by patients. In contrast, a staff member who truly knows and believes in the value of the treatment being provided by the practice, will send this message to the patient visually, vocally, and verbally. Once again, we come to the matter of instilling in staff members a belief in the practice and educating staff members as much as the patients about the benefits and value of treatment.

One of the best ways to achieve this is to clinically treat team members. If at all possible, staff should have treatments rendered by the dentist. It is extremely powerful for a patient to hear a team member say to a patient or prospective patient, "The doctor made a bridge for me last month, and it's so comfortable. It's easier for me to eat now. You'll be so pleased with your results!" or "The doctor gave me an injection last week . Her touch is so gentle and she's so skilled that I couldn't even feel it!" Patients consistently remark that staff comments like these are very meaningful and help to build trust for the practitioner.

Some staff members say, "Well, I know that our practice provides excellent clinical treatments and service for our patients, but I feel bad when there is a patient who I know really cannot afford it." If team members feel this way, they may need to evaluate how they project to patients. They need to instill confidence in the patient for having made the decision to accept the treatment. Patients want to hear that. They want to know, "Yes, this was the right thing for me to do." "Buyer's remorse" can sink in if the patient makes the decision to accept treatment, feels good about it, then has a staff member unwittingly undermine that decision. In effect, that is undermining both the patient and the practice.

THE POWER OF POST-TREATMENT CONSULTATIONS

A brief post-treatment consultation or discussion can help to reconfirm to the patient that the treatment was successful and the right decision for the patient to have made. Asking the patient a question like, "Have I met your expectations?" can aid in this process by opening a discussion about the benefits of treatment. This can also be an effective time to request referrals from those patients who are particularly enthusiastic. If the patient presents any concerns to you at this time about the treatment, it affords you the opportunity to investigate the situation and determine avenues to reach patient satisfaction.

I was posing as an undercover patient in the office of a general practitioner who had hired me. This doctor had never seen me before so he did not know that I was the "mystery patient". He had proposed two unrelated treatments which I did recognize were needed. The exam was coming to a close and he had not quoted a fee to me. I had no idea when I would find this out so I asked, "What are these two procedures going to cost?" At this point, the doctor rose from the chair and indicated, "Mary will give you that information at the counter."

The assistant directed me towards the counter where Mary looked at my records and then checked her computer monitor. She announced loudly and clearly, "The fee for the crown would be $X." The fee was higher than I had anticipated. My mouth dropped and I gasped slightly. The gasp was related just as much to the matter-of-fact manner of quoting the fee in front of other patients as to the amount of the fee itself! Then I asked the fee for the splint that was recommended and of course, that fee was also quoted well within earshot of other patients. I received no statement for the fee paid that day. I received no written treatment plan for the proposed treatment.

I have no doubt that based on patient attitudes heard in focus groups, most patients would have found this a very uncomfortable and insensitive situation. Mary then suggested, "Would you like to set up your next appointment?" Given the above situation, what do you think most patients would say? "I'll have to think about it and I'll call you." That's what I said, and that's what many would say. As I left this office, I had no real sense of the value of the treatment, but I did have a better understanding of why this doctor had complained about low treatment acceptance and patient retention rates.

From the patient's point-of-view, what was wrong with the scenario above?

• Nearing the close of the clinical exam the doctor should have communicated the manner in which the fee would be disclosed to me. It should have been communicated with confidence and in a manner that instilled patient trust for Mary. Ideally, Mary should have been in the room at the time this statement was made.

• Disclosure of the fee should have been made in privacy. This is an *absolutely crucial matter.* Payment of fees is a sensitive issue for patients. They talk about this in focus groups. They do *not* want this addressed in a public area where there are other patients. They feel most comfortable when they are with one person in an area that is out of earshot of others.

• Mary should have provided me with a printed treatment plan indicating the proposed procedures and the fees for such.

• Mary should have used the term "investment" rather than fee and she would have offered alternate payment plans in helping me find a way to accept treatment.

Dentists Should Not Quote Fees

Ideally, the person who handles financial matters in the office should be present when the doctor is finishing the discussion on the proposed treatments. After giving the patient the opportunity to ask questions relative to the treatments proposed, the doctor should then turn to the staff member and indicate to the patient, "Mary (the financial staff person) totally understands the treatment that we have been discussing. She is going to discuss with you your investment for the treatment and will be able to answer all your questions in relation to this."

It is important to have a staff member conduct this portion of the treatment plan/fee because patients are frequently uneasy talking about these issues in the presence of the dentist. They don't feel comfortable and they may not even ask questions that need to be asked. Most patients are really relieved when the doctor gets up and leaves the room!

Once the doctor has left the room, it is the responsibility of the remaining team member to continue the discussion of the treatment plan and the issue of fees. This individual must be highly knowledgeable about restorative and clinical issues and must understand what is optimal dentistry for this patient. She/he also must be sensitive to patient issues that could possibly interfere with treatment acceptance.

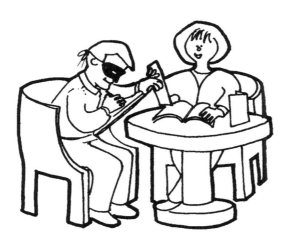

When we discuss fees and treatment plans with patients in focus groups we often hear comments like this, "Too many dentists are dogmatic about the treatment. I don't like it when they take the attitude, 'this is what you need to have done; there's no other way to do it, and here's the fee.' I may resist treatment just because of the dictatorial way this was stated!" It is crucial for the financial team member and the dentist to recognize the challenges that patients are facing financially and how this may affect treatment acceptance. The income of the average person is shrinking and the only way many can accept treatment is by investigating alternatives with the team. The patient only will consider this if the involved team members show some flexibility in offering alternate payment plans and phase treatment.

Repeatedly, patients have said they wish doctors would offer phase treatment. How they typically state this is, "I'd feel better if the doctor would prioritize the steps of treatment so that I could take it a step at a time." These patients are saying that they are far more receptive to treatment if they can do it in steps and pay for it accordingly. In this way, the treatment is within reach and feasible. This is not to imply that treatment shortcuts be taken. Phase treatment does not mean compromise in your treatment; it means structuring optimum treatment in logical steps. The more that you can prioritize treatment, the more you can organize the treatment plan in steps, the more receptive many of your patients will be. Consequently, the likelihood for treatment acceptance will rise.

Patients have indicated a similar preference in relation to different treatments that are presented at the same time. For example, if a dentist presents to a patient a need for both a bridge and a crown, many patients would like to have those two treatments prioritized. As one man put it,

Tell me which one I should do first. I'm probably not going to be able to afford them both at the same time. Letting me

*know the order of importance and when
treatment should be completed will help
me understand. Then I can think about
how I'm going to pay for it.*

Again, prioritizing treatment and discussion of payment alternatives is truly valued by patients.

Having stated this, it then becomes critical that the individual who presents the treatment plan and fee must know what the steps of phase treatment would be. This person must have the clinical understanding that facilitates this kind of discussion. Given such a discussion, it is probable that the patient will see the practice as one that respects and values him/her. After all, the practice wants to find ways to provide this patient with the very best treatment in a manner that is achievable for the patient.

It is also extremely important that this person communicate in a manner that indicates confidence and credibility. Eye contact, body language, vocal quality all need to reassure the patient that the team member is highly competent to discuss these topics. At the same time, she must recognize the behavioral style of the patient (See chapter on behavioral styles) and communicate in a manner that will earn endorsement from the patient.

Her conversation might start with, "Well, let's review what's been discussed and what needs to be done." Prior to the fee being quoted, it's important that the patient totally comprehend the treatment, the value, and benefit of such. Once this is understood, the financial person can quote a fee.

PAYMENT PLANS

Obviously, the ideal situation for the dental practice is for the patient to write a check for the full fee at the time that the service is provided. Only a very small percentage of patients are able and/or willing to do this. What are the options? You must have in place alternatives so the patient is encouraged to accept treatment.

I was having my teeth cleaned by a dental practice that I had selected from one of the several dental plans that I joined for research purposes. I was apprehensive about the office from the very beginning based on my initial telephone call. However, I was curious if they would be able to exceed expectations! The dentist not only conducted the clinical exam, but he also cleaned my teeth, all in a record setting—35 minutes. I have a retainer on my lower front teeth and I remarked on the awkwardness of flossing. He then showed me how I could angle the floss and *not* have to use a threader or go underneath the retainer!

Following the exam and cleaning, I went to the front desk and removed a credit card from my wallet to pay. I quickly learned that this office accepted no credit cards. Nurse Ratched had been transplanted from "One Flew Over the Cuckoo's Nest" to this office. Her steely eyes said it all. She couldn't believe I'd come to a dental practice without checks or cash to pay for the treatment. On the other hand, I was very disappointed that they didn't accept credit cards. From the patient's point of view, this practice was making it more difficult for me to do business with them. Considering my experience with the practice so far, I shouldn't have been surprised.

Patients expect you to accept the major credit cards, Visa, MasterCard®, Discover®, and American Express®. Patients do want this and if you do not offer your patients this option, it *will* affect your treatment acceptance rate.

I was very impressed with the experience I had in the office of another doctor who had hired me to evaluate her entire practice. This doctor had never seen me before but had received my name from one of her colleagues so I was anonymous to her and to her team when I arrived for my appointment. This was an office where every member of the team had a very high level of communication skills. This was evident from the first phone call all the way through to the close of my appointment.

Also I was impressed with the flow and the orchestration of the appointment by the staff in this office. On conclusion of the clinical exam, I was walked to the front desk by the assistant. She introduced me to Leigh, the financial coordinator who then invited me to a consultation room where "we could discuss the treatment plan more comfortably." The consultation room was located directly across the hall from the reception desk. Here, Leigh gave me a computer printout treatment plan. It had printed out while I was walking from the treatment room to the front desk. Leigh communicated in a very caring and sincere manner. She reviewed the treatment plan and made sure that I understood the benefits of the treatment. She then explained the fees to me.

I expressed concern about being able to afford the treatment and she indicated that the office offered a couple of other alternatives that I might be interested in. The first was paying by credit card and the second method was one which I had not seen before. It was a system called "PrideDirect" from The Pride Institute in Greenbrae, California.[2] This was a patient payment plan whereby the patient's checking account is automatically debited one to two times a month based on patient preference. There is no interest charged on this, just a minor transaction fee with each debit. This was a most impressive plan and one that I felt very comfortable with as a patient. Knowing the attitudes of today's dental patients, I felt that it was a very viable option for many patients and I was surprised that I had not seen this type of plan before.

The staff member in this office was exceptionally well versed on the plan and was able to communicate the benefits in a patient-friendly manner. What I found particularly interesting about this option was the apparent flexibility that the practice could provide the patient. The staff member openly initiated a discussion with me on what a feasible payment per month might be for me. When an office is able to offer options as this one did, patients will be more responsive to accepting treatment. It is also more likely that the patient will perceive the office as one that cares enough about its patients to have such a plan in place.

FEE DISPUTES

It is not uncommon for a patient to leave the care of a practice due to dissatisfaction with fees or because of possible fee disputes. It is also not uncommon for disputes between patients and practices to result in malpractice litigation. Clear disclosure of fees must be given to patients prior to treatment and there must be acknowledgment on both parts as to the agreement. It is best practice for the office to offer the patient a written statement of charges.[3]

From the patient's point-of-view it is certainly preferable to have a written statement or treatment plan with the fee in black and white. It is human nature that if a person is quoted a range of fees, they tend to remember the lower end of the fee scale! For example, if a team member says to a patient, "The crown will cost anywhere from $525 to $650," patients will remember $525. Be very careful about quoting ranges; once you know what the fee will be, then get it down on paper. There is also a perception of importance when one sees information in print versus remembering it floating through the air.

From one office I received a very detailed treatment plan which included a description of each procedure, the outcomes the patient could expect, and the benefits of the treatment. The fee was included in the treatment plan. I had never seen a treatment plan so specific and so detailed. My perceptions of the practitioner and the practice rose and my expectations of the quality of the clinical skills increased as well. The perception of treatment value increased and consequently the fee was validated.

CHARGING FOR BROKEN APPOINTMENTS

We have discussed in focus groups the issue of billing patients for an appointment time slot which they had missed. Discussion of the subject matter inevitably incites strong responses from patients. I've asked them, "Has there been a time when you have missed an appointment and you did not call the office?" In every focus group we've conducted we've had at least one participant who has indicated that this has happened. The vast majority of patients are aware of policies regarding cancellation in less than 24 hours prior to appointment time. Also, most of them have seen signs posted in offices indicating that the patient will be billed if the appointment is missed without proper cancellation.

However, when it comes to receiving a bill for a missed appointment, patients respond strongly. A significant number of patients in focus groups have said, "If I were billed for an appointment that I had missed because of something that was out of my control, I probably wouldn't go back to that office again." Not all the patients felt this way, but a significant number of them did feel very strongly.

Bill, a middle management executive with a major corporation said, "Not only would I not go back, I wouldn't let anybody in my family go back to that office either!" He went on to verbalize the feelings that we've heard expressed from other patients, "I've been a good patient of this office, I'm always there on time, I've had a lot of work done. I've waited when their office is running behind. If I have one problem that I need their understanding on, then I expect to get it or I'll go someplace else."

Male patients communicated more vehement feelings about this subject matter than females did. In fact, a few of the female patients were understanding and said that they would be willing to pay the office visit fee if it were something over which they had had control and if they'd had the opportunity to call the office earlier. The male participants understood the reasoning behind having such a policy, but they were less likely to be compliant about the matter.

You might have the sign at your front desk as a message to your patients, but think long and hard before sending a bill. If it should go to a patient you want to keep in your practice family, I certainly would advise against sending it!

USUAL, CUSTOMARY AND REASONABLE

UCR is the nemesis of the fee-for-service dentist. What do patients really think and how can you manage the impression of your practice in relation to this issue?

This is a complicated matter and one that is influenced by the patient's perceptions of value within the practice, their understanding of the healthcare marketplace today, the patient's dental IQ, and the skills with which the practice has educated the patient. It is difficult to manage many of those factors; however, you certainly can have an impact on the patient's dental IQ as it relates to this issue. If you effectively educate the patient about UCR and raise that patient's dental IQ to the next level, it is possible to have that patient desire treatment which is beyond the *usual, customary* and *reasonable* because there is a greater appreciation for high quality treatment.

Usual, customary and reasonable strike fear in the patient's mind as well. In focus groups, patients have indicated their concerns, "Have I been taken advantage of?" "Who do I talk to about this—the dentist, the staff, or the insurance company?" The questions go on and on and on. What they are expressing is an unsettling feeling of being in the middle and not being privy to the underlying reality. So they often believe that the "real and fair" answer lies somewhere in between the two extremes. The more you can educate a patient prior to this issue arising, the better you will be able to manage this challenge.

I have seen in several offices, printed material that aids patients in understanding their insurance coverage. Some of these pieces have been exceptionally well developed with very clear-cut explanations to patients about terms like UCR as well as information on assignment of benefits and denial of benefits or disputes over coverage. The best collateral piece I've seen along these lines was a small folder, "To My Dental Insured Patients". This was given to each patient of the practice who had dental insurance. Because this educational piece was printed on a heavier stock paper, there was a perception that, "This is something I should keep; it is valuable". Even a minor factor like the type of paper can influence the patient's perceptions. In other words, this practitioner thought enough of the patients to produce this tool which would be of help in understanding insurance issues. It is a valuable document to keep.

I've seen other pieces that list "Facts You Should Know About Dental Insurance." Some of these pieces have listed clear-cut explanations and examples of how UCR is determined and how it affects coverage. It is far better to discuss this issue early in the relationship than to deal with patients' misconceptions later.

A patient wrote to *Consumer Reports* magazine complaining that a health insurer refused to pay part of a bill, claiming the charges were "more than reasonable and customary". A response from *Consumer Reports* indicated, "If you feel that you have not been reimbursed fairly, challenge your insurer. Most insurance contracts contain a provision for appeal. If you find your policy difficult to interpret, your state's insurance department should be able to help you. Finally, if there's a lot of money at stake, you may want to consult an attorney."[4]

So, the responsibility is yours. If you want to stave off the patient concerns about your fees and UCR issues, you must:

1. Effectively educate the patient and raise the dental IQ as to the value provided by your office. Ensure that the patient knows how your office is different and recognizes the level of quality provided.

2. Prepare the patient for possible insurance company communication in relation to UCR. Prepare written information to help educate patients and offer the information in a patient-friendly manner.

3. If you produce a newsletter or promotional piece for prospective patients or patients-of-record, include information on this topic. When patients are educated by you in this continuing manner, they will better understand your position and their alternatives, if and when they are presented with an insurance problem.

4. In the event of a dispute with the insurance company, are you in a position to assist the patient in any

manner? Patients will ally with you if they see that you are on their side and wish to assist.

Most importantly, manage this issue with all new patients as they are indoctrinated into the practice family. Wait too late to do this and you can lose the faith of your patients.

THE LOCATION OF FEE DISCLOSURE

The ideal location for case presentation and fee disclosure is one of the following:

- In the treatment chair with the patient in the upright, seated position and with bib removed. The doctor should be seated facing the patient at the patient's eye level.
- In a separate consultation room.
- In the doctor's office in an informal seating area at a round table. Ensure that any participants in the discussion are able to be seated at this same table.

Choice of case presentation location can be dependent upon the demographics of the patient in question and the type of treatment being proposed. Consider the possible preferences of your patients. Business people and/or higher educated, upper income individuals will be more responsive to movement to a consultation room where they may feel more on equal footing with the practitioner who is presenting the case. An exception to this is if the case presentation is what the patient might consider to be an ordinary or standard procedure.

In our patient focus groups, we found that patients in lower income groups and/or lower educational levels tended to feel more responsive when a treatment plan was presented to them in the treatment room. These patients have indicated that moving from the treatment room to a separate consultation area tended to instill concern that they were going to be presented with higher fees or with bad news about their conditions.

All patients in all demographic groups indicated similar feelings about case presentation if there were a very high trust level in the patient or the practitioner. Patients who indicated high trust of their dentists said that the location of the case presentation was not an issue. For example, one of our focus group participants had been a patient of her doctor for over 27 years. When confronted with the concept of case presentation for two crowns, this patient said, "I trust my doctor so much it doesn't matter where he gives me this information. If he says I need two crowns, then it's not a matter of *if*, it's a matter of how will I pay for it."

If you have a consultation room, it would be wise to have a friendly *interview* with new patients in this room on the first appointment. In this way, the patient becomes acclimated to the environment in a very low-risk, non-threatening situation. Then subsequent *trips* to the consultation room will not be associated solely with fees!

THE BOTTOM LINE: SUCCESSFUL FINANCIAL ARRANGEMENTS

Confident communication in relation to fees and payment plans is crucial. Hugh Doherty, DDS, a Certified Financial Planner and retired dentist is a highly respected authority on the subject of financial control in the practice. He offers these important tips on successful financial arrangements with patients:

- Develop a financial policy with written scripts to overcome every obstacle that patients present to staff members who collect money.
- Ensure that firm financial arrangements are provided to patients in written form.
- The person collecting payments must be kind, gentle, empathetic, but most of all businesslike and professional in attitude. Not everyone collects money well; be sure to have the right person in this position!
- If you are going to extend credit, be sure to conduct a credit check with a firm like TRW.
- Streamline patient financing options for greater treatment acceptance.

The bottom line from Dr. Doherty: Maintaining a successful practice in this rapidly changing environment requires flexible payment options to increase patient affordability. Practices not offering flexible arrangements have traditionally incurred excessive labor costs. Maintaining a successful practice, requires a good conversion rate (treatment acceptance). The key to a good conversion rate is making patient treatment affordable with monthly payments.

TOP TIPS:

1. Fully educate the patient to treatment prior to quoting fee.
2. Provide a private area for fee discussions. This is absolutely *imperative*, fees should *never* be presented to patients within earshot of others.
3. Have a highly knowledgeable team member trained to present the treatment plan and fee.

4. Offer alternate payment plans to patients, including credit card payment.
5. Prioritize treatment plan to increase treatment acceptance.
6. Explain UCR to insurance patients early in the relationship.
7. Conduct a post-treatment consultation with patients to reconfirm value of the treatment and ensure patient satisfaction.

REFERENCES

[1]Frazer, Jr., DDS, Bob. "The Right Time To Discuss Fees—
Part II," *Dental Economics*, Feb., 1996.

[2] "PrideDirect" is a service offered by The Pride Institute
Greenbrae, CA. Information is available through (800) 925-
9993.

[3] Morris, JD, William Otis. *The Dentist's Legal Advisor*,
Mosby-Year, Inc., St. Louis, MO, 1995.

[4] _____, *Consumer Reports*, Yonkers, NY, November,
1991.

20

Patient-Friendly Practice Marketing

"The way to gain a good reputation is to endeavor to be what you desire to appear."

— S O C R A T E S

During the morning break at a meeting where I was speaking, I overheard two doctors discussing direct mail. One of them said, "Yeah, I'm thinking about doing one of those mailers that goes out to all the zip codes in my area. I've seen the numbers, and the costs are pretty low considering how many homes you reach." The tone of his voice, the attitude he took while talking about this and the balance of the conversation that I heard made me think, "Here's another doctor who is going to throw money at what he hopes will be an easy and quick fix to get bodies in the front door." Is this marketing? Of a sort. Is it effective marketing? It's doubtful. In the discussion, I heard no reasons that indicated understanding of the market or of the needs of the market.

The effectiveness of your marketing depends in a large part on understanding the attitudes and perspectives of your patients. You must truly understand the mind set of your patients. What is appropriate marketing for you depends on your locale, your client base, their socio-economic levels and so on. Every community is different. How well do you truly understand your patients? There are numerous books on this subject that can provide you with endless ideas on how to market to patients. Be careful in the approach you take. What may sound good to you may not be effective for *your* patients.

GAINING A PERSPECTIVE OF YOUR MARKET: ADVICE FROM AN EXPERT

One of the most important steps you can take in determining what will be the most productive and cost effective marketing for you is to conduct a needs analysis of your market and to understand the demographics of your area. Joe Lancellotti is a marketing consultant who has extensive experience helping dental practices dynamically position themselves in their markets. He emphasizes the importance of developing a solid marketing plan. In his strategic planning sessions with practitioners, Lancellotti suggests that the wise practice evaluate the strengths, weaknesses, opportunities and threats that affect the lifeblood of the practice.[1] Any successful marketing plan is built on a solid foundation and understanding the market must come first. Once understood, you can devise the tactics to effectively reach your target markets.

"You don't need to wait to do a full scale market needs analysis", says Lancellotti. He suggests, "the easiest way to begin your investigation is through addressing the five W's:

1. **Who:**
   - Who are your current patients?
   - Who are your potential patients?
   - Who are your competitors?
   - Who are your key team members?

2 **What:**
   - What products and services are you offering to consumers in your market?
   - What is your estimated share of your market?
   - What are the most effective systems you use in the practice?

3. **Where:**
   - Where do current patients live?
   - From where will you draw future patients?

4 **When:**
   - When do you experience your best months?
   - When do you experience your worst months?

5. **Why:**
   - Why do patients come to your practice?

Lancellotti states that of the five W's the last, *why,* is the most important. Do you really know why patients choose your office as opposed to other dental practices in your community? I certainly agree that this is the most important question of the five. Can you definitively list the top five reasons? Are these the *best* reasons for patients to come to your office? If not, perhaps you have not communicated your greatest strengths effectively enough to your patients.

PLAINSPOKEN TRUTH FROM THE PATIENT'S POINT-OF-VIEW

Here's the patient's reality. This is a picture painted with a very broad brush. I propose here some general statements based on extensive feedback we have received in focus groups. The balance of this chapter will provide more information and illustrations to back up these points:

- Patients respond to internal marketing more positively than external marketing.
- Perceptions of clinical excellence by a practice are in inverse proportion to the amount of external marketing conducted by that practice as perceived by high-income, highly educated patients.
- Patients who are attracted to discounted dentistry or who use coupons because of discounts or specials do not perceive the quality of dentistry to be as high as if they had paid full fee.

I do have a bias against extensive, expensive external marketing. These perspectives are not mine alone, however. Because of the number of patients I survey, I am strongly influenced by the attitudes and preferences I hear from them. Therefore, my attitudes are closer to midstream than being on either end of the scale.

PATIENT FRIENDLY MARKETING FOR THE SQUEAMISH

I can see it, feel it, and hear it. In the team meeting following a mystery patient visit I also address the most effective forms of internal marketing to patients. That's when it starts. It starts with crossing and uncrossing the knees, squirming in the chairs, eye contact avoidance, and a lot of *yes, buts* . . . Many dental teams do not feel comfortable with the idea of marketing. The verbalized message I hear is often, "Well, I don't really feel at ease in *selling* the practice to patients; I'm afraid they'll be offended." Some staff members say, "I don't want to come on too strongly." The issue is frequently wrapped in the word *uncomfortable*.

This is an enormously important subject and one that needs to be addressed openly in any office that harbors this concern. Sometimes a challenge like this can be managed with a fresh outlook. I suggest that if you *don't* market your practice, then you may be doing your patients a *disservice*. This statement must be tempered, in that the marketing must be handled in a patient friendly manner and it must be practice friendly also! Take the following example that illustrates the concept.

We conducted a survey of patients for a private practice. A segment of the survey was designed to determine the patient's knowledge about services offered. Patients were given a list of services and treatments, all offered by the practice. Patients were asked:

1. Which of these services/treatments are currently offered by this office?

2. Which of these services would you like to know more about?

The responses were startling. We learned that a significant percentage of the patients did not know the office already offered some of the services and treatments for which patients wanted more information. I'll put this another way. A serious number of patients were unaware of what the practice was already doing. These same patients were interested in getting additional information on these treatments! You may be wondering, what were the treatments? Those at the top of the list were: anti-snoring devices, bonding, veneers, and whitening. Some patients even wrote comments at the end of the survey like, "I'd like more information on anti-snoring devices for my husband/wife." (The request was consistently for the spouse!)

The point I make is not relative to specific treatments but to the need to provide patients with information which they will appreciate and find valuable. Patients of this practice might have gone elsewhere for these services because they didn't even know they were offered by the practitioner. Likewise, you have a responsibility to provide your patients with the information that may be valuable to them. Don't prejudge what services you think the patient would find valuable. Give them information. Educate your patients. Raise the dental IQ of the patient. Market in a patient friendly manner. Making opportunities happen starts then.

Third-Person Credibility

In advertising, a frequent way of building credibility with a reader or TV viewer is through the concept of third-person credibility. This is a method by which an advertiser speaks to us through a third party. This third party is one that typically has a high profile and is well respected. An example of this concept might be the following fabricated scenario:

> *Michelin Tires may want to market direct-*
> *ly to us. However, they recognize that*
> *direct marketing is not nearly as credible*
> *as a referral from a trusted individual.*
> *Consequently, they choose a public*
> *spokesperson who is knowledgeable, ethi-*
> *cal, and well respected. In this case*
> *Michelin Tires might choose someone like*
> *Paul Newman, who as a race-car driver*
> *has knowledge about the subject of tires.*
> *He is recognized readily due to his movie-*

*star status and is known for his high
ethics. When Paul Newman speaks to us
about Michelin Tires, we want to believe
him. The message is more palatable and
credible coming from him than coming
directly from the promoting company.*

Let's take this into dentistry. Third-person credibility is extremely powerful when relating what other patients say about the practitioners, the practice, and the treatments offered. This concept should be discussed and understood by every team member. This also requires understanding your client base, how they *do* feel about you, what they *do* say about you. Effective use of this concept also requires that the staff have very strong, "gut-level" beliefs in the entire practice. When using third-person credibility, the communication must be made from a place of great belief. Otherwise, it can be perceived as an attempt at being manipulative.

An example of positive use of third-person credibility in the dental office might be:

*A patient-of-record has had a clinical
exam during which dental implants were
discussed and proposed. The patient is
mulling this over out loud at the counter,
while the team member prepares the
patient's statement. The front-desk person
comments, "We just had two patients last
week who were talking about how pleased
they were with their implants. Both of
them were talking about how much more
comfortable it was to eat and how good
they felt about their appearance. It is really wonderful to hear patients talk about
what a difference that these implants can
make in their lives."*

This is a very low-key, understated way of promoting treatment in a patient-friendly manner. It builds confidence for the patient. It is a message that patients want to hear and it gains importance when the staff member is quoting other patients.

INTERNAL VS. EXTERNAL MARKETING

A business was failing and a consultant conducted a survey of company clients. On conclusion of the survey, the consultant suggested, "Start advertising and use three media: radio, direct mail, and courtesy. The first two will cost money, the third is free but is the most important."

Patients we've surveyed express greater receptivity to all forms of internal marketing than to any form of external marketing. Focus group participants frequently blur the line between marketing internally and customer or patient services. As one group participant put it, "What's going to keep me coming back to an office is the quality of service. Can I depend on these people? Do they really care about me, or am I a number? Of course I want them to be technically proficient, but I *do* want the service to go along with it."

It was the service, he went on to say, that would keep him going back to the office and would increase the likelihood of his giving referrals to friends. He related a very frequent comment— patients like to feel proud of the offices that they refer. Patients who refer friends or family to your office, want these referred patients to leave your practice with a "WOW" feeling. It's like a pat on the back for the referring patient.

Having heard patients talk about this subject matter at length, I am convinced that those doctors who spend a significant amount of money on external marketing might do well first to look more closely at the practice. The money that is going out from the practice might not be cost-effective and might actually be working against them. Instead, I suggest that every dental practice take a long hard look at internal forms of marketing. These will have a more immediate impact on all patients, result in increased referrals, and be more likely to aid in significant patient retention.

ADVERTISING

On the whole, advertising was looked upon skeptically by a significant percentage of focus group patients. This was true in all demographics, but the most dramatic responses were those from high socioeconomic groups. Many verbalized their feelings like this, "There is a reason that the doctor is advertising. He or she doesn't have enough business and is trying to cover overhead by getting new patients. That might make me worry about quality and *why* they need to advertise." If your goal is to seek a highly sophisticated patient base, then advertising and direct mail marketing generally will not appeal to this group.

Some of the patient thoughts about why a dentist would advertise included:

- This is a young doctor who is just getting started.
- This is a doctor who doesn't have enough patients and is actively trying to grow the practice.
- This is a doctor who can't keep the patients he/she has.

One middle management advertising copywriter noted,

> *My guess is that the ones who advertise in newspapers or flyers are either new dentists who are trying to build a practice or an established dentist who is on rocky*

*ground financially. In any case I don't
want to go to that office.*

This person also remarked that the only way she
might even look at the ad was if it were well designed
graphically, but that in many cases the actual copy seemed
to be written for a less sophisticated audience.

Patients have mixed feelings about the idea of the
dental practice advertising its services. There is one basic
truth that arose regardless of socioeconomic group: there
was a basic skepticism about practices that advertise or use
flyers to promote their services.

You might ask, "So what's the difference between
patient perceptions of a newsletter vs. perceptions of an
advertising flyer? Do they fall in the same grouping in the
patients' minds?" No, they don't. Patients perceive "soft"
marketing—that which is presented in an educational and
patient friendly way—is more professional and appealing
than any form of "hard" marketing. A newsletter is seen by
patients as a form of soft marketing. A flyer is understood
to be direct marketing with a sole purpose of soliciting
new business.

It was interesting that even though the lower
socioeconomic groups recognized this reality, many
indicated that because of the lower fees they would still
take advantage of the services. Therefore, though they
might be skeptical about the doctor or the practice, there
was some degree of acceptance because of the cost
savings.

This same demographic group often remarked on
the photos that were used as well as the coupons that
were included. In one focus group, as the patients viewed
flyers and promotional pieces, they expressed some
amusement at the photographs indicating, "Well, she's a
model, I know the doctor didn't do her teeth!" Another
patient looked at a doctors picture and commented, "Do
you think the doctor's going to look that happy in person

when I come in with this coupon? I doubt it, because I'm not paying the full, regular amount!" The more educated and the higher socioeconomic group of patients were even more skeptical about the clinical skills and the cleanliness of these offices. Their collective thinking was along these lines, "If the office is spending money on a flyer that looks like this, they obviously need patients. Are they cutting corners somewhere?"

As most consumers today, I receive mailers with promotions of dental practices. Periodically I make an appointment or conduct a "drop in" visit. My interest is in determining how congruent this practice is with their image on paper. I received an unusual promotional piece in the mail. It was a four-color piece that included coupons and numerous pictures of the office, the doctors, and the team. I was intrigued with what I saw on paper and made an appointment. The entire team looked so friendly and energetic in their pictures; I hoped this also would be the reality.

I was pleasantly surprised with the office when I arrived. The location was convenient, the building was well maintained and attractive on the outside, the decor of the facility was pleasant, and the receptionist was welcoming. My appointment was for a cleaning and a clinical exam. The hygienist was friendly, although almost too "chatty". It was the dentist who concerned me. He was not congruent with what I saw in the photograph. The "friendly doctors" who would help eliminate any "anxiety or patient concerns" did not seem to be in evidence during my visit. The doctor who was smiling so agreeably in the photograph was not so agreeable in the visit! He communicated in an abrupt manner with the assistant who was in the room during the exam. I recognized her from the picture and she was certainly not smiling during this exam. The doctor's focus was on the file and there was little warmth from this man.

The likelihood was great that patients who might enter this office based on what they saw in the flyer and based on the positive first impression on sight, might feel let down with the coldness experienced during the clinical exam.

Walk your talk. Be consistent. This office lost credibility because they were not in reality who they presented themselves to be on paper. As you look at putting yourself together on paper your first responsibility, from the patient's point-of-view, is to "be real". Don't present yourself as something that you are not.

Think long and hard before putting a lot of money into direct mail pieces. Will you be making the statement you want to make about your practice? Will you be attracting the type of patients you want to your practice?

THE SPECIAL THAT IS NOT A SPECIAL

A trend that I see in dental practice marketing that concerns me relates to some "specials" that are offered. In many cases, these specials are not really specials! Frequently, an advertisement, flyer, or coupon may offer a consultation that is "valued at over $125.00." But the reality is that throughout the profession it is recognized that consultations of the type being marketed are not typically fee-based. This is misleading to patients. I find the practice questionable and have asked about some of these marketing pieces in patient focus groups.

Let's take, for example, promotion of an orthodontic consultation for prospective patients. Those focus group participants who had been through orthodontic treatment or who had children in orthodontic treatment recognized that most often the initial visit with a prospective patient is on a no-fee basis. These patients responded very negatively to this promotional technique. Patients who were not familiar with this concept responded far more favorably. The point is this, you might get the patient in the door with this concept, but once the patient becomes more aware of the reality, the use of this promotional approach may reflect negatively on you and the perception of your ethics.

Picture this, an individual receives your coupon or flyer by mail that promotes such a "special." It looks like a good deal to the reader and she mentions it to her neighbor. Her neighbor comments, "I'd be careful about that, nobody charges for that type of appointment. If you are interested in a consultation for braces, you can go to any doctor you choose." Ask yourself, how would you respond at this point?

YELLOW PAGES AND MAGAZINE ADS

In a written survey we conducted of dental patients in 1994, we asked about the most effective way of locating a dental office that offered high clinical skills. This survey was followed by extensive focus group analysis. It was not a surprise that personal referrals by friends and family led the list and print ads fell to the bottom of the list, along with flyers and mailers. Those patients who used Yellow Pages for dental selection fell into one of three categories.

• Patients who were selecting an office with a convenient location.

• Patients who were seeking an office that offered emergency treatment, extended hours, acceptance of credit cards, multi-lingual staff, or assorted other specialized treatments or circumstances.

• Patients who were seeking a telephone number for a dental office they had already selected.

Some dentists hurt their practice image by their design of a display Yellow Page advertisement. That is, they opt to promote treatments, location, emergency treatments, etc. as their primary attractions. These may be key factors in getting a patient's attention for a specific situation; however, they do not effectively market the practice. Consider what kind of patient you want to attract. Are you seeking loyal patients-of-record? Are you wanting to develop relationships with your patients and thereby build your practice through referrals? Or, does your advertisement result in a revolving door of "one-shot" patients? Again, the type of patient with whom you are going to build a long-term relationship is not one who is frequently reached via advertisements; there *are* always exceptions that prove this rule. Taking the devil's advocate position however, many patients will look at advertisements with a questioning mind.

Every city I visit as a speaker, I peruse the Yellow Pages in my hotel room. I am amazed at some of the ads that I see! Suffice to say, if you are going to create a display ad, have it designed professionally. The larger the advertisement is, the more crucial this is. Bear in mind, patients perceive dentistry as an honored and highly respected profession. Ads of questionable taste or judgment will reflect on the patient's perception of the practitioner's clinical skills.

If you are considering advertising in a magazine, carefully study the readership of the publication. Does it represent the profile of your client base, or of your targeted client base? The most tastefully displayed ads in magazines I have seen have appeared in the city or regional magazines, like *Texas Monthly*. Such publications typically attract a middle-to-high socio-economic group. Study some of the advertisements that you see in these publications. Particularly, look at advertisements for organizations that are involved with the creative arts, interior design, high-end furniture stores, etc. They can provide insight into the kind of graphic design that are effective in a display ad. More often than not, advertisements lean toward the "too busy in text and graphic elements." If you are going to advertise, keep it simple, keep it clean; it has a more tasteful appearance.

MARKETING OPPORTUNITIES THAT FLOAT BY—CARPE DIEM!

Every practice I visit I experience the "lost opportunity". These are the situations that are either passive and relate to the office environment or active and relate to communication issues. The passive environmental opportunities might be as simple as an office not having its brochures or newsletters on display and available to patients in reception. Examples of these opportunities are spread throughout this book.

It's the active, or communications opportunities that can be the most significant and, if I were the practitioner, would concern me most. I think of these as "vapor moments." They float through the air and the moment is lost. Typically team members are so involved in procedures, clinical or nonclinical, that they are unaware that the moment has even passed! Sometimes I throw out "opportunity bait" to see if it will be recognized; and all too often it is not. I promise you that opportunities abound! This is the part of my work as a mystery patient that I love the most. These countless little unseen opportunities are like unpolished gems lying just under the surface. You just need to see them and polish them up a bit! They are happening every day in your office and so many of them are slipping by. Recognizing them comes first, then the team must know how to capture the moments and act on them in a patient friendly manner.

Here are some examples. Test these on the rest of the team and (1) see if the opportunity is recognized, and (2) how the team would capture the opportunity in a patient friendly manner:

• A new patient arrives for an exam. She and her husband have just moved from another state and they have school-age children. She was referred to the doctor by one of her neighbors. Yours is a family practice.

This one is rather obvious, yet no matter how many times I've posed this same situation as an undercover patient, I've never had any team member verbalize an invitation to other family members. (I promise that it's not because I've played an obnoxious patient!)

This amazes me! This new patient should be warmly welcomed to the state and the practice. As a part of building rapport with a patient it's natural to communicate interest in the individual without being perceived as prying. Also, most parents are delighted to talk about their children given the opportunity. A warm invitation to the rest of the family with reassuring words about the team's skills with children would be typically welcomed by a parent.

• A patient calls and inquires about the practice and the doctor. The caller relates a few details about painful experiences in past dental offices and expresses his fear of injections and associated pain. He is tentative about making an appointment, saying he'll think about it and will call back later.

Invite the caller to come by the office. Frequently a brief visit can turn a visitor from a prospective patient to a new patient. Numerous readers, no doubt, are groaning with this one, "No way can we handle this kind of situation!" Here's the reality: in the majority of cases, callers won't come in! But the fact that you offered is rare and remarkable—just through the invitation you've set yourself apart. If the patient does want to drop-in, then set a time preferably during your slower hours. Rapport can be built more easily face-to-face than on the phone. Also, we have found in focus groups that a fearful patient who finds a practitioner with whom a trusting relationship can be developed is a very loyal patient and one likely to refer to others. This investment is worthwhile.

• A patient indicates an interest in having her teeth whitened. She brings it up when she sees your counter card about the treatment at the front desk. She asks for brochures but your supply has been depleted and you don't have one for her to take with her. This is a long term patient of record who has a high dental IQ and is willing to invest in such treatment.

"That's easy!" you might say. But do you go past the obvious into a patient friendly way of marketing the practice? This requires a more detailed process than the two examples above. Here are the steps you could follow in this situation:

(1) Offer to mail a pamphlet as soon as your supply comes in. Be sure it is stamped with your name and phone number on the back.

(2) Ask the patient if she would be interested in seeing some photos of results with other patients (Show results that increase interest and desire, instead of showing the "tools of the process")

(3) If a team member has experienced this, address the way she/he felt on completion of the process, or relate the responses of other satisfied patients.

(4) Mail the brochure and be sure to attach a personalized note to the patient. Indicate you'll follow up with a call to answer any questions the patient might have (and to hopefully schedule an appointment.)

(5) Call the patient within five working days of the patient having received the pamphlet. Tell the patient you're calling to follow up on the questions that the pam-

phlet might have raised. In the context of the conversation, raise the issue of making an appointment to start the process. The thrust of the conversation needs to be service-oriented, the thinking being, "I want to provide you with information and ensure that you have your questions answered about this matter that you have expressed interest in." This must be handled adroitly to ensure that the patient believes that you are attending to the patient's interests and not solely the interests of the practice!

This same process could be followed with a prospective patient who indicates an interest in this treatment. In this case, also include any other collateral materials you may be able to offer about the practice—a newsletter if you have one. In your note indicate an interest in treating the individual as a regular patient.

WHERE'S WALDO®?

Where's the opportunity for you and for your practice? It's like the children's illustrated game of "Where's Waldo®?" How many drawings of this character can the child find hidden in the elaborate illustration? Likewise, can you see the opportunities hidden in each patient interaction?

In every phone call, in every patient visit, and with every team member, realize:

• There *is* an opportunity. Sometimes it will present itself, sometimes it must be sought.

• Once the opportunity is recognized, decide how it can be developed and acted upon in a patient-friendly manner.

PATIENT PROTECTION AS FRIENDLY PROMOTION

There are opportunities that may not be seen as "typical" marketing situations. Recognizing the opportunities that exist surrounding the issues of patient protection are exceedingly important for the entire team. Often the office looks on procedures related to sterilization and infection control as just that, procedures. Rather than being seen as mundane, they might be viewed in a new light. If the team members could take off their "clinical hats" and view the office from the patient's point-of-view, they would recognize that there are a multitude of educational and promotional opportunities presented here.

A general dentist had hired me to come in under cover and to experience the office from the patient's point-of-view. I was having my teeth cleaned by the hygienist. She had placed on the tray in front of me a slim, hinged, metal box that contained the instruments. A large percentage of the offices that I visit use individually wrapped instruments. Patients in focus groups recognize sterilized equipment when the team member rips open a sterilized bag in front of them. This metal tray might not be as readily recognized by patients. Therefore, I asked her about it and I was curious whether she would recognize the opportunity within my question.

"What's the deal with this box?" I asked. "I've never seen one of those before." What's important about recognizing this type of question is that it may also be an indicator that the patient is concerned about sterilization and so the education of the new patient is particularly important here. She responded, "It's just a container that helps us organize our instruments and lay them out so that they may be picked up more easily." Not one word was mentioned about sterilization. That was the end of that conversation! She moved the discussion in another direction at this point. I was amazed.

This was an opportunity missed. Instead, she could have taken this as an opportunity to promote the high level of patient protection offered in this office. Combined with effective patient education she could have built my confidence in her, the doctor, and the entire practice. But it was a "vapor moment," not to be recognized and not to be retrieved.

In the staff meeting that follows a mystery visit I typically discuss the opportunities that occurred during my appointment and the opportunities that exist in general within the practice. The purpose is to raise team awareness that these opportunities *do* exist and that they must be acted upon in the most effective manner for both the patient and the practice. In this staff meeting we discussed this specific opportunity and how each team member plays a part in raising the patient's awareness level, the patient's dental IQ, and promoting the practice in a patient-friendly manner.

One dentist exhibited a very high awareness of promotional opportunities in the area of patient protection. Dr. Mitch Moore of Austin, TX related to me that a patient visited his office and commented on all of the steps his office took to ensure patient safety and a sterile environment. The patient was so impressed that he commented to the doctor, "You really ought to invite someone from the press out here to see your office. With all the concerns about patient safety today, I think that you'd get a lot of interest."

The doctor wisely responded, "It would probably mean more to the press if that suggestion came from a patient, rather than the doctor!" With that, the patient contacted a local television station with his suggestion. The TV station sent a crew to the dental office, interviewed the doctor and video taped all of the different ways in which a patient is protected in this office. The segment was newsworthy, and the TV station was providing an educational opportunity to its viewing audience.

Dr. Moore received numerous positive, inquiry calls following the showing of this news segment. He also requested a copy of the tape for use in his office. Using video hookup to his intraoral camera for patient education, he made sure that all new patients who entered the practice were shown this video to help them understand the level of care provided and the level of patient safety in the office. With continued use of this video, Dr. Moore has noted a significant increase in new patient referrals. This is certainly a testimony to the effectiveness of high standards of patient protection and excellent patient education. This is marketing in the most positive sense for patients and for practice.

NEWSLETTERS

In our focus groups we've shown patients many types of newsletters from dental practices. Their responses vary quite widely on this based on the demographic group and even within a group. However, there was one issue which came up with all groups—and that was the matter of newsletter cost. Regardless of the group demographics a comment that was frequently made was, "They're producing this newsletter and they're sending it out to all their patients but I'm paying for it." A comment which would frequently fall on the heels of that statement would be, "Why don't they just forget the newsletter and reduce the fees!"

You can bet your patients won't express this to you! Once we got past that point we would discuss the pros and cons of the practice having a newsletter and the do's and don'ts of what should be in the newsletter. We would ask patients, "How many of you would read the newsletter?" A common response was, "It depends on how long it is and the content."

In order for patients to feel the newsletter is cost effective, it must be newsworthy to them. What news do you have to offer your patients that aids in justifying the costs of your newsletter? What do you *need* to tell them that will be helpful to the patients. This could be something related to your office, your location, or current dental issues. Have you recently added equipment which will be of benefit to patients? If so, tell them, but tell them in such a way that they understand the benefits to them instead of thinking about the cost of the equipment to you. For example, "One of the benefits of our new intraoral camera is that it will offer faster communication with your insurance provider. When they can *see* the condition, the likelihood of coverage increases."

Another example would be if there is road construction going on near your property, can you forewarn patients about this and offer an alternative route to take to your office. This is helpful information and patients will appreciate your thinking about it and meeting their needs ahead of time.

These may be little things but they are the little things that say you can anticipate the patient's concerns and you want to alleviate any anxiety before it occurs. If you have conducted a survey of patients in your office, your newsletter is a wonderful place to inform patients of the results. Let them know what you learned and how you are going to act upon it. The bottom line is this:

- Make sure that you include information the patient needs to know and (for the patient) justifies the cost of this collateral piece.

• Address topics that relate to your practice and to patient health. (Fig. 20-1)

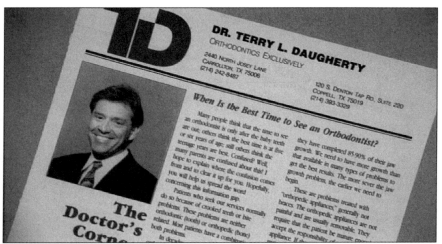

Fig. 20-1 An effective newsletter has a clean look, is visually pleasing, and easy to read. It's sent to current and prospective patients, and placed in the reception area for pass-along and referral purposes. (Courtesy Terry Daugherty, D.D.S.)

The topics that made the most sense to patients were health related and most especially, oral health. Patients particularly appreciated educational tips that were short, snappy, easy to read, and gave them valuable information they could use. One newsletter had incorporated a *USA Today* type graphic that addressed a single topic, showed related statistics, and had a patient tip along with it. The patients really liked this approach because it was easy to read, fun, and patient-friendly.

They did not like hard promotion. They commented that soft promotional approach would be appropriate and understandable. However, this is much like the issue that was addressed in *on-hold* informational tapes. The same topics that they responded to well in the *on-hold* tapes are also appropriate for inclusion in newsletters.

The topics that you cover need to make sense to the patient. As a healthcare provider, you are seen by your patients as an expert in the area of oral health and a highly knowledgeable and aware professional in the areas of health overall. These are the topics which will make the most sense coming from you in your newsletter. They are the areas in which you have the greatest credibility with your patients.

Another marketing concept relating to newsletters is their use with referring offices. Specialty offices should forward or deliver additional newsletters to the offices of their referring general dentists. The referring office may effectively use these to aid in educating their patients and as an informative tool to introduce a patient to your office prior to, or in conjunction with, treatment. In this manner you are helping your colleague and also increasing the confidence of the prospective patient toward your practice. This same approach may be taken in relation to brochures.

Outflow = Inflow: What Do Patients Think?

Some experts think that as long as patients are receiving materials from the office then they "have a dentist". The marketing philosophy at work here is, the more the office sends *out*, the more patients will come *in*. Some doctors believe that it is not important that the patient reads the newsletter, but that it identifies the patient as "part of the family."

It's an interesting concept, and one that may work with some mainstream businesses. However, when queried about this in relation to the mailing of newsletters, birthday cards, etc., there are typically a number of cynics in a focus group. They make statements like, "Why don't they just save the money and stop increasing our fees," "I know the birthday cards are just pumped out by the computer—it's not such a personal statement to me." Male patients typically offer these responses more than female patients.

More meaningful to both genders is the quality of service and care provided on the phone and during appointments. If the patient feels special to the practice it is more meaningful than being a part of a mass mailing. If you are able to instill that *special* feeling in your newsletter or birthday card, wonderful! If inquiries or referral calls increase after such a mailing, great! If you get a high percentage of positive comments following such a mailing, then don't change a thing. Your approach works for you and your patients.

But if you get no such response, then think twice about it. You may be investing in something that is not cost effective for you. Worse, if your mailings are too frequent, you may irritate patients or place concerns in their minds about costs of these items in relation to your fees. There's the pro and con of the issue from the patient's point-of-view. Make the decision based on your market, your clients, and your practice. A piece that offers valuable information, is patient friendly without a lot of technical terms, is well designed and does not look terribly expensive, and is mailed no more than two times a year may be an effective way of staying in touch with your patients.

THE COMMERCIAL NEWSLETTER THAT YOU CUSTOMIZE

There are also newsletters that can be purchased for practice use. Some are ready to mail and may be stamped or imprinted with your practice name and address. Others may be a shell with the outside preprinted and the inside for customization by the practice. Either of these methods can offer a high quality look that would probably be far more expensive for you to create on your own. As with anything else, there are pros and cons to the concepts. The newsletter that is totally preprinted doesn't speak to matters specific to your practice or patients. I've seen some of them that are quite beautiful with four-color photographs, interesting articles, and are printed on quality paper. However, they are not effective in marketing your specific practice. You can place them in your reception area, but they don't have the "pass-around" referral quality that a customized piece has. The commercial newsletter you customize is more effective in promoting your practice. If you want to use your newsletter as a serious marketing piece, then create your own.

USE AND PLACEMENT OF MARKETING PIECES

Development of a brochure is discussed at length in chapter 10 on practice identity. Once you have the piece, what do you do with it? Obviously it should be sent to all prospective and new patients, but I experience numerous situations where an office has brochures and doesn't get full use from them.

You may have a marketing piece that was extremely expensive to produce and you don't want to be arbitrary about its use or you may want to control the dissemination of the material in it. Then consider creating a less expensive, one page bio/flyer that can be offered more widely and increase your reach. It could be one sheet printed on one side and offer basic information on your office. Just make sure that it is well designed and congruent with your office and consistent with the balance of your collateral materials.

These pieces need to be:

- Placed in a highly visible, stand-up pamphlet holder in your reception area.
- Positioned at the reception counter and available to visitors as well as patients who are leaving.
- Offered to referring dentists or any type of office that may refer to you; this is far preferable to the referring office than just handing out a business card.
- Included in any welcoming packet sent to patients.
- Offered to patients who mention possibly referring another person.

Newsletters should be made available in the very same manner. Overprint newsletters for these very purposes.

WELCOME PACKET

Many offices send a welcome packet to new patients. The timing of the packet should be sent so that it reaches the patient prior to the first appointment. The purpose of the packet should be to introduce the patient to the practice, to instill confidence in the practice, and to help the patient look forward to this first visit.[2] From the patient's perspective, those are the most important criteria relating to this packet. Any other purposes for mailing this packet should be secondary to those stated above. In other words, the purpose of the packet should *not* be primarily to send the new patient forms so that you can have them made out prior to the appointment. That may be a goal of yours but it is not the primary goal of the patient. This also should be a secondary goal of the practice.

The feeling that the patient has upon receipt of the packet should be: "This office is warm, welcoming, and recognizes the importance of its patients. I feel valued by them." A very important response by the patient upon receipt of the packet is also hopefully, "I can already tell that this dental practice is different and special."

Elements to be included in the welcoming packet are:

- Customized welcoming letter
- Practice brochure
- Appointment card
- Business card
- Infection control information (generic brochure or educational material from your office)
- Patient history/information form
- Optional: newsletter
- Optional: self-addressed stamped envelope if you request forms to be mailed back to you prior to the appointment

If the patient asked questions about specific treatments on the phone, be sure to include an informational pamphlet on the subject when you send the welcome packet. The benefit of doing this is:

- It tells patients you are really listening to them on the phone.
- It says you are interested in being of service and educating patients.

- It gets the patient thinking about the treatment more deeply.
- It can offer the perfect bridge to initiate further discussion with the patient during the appointment.

Make sure that *anything* sent to patients includes your name, address, and phone number. This includes any generic brochures like promotional or educational items on whitening, implants, and sterilization, etc. You may consider purchasing a stamp for the backs of these generic brochures though an adhesive label which has been professionally printed looks better and can be used on more items than just paper products.

Congruence and consistency is key in whatever you do in your practice. Patients are going to be looking at who you say you are on paper, who you say you are on the phone, and then evaluating their reality of these issues. Make sure in putting your presence on paper that you are presenting a practice which will be congruent when the patient visits your office.

ON-HOLD PROMOTIONAL TAPES

In seminars I conduct, the topic of marketing often is raised in relation to discussions of telephone on-hold promotional tapes. Because of the increasing interest by professionals in this form of marketing, we presented the concept to patients. (See chapter 11.) In several focus groups we played demo tapes to patients to determine their likes and dislikes.

One of the tapes took a pointedly advertising position. When the focus group patients heard, "Ask us about X-brand whitener. In just two weeks you'll see a difference ..." they groaned. One woman said, "With that comment, I'd turn the tape off in my head—the office just lost my respect because they sound desperate, like they're pushing treatments."

Another tape addressed the same topic but used a more patient-friendly, educational approach. "These are some foods that can stain your teeth: coffee, tea, blueberries . . . if you would like more information on this or on our whitening process, we'll be happy to talk with you about it during your next visit." Patients commented that this was interesting because it was informative, even though they understood that it was also promotional. They responded more positively because they weren't "listening to an advertisement," as one man put it.

Topics that are patient-friendly in *on hold* tapes include:[3]

- Dentist's background: education and experience
- Team background: education and experience
- Continuing education of the entire team
- Infection control procedures
- New developments in oral healthcare
- New office technology that results in higher levels of patient care or comfort
- Tips on dental care: these can include soft promotion of in-office treatments, but educational tips should precede the promotional information
- Achievements earned, awards or honors the practice may have won
- Office hours, location, directions to the office
- Updates on issues patients may have seen addressed on TV or heard on radio
- Practice philosophy and/or mission statement
- Introduction of new employees
- Affiliations with other organizations (ADA, local, state societies)
- Affiliations or sponsorships the practice provides (Supporter of local school team)

This list could go on and on. The important point is that the issues addressed must be patient-friendly and promote the practice in a non-aggressive manner. Blatant advertising can do just the opposite from what you intend. Patients said it best, "You can go over the line, if you push too hard. It seems unprofessional for a dental practice." Advertising and marketing are the flip sides of the same coin. Package your message so it's palatable to the patient; wrap it up in patient education and your message will be received more readily.

In discussing the issue of on-hold tapes I have been asked more than once by doctors, "What if we put the patients on hold just so that they can hear this tape?" Interestingly, patients in focus groups verbalized the fear of this. Some stated, "I am afraid when I hear that tape that they are putting me on hold on purpose!" We are dealing with differences in people, differences in the approaches on the tapes, and the length of time that patients are put on hold, as well. This is not a black or white issue, there is a lot of gray here. Ideally, patients would be put on hold so seldom, and for such a short time, that the only likelihood of their coming to such a negative response would be if they heard a segment of the tape that was particularly hard-hitting in terms of aggressive promotion.

EDUCATIONAL PRESENTATIONS

Offering programs to the general public, or even to your own patient base can be a highly effective means of promoting your practice in a patient-friendly manner. The exposure alone in promotion of the event can be helpful in getting your name to the public. When you present a seminar of any length to a group, you are seen as the expert and are likely to find an increase in inquiries as a result. Be aware that the type of sponsoring organization will have an impact on the type of audience and consequently inquiries you will get. Association with a high profile healthcare group or event can produce high quality prospects. (Fig. 20-2 and 20-3)

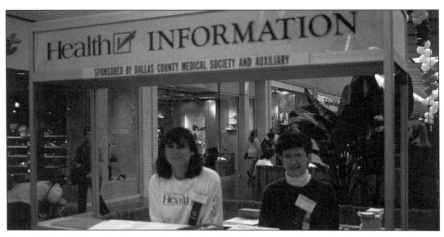

Fig. 20-2 This entry to a major health fair at an upscale, regional mall attracts prospective patients. Doctors are available for demonstrations and consultations. This creates community goodwill, increases public health education and information, and offers volunteers opportunities to connect with prospective patients.

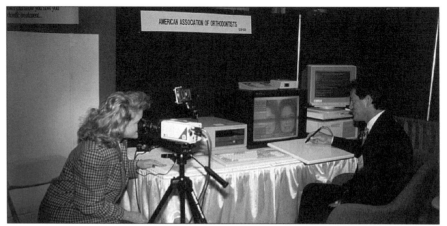

FIG. 20-3 Patients experience "imaging" in the booth sponsored by the American Association of Orthodontists.

Although you may not at first feel comfortable with this option of marketing your practice, you need to know that:

1. The anxiety you may feel CAN be overcome. There are plenty of resources to help you handle this and get those butterflies flying in formation.[4]

2. It is a highly effective means to promote your practice and one that can be a very worthwhile investment of your time. Dr. Frank Edwards, marketing guru, states that the combination of a strong brochure and a good presentation can be the most effective means of promoting your practice.[5]

Your presentation needs to be to the point, educational, but also give you the opportunity to showcase your interpersonal skills. You want the audience to leave knowing that you are a sincerely caring practitioner who has the needs of the patient in mind. Prospects who talk with you after the program will be judging your sincerity by how you respond to them in a one-on-one basis.

I attended a public seminar that was held in conjunction with a citywide event at the local convention center. A doctor offered a seminar on dental implants which I attended. He had excellent slides, discussed his experience with this treatment, encouraged questions from the audience, and showed his caring attitude via the sensitivity of his answers. He also exhibited a sense of humor which kept the audience involved and interested; it made him more approachable and likable.

This event attracted a significant number of patients in the senior age groups. His seminar was well-attended, with a number of individuals talking with him on conclusion of the program. He also had collateral materials available for all to take home. These handouts were educational in nature and subtle in promotion—a patient-friendly way to approach such an opportunity.

For those who treat a high percentage of children, school programs are an excellent way to connect with prospective patients. Sending materials home with students can aid in increasing parent interest.

An organization that has achieved a high degree of success in educating young audiences is the Dental Health Theater in St. Louis. MO. It is sponsored by the Foundation of the Greater St. Louis Dental Society. The theater conducts informative and entertaining presentations for school groups. The variety of presentations includes puppet shows, film clips, and oral healthcare demonstrations in a setting of mammoth size fiberglass teeth.

Although the above concept and environment is certainly unique, application of some of the concepts and topics presented to these audiences could be applied by many dentists. A visit to this facility could be especially inspiring for the family or pediatric dentist.[6]

VIDEOS

Technology is slowly making its way into marketing the practice. That does not mean printed matter is going out of style! Printed collateral pieces are easy to use; they can be taken anywhere; they can be accessed and read without need of any electronic equipment. However, new forms of communication are affording the dental practice more opportunities to show patients the facility, introduce the team members, and educate the patient.

Leading the way in practice promotion is the "video brochure." This concept has been used in other fields, professions, and businesses for some time; however, it is relatively new in the area of promoting the dental practice.

Dr. Terry Daugherty, an orthodontist from Carrollton, TX produced a highly effective video brochure for prospective patients and referrals. The prospective patient who may be considering this practice, has the opportunity to see the office and the staff at work. A most impressive aspect of this video brochure is the inclusion of actual patients who discuss the excellent outcomes of their treatments, the impact on their lives, and their feelings about the practice team. Hearing and seeing patients who represent various demographics is a very powerful way to get your message across in a highly credible manner.

In addition, Dr. Daugherty speaks directly to the viewer about his philosophy of orthodontic treatment and his feelings about working with his patients. Most importantly for the patient, he addresses results and patient benefits.

In under ten minutes a prospective patient is able to gain an in-depth understanding of this practice and the benefits of orthodontics. The approach in the video is one of educating the prospective patient and answering typical questions rather than promoting treatments. However, the outcome of viewing the video is that it does promote treatment, and it does so in an educational, patient-friendly manner.

This type of promotional vehicle is particularly effective for the practice that may be offering long-term treatments such as orthodontics or those treatments that require significant financial investment. In focus groups, patients who commit to long-term treatment with a practice feel very strongly about selecting the appropriate office, practitioner, and staff. Consistently, these patients refer to the importance of being in sync and feeling a commonality with the practitioner. When they have an opportunity to view a video like this, it helps them understand the office in a way that cannot be communicated on paper. It is very important that the practitioner and team members who are going to be seen on this video communicate in a positive and warm way to the viewers. An understanding of behavioral styles and communication in general, will be extremely helpful in connecting with viewers and gaining treatment acceptance. (See chapters 14 and 15.)

At the same time, the practice that produces such a video will need to be aware of perceptions of professional fees by the viewing audience. Because this medium is a sophisticated form in which to promote a dental practice, some patients will perceive this as an indication that the practice or the treatments will be expensive. Consequently, it will be important that the video be appropriate to the widest demographic group that they hope to reach in terms of socioeconomics. If you wish to reach a wide audience, then make sure that that audience is represented in one way or another in the video. That representation could be via actual video tape of patient interviews, as in Dr. Daugherty's video or it could be in still photographs used throughout the video that represent patients of different ages and cultural groups. This visual message is far more powerful than any spoken or written words addressing the same subject. Bear in mind that patients feel most comfortable with a practitioner who is down to earth and they may well make decisions on that basis.

A practitioner who has used videotape to promote the practice in a different way is Dr. Mark Friedman of Encino, CA. Dr. Friedman is a nationally recognized practitioner in the area of aesthetic dentistry. He is also known for having developed a cutting edge office in the area of infection control.

Dr. Friedman has produced a video tape that introduces patients to the practice and educates patients as to safety practices in his office. Because the design of his office is so unique, this introductory video helps patients understand and value the office design and the procedures that ensure patient safety. The video shows patients the high tech treatment areas and sophisticated infection control environments which maintain the highest level of sterilization and patient safety possible. Patients are educated about the infection control procedures in this office. In addition, viewers are able to see Dr. Friedman treating a patient during a procedure.

The patient is shown wearing a headset and viewing a soothing, relaxation video. The underlying message to the viewer is, "You will be comfortable and at ease in this relaxing and safe environment." Although the video has been produced in order to help the patient understand the dental practice environment, the outcome is that patients realize they are in a truly unique practice. This is a twenty-first century office and after patients view the video they will understand the benefits to them personally. This piece is used with new patients; however, it could also be used in introducing the office to a prospective patient.

Dr. Friedman makes an extremely important point in relation to the use of a video, "In any collateral piece, whether it is a video tape or a brochure, the cover must be designed so that it is compelling. The patient has to *want* to know more." This is an extremely important point. If you are going to invest time, money, energy, and effort into the production of a video, you must make sure that patients will view it. The slip case of the video needs to grab the patient's attention. Also, Dr. Friedman suggests that the label on the video front and the video spine be attractively designed and include an attention-getting title. So often videos are separated from the covers and without an arresting label, this precious promotional piece can become anonymous to the patient.

Some final tips regarding video brochures:
- Keep it short! The shorter the better—under 10 minutes is an absolute must. Six to eight minutes is even better.
- Include patient testimony. Let patients hear other patients talking about your office and treatment. Be very judicious in your choice of patients and their abilities to communicate effectively.
- Create a title that is patient-centered and exciting.
- Create video cover labels that are visually attractive and enticing. If possible, use color and graphics.

A final caveat in relation to the production of a video tape like this: don't attempt to make this tape yourself! It will likely look "homemade" and patient perspectives may be that you tend to cut corners. If you're going to take on this project, do it right. As with Doctors Daugherty and Friedman, have the project done by a professional team that has created such demo tapes before. Take a look at the production company's work. Make sure they understand who you are and what you're really trying to say. You will be creating a piece which, once mailed or given to patients, may not be retrievable. It will live on after you and you need to be proud of it!

Also, this is not an inexpensive project. So it is crucial that the end result be one you can use for a long time, or that will result in enough new business to be cost effective. Make sure you are disseminating a quality product that accurately represents your practice, or *don't do it!*

OTHER PROMOTIONAL OPPORTUNITIES

The opportunities that you have to market your practice are endless. They could easily fill five books the size of this one. The purpose of this book is not to teach marketing concepts, but instead to provide insights into how patients feel about select issues discussed in focus groups. What follows are some of the concepts that have been raised in focus groups and the associated patient attitudes about them.

• **Advertising Specialties:** Patients like it when you provide "freebies." When offered as a gift to a patient, it helps the patient feel valued by the practice. Advertising specialties include any items imprinted with your name or practice information. These may include toothbrushes, pens, magnets, calendars, etc. The benefit to you of offering advertising specialties is the prospect of having your name in front of the patient on a consistent basis. If you are going to provide the patient with an advertising specialty, which is clever or cute, but ends up in a desk drawer, you are not investing your money wisely.

Patients have almost come to expect receipt of a toothbrush in conjunction with a hygiene visit. Make sure that you offer one that is imprinted with your name because patients do look at it daily. There are all types of toothbrushes available on the market today; some of them very high tech and highly engineered. If you want to add importance to this offering and increase patient perceptions of you as an educator, then don't just hand them the toothbrush. Give it some significance. Explain any special properties or benefits of its design that will aid in the patient's oral hygiene. If you offer several styles of toothbrushes, then make sure the patient knows you have selected a particular type of toothbrush just for him or her. This may seem a minor matter, but it is significant to a patient because you are doing something different. You are making what has always been an ordinary experience more important. You become more important in the process and you communicate a value of the patient. It is little actions like this when combined with others that create a fine edge and set you apart. What may seem insignificant to you may not be insignificant to your patient. I've only had this type of experience once. A hygienist, who was an excellent communicator and educator did this and I was extremely impressed. She increased my belief in her and in the practice as well.

Another office I visited had a number of attractively designed magnets laid out on the counter where patients paid their bills. Obviously these were for patients. However, it appeared that patients just helped themselves to these rather than being offered them. I wanted to see if this small token might be given significance.

While I was getting ready to write my check I picked up one of the magnets and made a point of studying it where the staff person could observe me. She said nothing. So I threw out a piece of "opportunity bait" to her saying, "These are really neat looking magnets." I had hoped that she might offer me one. No such luck. She responded with, "Yes, they are!" So I moved to the next level, "Can I have one?" "Of course," she countered. "They are for our patients." Again, this is a small matter. However, she could have helped me feel really good about this moment by making it special and helping me to feel more valued in the practice.

I would suggest that the magnets remain behind the counter and that each patient be offered one as a gift. If she had said something like, "We really appreciate you as a new patient in our practice family and we'd like you to have one of our magnets. You can put in on your refrigerator and you will always have our number handy. Also, I want you to know that our special emergency number is on here so you will always be able to reach us." What a difference in the way this would be received by the patient between the first scenario and the second. Now the patient is likely to feel more valued and cared for by the practice.

In another office when I was writing my check I saw a stack of coloring booklets. These could have been used for young patients waiting in reception. However, based on their placement, they were more likely given as a gift at the close of the appointment. I threw out a bit of "opportunity bait" to the staff member at the counter with, "My sister has small children who absolutely love to color. They come to my house and we end up with coloring books and crayons spread all over the living room floor." The staff member responded with, "Yeah, I've been there, I know how messy that can get."

Another opportunity lost. This could have been a connect with either my sister's family as possible patients, or an opportunity to communicate patient value and build relationship. She could have responded with, "Well, let me give you a few of these for your nieces or nephews. You could pass them on to them, or next time they come to your house, you can be ready for them!" What happened was she had applied the situation to herself and her own life instead of thinking, "Is there an opportunity here? How can I connect this patient's statement with marketing our practice?" The staff member could have even added, "Dr. Jones is absolutely wonderful with children. How old are your sister's kids?" Then this might have continued the discussion in a direction to effectively market the practice.

• **Gifts For Referring Patients:** Most of the time when I call an office to make a new-patient appointment I am asked a key question, "Whom may we thank for referring you to our office?" This is also a key message for the caller. It says that you value your existing patients and do want to thank them for the referral. For the aware caller, it indicates that you were smart enough to track your source of new patients. Once you know who the referring patient is a *thank you* is certainly appropriate, whether or not the individual makes an appointment. Patients like to be recognized for giving referrals to your office. Acknowledgment of this sort indicates that you recognize the patient's importance and that you value that patient.

Patients have mixed responses in focus groups as to what is an appropriate gift for a referral. Some say, "This is not necessary at all. Just give me a call and let me know that the referral is appreciated." Other patients value a gift. We've asked patients what is an appropriate gift. "Appropriate" has an extremely wide range. There did not seem to be any trend in what was considered "most appropriate" except for one concept. Almost all patients responded to the idea of a gift certificate. The most enthusiastic type of gift certificate was one that provided entertainment or pleasure, such as gift certificates to movies, video rentals, fast-food or regular restaurants. As I heard patients talk about this, it made a great deal of sense to me because the patient then associates a pleasurable time that was offered by the dental practice. On the other hand, some patients verged on being offended with the idea of a gift for a referral. This stated point-of-view was, "I don't feel comfortable accepting a gift for something that I feel was a simple act of kindness, passing the doctor's name on to a friend or family member." Patients who felt this way were often concerned about how the family member might interpret this. Would they think that it was a "bribe" of sorts?

Because of the wide range of responses to this concept, I suggest that each individual practice find out from your own client base what is appropriate in your community. This can be done most easily by a survey or focus group of your own patients. Ask them! Find out what *they* think is appropriate, then take their suggestions to heart. Whatever the outcome may be, know this: Whether you give a gift for a referral or not, your patients will always appreciate and respect a hand-written note from the doctor acknowledging the value of trust shown by the referring patient. For some patients this is enough and it is very meaningful when it comes from the doctor.

• **Patient Education Materials:** I have addressed the subject of patient education throughout this book. It is an exceedingly important subject in relation to patient perception of the value of your practice. It can also be an important form of marketing your practice.

I visited undercover the office of Dr. Norton Bicoll of Dallas, TX and inquired about the practice. Sheila was at the front desk. She not only introduced me to Dr. Bicoll, but on my departure, she gave me a couple of patient education sheets.

I learned later that these pieces are given to patients on a regular basis. They are created and duplicated in the office. Some have to do with regular oral healthcare, such as those I received. Others are given to patients following a treatment and inform the patient what to expect following the procedure as well as proper care following treatment. The pieces are not created as promotional pieces; they are to provide guidance and help to patients. But this is one of the ways that this office differs from others. It offers more; it cares for the patients beyond the appointment; and it continues to educate the patient.

This type of educational piece can be inexpensively produced and its message of patient value far exceeds the financial investment. Why not produce such a piece on a quarterly basis and have them available for every patient who comes into the office? It doesn't require postage and you are doing something unique that truly helps your patients.

- **Patient-Centered Events:** Consider having an open house or annual party for your patients and guests. This is a wonderful way to communicate patient value and to build a sense of family and community within your practice. It is also a great way to aid in building a cohesive team and communicating value of the team to the patients.

What type of event should you plan? I have seen and experienced many different types of get-togethers for patients. Sometimes they revolve around a significant date, such an anniversary of the practice. Other times it may be an informal barbecue or lawn party.

The Reisman Group of Dallas, TX, hosted a twentieth anniversary celebration for the practice. This open house was held in the office. It was conducted on a Friday afternoon and extended into the early evening hours. (Fig. 20-4) The event was catered with beautiful displays of food and fruit available throughout the office. Staff aided in hosting this function and guests included patients and friends of the practice, as well as colleagues. There was a clear sense of camaraderie felt among the entire group. This was not only a milestone celebration for the practice, but also was an opportunity to communicate to patients their value and significance within the practice family.

- **Patient Recognition:** I've been in numerous offices where bulletin boards are used to acknowledge and highlight patient activities and honors. These are extremely successful in many family practices where the practitioners treat a large percent of the children. Nothing delights a parent more than to see a photograph or an article, letter, or artwork from his or her child posted for the world to see. Even if one doesn't have a child, this is a message of a caring, warm practice family. Use of this type of marketing device must be congruent with the image of the practice.

Patients have talked about this in focus groups, particularly those who have school-aged children. This is very meaningful to these parents to know that the office team takes an interest in the personal lives of their young patients.

COME HELP US CELEBRATE OUR 20TH ANNIVERSARY
(1976-1996)

We couldn't have done it without you!

Friday, September 6

OPEN HOUSE   5-9 PM

RSVP by August 30th if you're coming

The Reisman Dental Group
Drs. Reisman, Roberts & Team

Medical City Dallas
7777 Forest Ln., Suite C-104
Dallas, TX 75230

Tel 661-4990
Fax 661-4993

Fig. 20-4   The Reisman Group celebrated its 20th anniversary with a patients open house. (Courtesy James Reisman, D.D.S., F.A.G.D.)

But recognize that adults are not exempt from favoring this type of promotion. An adult patient who has received public acknowledgment of an honor or an award appreciates your recognition of this and also likes to see it displayed.

• **Marketing The Team:** In a manner very similar to that listed above, patients enjoy knowing more about the team members who treat them. It helps the patient feel a part of "the family". Having a bulletin board or an area where there are informal pictures of team members is a powerful message to patients. It says, "We like each other, we respect each other, and we can have fun with each other." This is a message to patients that practitioners are people too, and want to be seen as such. The more we know about each other, the more we are able to build a relationship. Again, the use of this type of marketing device must be congruent with the practice.

THE A#1, SOLID GOLD, PULITZER PRIZE WINNING MARKETING "TOOL"

It's really no secret. Ask any patient. The very best marketing "tool" a dental practice can possibly have is an efficient, cohesive team with savvy people skills. When patients enter an office where the staff has strong belief in the practice, where the team members truly like and respect each other, and where they are knowledgeable and genuinely care about the patients, it's the biggest *WOW* any patient could hope for. Putting effort and energy into development of this kind of team is one of the best investments any practice can make.

Top Tips:

1. Never mail anything to a patient-of-record or to a prospective patient without some type of personalization or note. Use the patient's preferred name and sign it with your name. This is crucial, even if you're just jotting on a Post-it note and attaching it to a form or a pamphlet.

2. Recognize those patients who opt to look at patient education material in the reception area. This may be an indication of: a fairly high dental IQ, interest in particular treatments for the patient or a friend /family member.

3. Use educational pamphlets to educate the patient and market the treatment in a patient-friendly manner. Mail pamphlets on specific treatments to patients who inquire by phone. Be sure to follow up with a discussion and request for questions when the patient arrives for the next appointment.

4. Seek the opportunity. This can be fun!. Challenge yourself to seek out and act upon all opportunities in a *patient-friendly* manner. Often this crosses over to providing service and building relationships with patients; that is also an internal form of marketing the practice and a very important way to do so.

REFERENCES

[1] Mr. Lancellotti of Camelot Professional Services also offers his planning strategies in the audio album, "Successful Strategies for Winning Patients and Keeping Them Forever. . .Profitably," Camelot Professional Services, E. Brunswick, NJ, 1994.

[2] de St. Georges, Jennifer, "The Welcome Package: A Must For New Patients," *Dentistry Today*, February, 1992.

[3] Some of these concepts were provided by D. Wayne Blankinship of Custom On Hold Services, Inc. Of Bothell, WA (800) 950-8996. This is one of several such companies that takes a patient-friendly approach to soft marketing.

[4] I personally know that *anyone* can overcome this fear. I overcame an incapacitating fear of public speaking and found that not only do I love it, but it is a strength. Many community colleges offer courses on public speaking. Toastmaster's International has chapters in town and cities from coast to coast. For more personalized guidance, there are public speaking coaches who can offer one-on-one assistance in overcoming anxiety, crafting a speech, and gaining audience interest. For example, Karen Cortell Reisman, MS, is a public speaking coach and consultant from Dallas, TX, (972) 490-8676, who helped me overcome early anxieties. She assists dentists nationwide in developing and fine-tuning their skills. Additional information on overcoming anxiety and gaining confidence in public speaking is available in the audio, "Speak Out with Clout" through Suzanne Boswell Presentations, (972) 243-2086.

[5] Edwards addresses this topic very well and includes sample presentation outlines in his excellent book, *Marketing Professional Services,* by Frank Edwards, Ph.D., Louis Allen Associates, Inc., Louisville, KY. Additional presentation information may be found in the ADA booklet, "Winning Patients Through Powerful Presentations." This is available through ADA's catalog department.

[6] More information may be obtained by contacting the Dental Health Theater, 727 N. 1st Street, St. Louis, MO 63102; (314) 241-7391.

21

After the Appointment Is Over

"It just shows what can be done by taking a little trouble", said Eyeore.
"Do you see, Pooh? Do you see, Piglet? Brains first then hard work."

—From *WINNIE THE POOH* BY A. A. MILNE

What happens following patients' visits to your practice influences their perceptions of your practice, the likelihood of their sending referrals to you, their discussions about you with their friends and family, and whether they will return to your office. Some might say that once the patient has reached the Post Appointment phase their perceptions are set; you can no longer influence their thinking about your practice. Not so. The reality is that you are still in the position to improve relationships with the patient and increase positive perceptions of your practice based on your actions.

When it comes to retaining your patients you must be persistent, in a patient-friendly way. Building long-term relationships with patients does not happen by itself. It is a process that requires consistent investment on the part of the entire team. The cartoon character, Ziggy®, said, "The road to failure is actually the path of least persistence!" It takes persistence to maintain the relationships with your patients.

PATIENT'S EXPECTATIONS VERSUS REALITY

Before discussing the Post-Appointment *WOW'S*, let's look again at the process the patient has already been through. One must understand the patient's experiences to know what type of Post-Appointment contact will be effective.

As we've seen throughout the patient process, consistency and congruence is crucial to gaining and retaining patients. In chapter 9 on selecting a dentist, we investigated the many ways that patients first view a practice. In the Pre-Appointment phase we saw that patients are making judgments about the practice before they ever enter the office. So many criteria are influencing their perceptions of the practice and their expectations of what may happen to them as patients in the practice. If the office has done an admirable job in presenting itself positively to prospective patients, then these new patients will have high expectations. These expectations will be based on whatever form of initial contact was encountered by the patient and this could be by mail, by referral, by telephone contact, by print promotions.

Let's just say that you have on your front line a wonderful receptionist addressing prospective patient questions and calls. This person really knows how to present the practice in a positive and realistic manner. She helps callers feel comfortable and welcome. Therefore they approach the appointment positively with high expectations.

What happens during the Appointment phase is key. It is the responsibility of the entire team to maintain the same level of quality both clinically and non-clinically that may be expected by this patient. Take a look at your front desk and ask yourself this, "Do we fall below, meet, or exceed the expectations that might be experienced by patients based on the way the business team presents itself?"

If your response is, "Well, we're okay on the phone but we're really much better face-to-face," then you have a more significant problem than you may realize. If your front desk is not communicating in the most positive way possible, then chances are good that you are "walking" some patients. In other words, they may never get to the Appointment phase because they go elsewhere. You've lost an opportunity when it presented itself and you may not have another chance at it.

On the other hand, if you said, "We are really terrific on the phone. The phone receptionist is absolutely wonderful, warm, friendly, welcoming, knowledgeable. The rest of the team doesn't have quite the same level of proficiency as this front desk person." This is also a matter of serious concern. After all, the patient is entering the Appointment phase with very high expectations and patients do not like to be let down. They don't want to think, "This practice is not who they present themselves to be." The bottom line here: consistency is crucial. Be who you are, walk your talk. Make sure that there is congruence throughout the practice.

Incongruence can occur if the front and the back of the dental practice are not in sync. It is the inconsistency that is frustrating to patients. It is crucial that the entire team understand the significance of this. Those terms, "the front" and "the back" communicate a great deal. They are a physical division in the office between clinical and non-clinical areas. If those two terms also represent a difference in philosophy or approach with the patient, there is a major cause for concern.

Sometimes in talking with team members, I envision a Berlin Wall that divides the office. When a staff member says to patients things like, "Well, I happened to answer the phone, but I normally work 'in the back,'" a patient's confidence can be shaken. "The back' sounds like the hinterlands, a distant and perhaps, forbidding place! I often wonder if a foreign language is spoken there (and sometimes it is!) When calling for the doctor, I've been told on occasion, "I'll tell her you called the next time she comes to 'the front'." Compartmentalizing the office makes the practitioner seem very inaccessible, a negative perception for patients.

The feeling that the patient has throughout the appointment must equal or exceed the expectation in the pre-appointment phase. Your challenge is this, if you exceed patient expectations in one appointment, patients want consistency from then on. They will want that same level of quality service in their next appointment.

In focus groups, patients discuss the importance of consistency and they communicate an unsettled feeling when there is inconsistency. Patients sometimes refer to this using the word "unstable." If the patient feels unstable in the practice or if the practice is perceived to be unstable to the patient, it may give rise to feelings of dissatisfaction and the possibility of the patient grazing to another office.

The Post-Appointment phase is the point at which patients really consider their feelings about accepting treatment or returning to the office at all. This can occur in a very concrete way with new patients because they are consciously evaluating how they feel about the office and how they feel about their decision to come to this office.

With the long-term patient-of-record, this decision-making process may not be as concrete or as quickly decisive.

Frequently it is a specific incident that may prompt the patient-of-record to evaluate his/her feelings and standing with the practice. Sometimes a gnawing discontent is tolerated until a specific event occurs that spurs action. Like the proverbial "straw that broke the camel's back," it could be a problem with billing or insurance or a team member who comes across in an abrupt manner, or a perceived lack of appreciation for the patient.

In situations like these, if the patient is presented with the possibility of a managed plan, this patient is at risk for leaving the fee-for-service practice or moving to another provider on their list. A strong, positive relationship has not been maintained and the patient does not feel valued by the practice. As many patients have commented in focus groups, "If I'm not getting the service that I'm paying for here, then why *not* go someplace else?"

In my seminars, I am frequently asked questions about gaining new patients. This is a major issue for dental practices today. But sometimes I feel a greater interest and concern from practices about getting bodies in the front door when there might be more emphasis placed on retaining the patients that the practice already has.

LIKELIHOOD OF REFERRALS AFTER THE APPOINTMENT

It's important to consider why patients refer friends, family, and colleagues to their practitioners. They refer when they are confident in the practitioner, when they see the practice as one that is well-run, when the patient is appreciated, and when they are proud of the practice and their affiliation with it.

If new patients make judgments about the office on their own and not by a referral, their perception may be based on just one visit. If it's a wonderful visit, if they are treated well, and if they perceive the practitioners to be caring, professional in demeanor, and expert, they may refer. If they had a difficult time during the visit, if anything during the Appointment phase has rattled their confidence, then they're not likely to refer. All of this seems rather obvious.

However, there is another factor that comes into play in evaluating the likelihood of referrals from new patients. This factor occurs when the patient is a referred patient. That is, if they received your name with high marks from a friend or family member, their expectations may be higher than if they had no prior information about you. This is the patient who is typically going to enter the office *expecting* good things—expecting to feel positive about the experience. Even if the expectation is considered only "acceptable," the likelihood of them giving referrals is still greater than the patient who came in off the street or from a promotional piece.

That patient who enters your office and has already had a positive referred introduction is more likely to be a long-term patient or to be a patient who refers to your practice. I was conducting a focus group with 10 baby boomers from a metropolitan area. Two of the patients in this group had the same dentist. These individuals were not seated next to each other and I hadn't noticed anything prior to the session that indicated they knew each other. During the session, when I asked the group to tell me what they really liked about their dental offices, both of these patients gave rave reviews to the practitioner and the team. Their trust level was exceedingly high. I asked them if they knew each other and they laughed. Sally said, "Well Arlene has gone to Dr. X for 27 years and she gave me his name 18 years ago. I've gone to him ever since." I asked Sally, "Have your referred Dr. X to anyone?" She indicated that she had referred the doctor to one family member and one friend both of whom remain patients of this practice. Here was an individual whose practitioner developed a relationship that resulted in long-term relationships with referred patients. Satisfied patients tend to breed satisfied patients.

I asked Arlene, the "original" patient, why she remained with this doctor when she had moved twice and she now had to go out of her way to reach the doctor's office. She responded, "I trust him. He's like family now." Sally was a teacher at a junior high school and she noted that this practice also took into account the needs of the patients. She noted: "He has office hours that can accommodate teachers. Not everybody can just take off in the middle of the day. Also, he has called me on a couple of occasions after hours when I had a difficult time with a toothache and with a crown. One time I had an emergency and he met me at the office that night. His wife came with him to the office and he introduced me to her in a way that made me feel important in his practice."

Here's where the long-term patient of record looks at your track record. How has your office been over the long haul? Are you consistent? Do you genuinely care? Or was the patient "courted" in the beginning and then the relationship trailed off to where the patient felt taken for granted. If a patient-of-record ever gets to the point where he/she feels taken for granted of if he/she feels "like a number" (patients do use this term in focus groups) you can certainly forget gaining referrals from them and the chances increase that he/she is at risk of leaving your practice.

Every day, every moment with your patients is an opportunity to maintain and build positive relationships. This continuing process is what is going to gain you referrals, gain treatment acceptance, and aid in patient retention.

POST-APPOINTMENT "*WOWS*"

Here are some concepts to consider that can positively influence patients following appointments. Bear in mind that the most important issue in all of these, the foundation of any Post Appointment message should be, "You are valued by this practice." When this message goes out to patients and they are not expecting it, when you are doing something extraordinary and not following rote protocol, that's when patients respond, "WOW!" The list that follows is a short one. Its purpose is to generate ideas within the entire team. This is a starting place for you to say, "What can *we* do for *our* patients that will differentiate us and communicate to patients that we truly appreciate them?" This is the fine edge of added value that makes a significant difference and can help to keep patients in your practice.

• Phone call after a difficult treatment: Without a doubt, this is one of the most powerful messages you can send to your patients. I'm frequently asked by seminar attendees, "Does it matter if the call comes from the doctor or from a team member?" Here's what patients say, "I couldn't believe it. *The doctor* called me that night after the surgery!" Yes, it is meaningful to get a call from a staff member, but the hard-core reality is that it is most meaningful to the patient when it is the doctor who takes the time to do this. Patients perceive that the doctor is important, and now the table is turning and the doctor is saying to the patient, "*You* are important!" This is not forgotten.

• Personal notes to patient: A handwritten note from the doctor or team member regarding an accomplishment of the patient. The note is most appreciated when it comes directly from the doctor. I doesn't have to be long. It could be a couple of sentences, but a handwritten note is extremely impressive to patients. Let them know that you recognize their accomplishments or their honors—or empathize with their difficulties or losses, as in a death in the family. This indicates an awareness and a sensitivity to the patients.

• Thank you's for referrals: This is a given. Patients want and appreciate recognition of referring patients to the office. Gifts are valued by patients from the practice. However, most important is that the acknowledgment is sincere. Yes, a phone call from the office thanking the patient for a referral is valued but not nearly as much as a handwritten note that includes a promise to fulfill the responsibility and trust placed in the practice by the referring patient.

• Patient anniversaries: When was the last time that you thanked your long-term patients of record for being a member of your practice family? What about those patients who have been with your practice for 10, 15, 20 years? Have you verbalized your appreciation and acknowledgment to them? This is crucial today. Acknowledge their tenure with your office the next time these patients come in for an appointment. But if you really want to WOW them, develop a method of tracking these patients and send them a *personalized* letter or memento on their landmark anniversaries with your practice. Consider sending a couple of movie passes with it. They will associate a pleasant experience with you. You can be sure that patients will remember this and value you more for valuing them!

Note: This "anniversary" approach is more unusual than a birthday card. Some patients in focus groups have said things like, "Hey, the office can just spit out the birthdays from the computer. I also get a card from my car salesman and my insurance salesman."

With the birthday card your goal is to say the patient is important. With the anniversary card you're saying the patient *and* the relationship with the patient are important. It's a stronger message and one patients are not expecting! They probably won't miss getting a birthday card from you; they'll be "WOWed" by getting an anniversary card from you!

• The "night before" call: When you have a patient who is going to experience a difficult procedure or a patient who is typically anxious or fearful, consider calling the patient the night before the treatment. A patient in a focus group brought this up. She indicated that she was going to have what she feared to be a "long, grueling, and painful treatment." She was very nervous about this and her concern was made even greater because she was a fairly new patient in this practice. She had been to the doctor's office only three times prior to the upcoming treatment. She said, "I couldn't believe it, this doctor called me the night before this procedure. He knew that I was very nervous because I'd made a couple of calls and asked questions of the staff. He phoned and explained what to expect the next morning. He told me that he would walk me through the process and he explained how patients typically feel. I felt like this doctor really cared and understood."

This was a very positive action and earned enthusiastic responses from the rest of the group; they indicated they'd never heard of a doctor doing this before. The group was "WOWed" over this. It is a powerful statement.

• Publication clippings: As you read publications, if you find an article that may be of interest to a patient tear it out and send it with a one line note from you. This is a remarkable statement to a patient because it's underlying message it, "I see you as a person, not just as a patient and I recognize your value as a person, not just as a patient."

• Appropriate apology: If a patient has been kept waiting, if a patient has had a difficult time, if the office has made an error, if the patient communicates dissatisfaction and with good reason, make an apology. Send them a note after the appointment, give them a percentage discount on an upcoming treatment or cleaning or send them a gift certificate or movie pass. The fact that it even occurred to you to do this and to acknowledge the situation will raise their estimation of you. Patients who experience this often turn out to be your biggest fans, and speak glowingly of you to others!

These are but a few of the ideas that you could implement in your practice to continue to communicate positively to your patients after the appointment and on a continuing basis. Brainstorm with your staff about specifics that are unique to your office and unique to your demographics—that will enable you to build and maintain relationships with your patients.

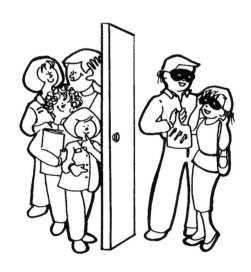

MY PERSONAL MESSAGE TO YOU

In my work with dental practices nationwide and in presenting to dental profession audiences across the United States and Canada, I have found that dental teams are a very special group of people. You are truly caring, compassionate professionals with a lot of heart. My view of the profession is confirmed by the sentiments of most patients we interview in focus groups.

At the close of each focus group we conduct, I pose to the participants, "If you could offer one suggestion to practitioners, what would that be?" Their responses vary based on their own experiences, and the most common offerings are referenced in the following chapter. But I would like to mention one that I hear from patients and I sense myself from many practitioners—a need to lighten up! I've seen you loosen up in my seminars and it's important for you to know that your patients want to see that side of you too! They *do* want you to take your profession seriously, but not yourself *too* seriously!

You do have to manage stress every day in the profession and a significant part of that stress is people-related. Every day you're juggling the challenges of dealing with so many different kinds of people and situations. Whether it's patients, peers, practitioners, friends, family, or foes a little "lightening up along the way" can help you get through the day with greater satisfaction for all. Yes, you've got to remain on your toes and balance your challenges as well, but I believe they can be managed when we put it all in perspective.

The writing of Theodor S. Geisel, more well known as Dr. Seuss, has offered me perspective on many issues throughout my life. Packed in his "simple" books are valuable insights that can help all of us. Although I didn't know him personally, in his passing I felt I lost a friend and an advisor. Fortunately his wonderful work remains to provide wise guidance in a delightful and welcome way. In his last work, *Oh, The Places You'll Go*, Dr. Seuss offers a common sense approach to people and life. This is a message that the child in all of us can learn from:

> You'll get mixed up, of course,
> as you already know.
> You'll get mixed up
> with many strange birds as you go.
> So be sure when you step.
> Step with care and great tact
> and remember that Life's
> a Great Balancing Act.
> Just never forget to be dexterous and deft.
> And *never* mix up your right foot with your left.

REFERENCES

[1]Geisel, Theodor S. and Geisel, Audrey S. *Oh, The Places You'll Go*, Random House, New York, NY, 1990.

22

Twenty-Two Top Tips and Topics From Patient Focus Groups

"It is better to know some of the questions than all of the answers."

—JAMES THURBER

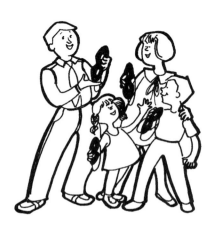

1he following are the top items that patients are concerned about and are interested in talking about in focus groups. At the close of each focus group we ask patients to tell us what message they want to send to dentists. The following issues are raised consistently by patients from all demographics. They deserve special attention by the entire team to encourage and increase likelihood of patient retention and treatment acceptance.

Chapters are referenced for insights into each area. Chapters that affect or influence the topic are listed and the primary chapter addressing the subject is in bold face type. Tips are listed in random order.

1. See The Patient As a Person. View the patient as a person first, rather than a "case". Patients respond to the team that recognizes individuality and uniqueness of patients, knows something about the patient and communicates interest in the patient's family, work or hobbies. This helps to build a strong bond and strengthens relationships with patients.
(Chapters 1, 2, 7, 9, 10, 11, 14, **15**, 18, 19)

2. Remain "In the Moment." When you are *with* the patient, *be* with the patient! Focus on patients during your brief time with them. Perception of how much you really care about the patient is manifested through your attentiveness to the patient verbally and nonverbally. Remember that the patient's "window of time" with you is very small; how you relate to the patient during the appointment is how patients perceive you to be all the time.
(Chapters 3, 7, 9, 11, **14**, 15, 16, 17, 18)

3. Pleasant and Comforting Decor. Create an environment within which the patient will feel comfortable, safe, and nurtured. Recognize that patients are making judgments about the cleanliness, sterility, safety, and professionalism of the practice in a large part based on the physical appearance of patient areas including reception, rest room, and treatment areas. Decor carries very special significance if the office promotes aesthetic treatments. Attend to the amenities that increase patient comfort and acknowledge an appreciation for the patient.

(Chapters 4, 6, **12**, 13)

4. Impeccably Groomed Team. This is extremely important to patients of all demographics. They judge office cleanliness and their own personal safety in the office partially based on the grooming and physical appearance of the team. Like decor, this area is especially important in an office promoting aesthetic treatments. Patients state that the appearance of each team member represents what is acceptable to the practitioner and may reflect on the clinical skills and quality of the practitioner.

(Chapters 13, **14**, 17, 18)

5. Value of Patient Education. This issue is important only if you want to retain your present patient base and gain referrals! The entire team must be involved in active patient education. Patients consistently describe the "ideal" dentist as being a good "teacher."

(Chapters 1, 3, 5, 8, 9, 10, 11, 13, 15, 19, **20**)

6. Communication and Patient Education on Infection Control. A misconception in the profession of dentistry today is that patients are not concerned to any significant degree about patient perceptions of infection control. They *are* concerned; they're just not talking about it! Patients say that they want the dental practice to bring up the issue first. Ensure that *all* new patients are educated about your infection control measures.

(Chapters 4, 6, 8, 9, 10, 11, **13**, 16, 17)

7. Offer Options, Alternatives and Prioritize Treatments. Make it easier for patients to accept treatment: give the patient choices and offer the

pros and cons of each. Patients say they want a part in determining the most viable treatment(s) for them. The concept of codiagnosis is favored by patients today.
(Chapters 3, 5, 7, 8, 15, 16, **19**)

8. Explain Procedures Before Treatment.

One of the reasons patients move away from a practice is that the practitioner did not advise the patient what to expect before and during treatment. Patients highly resent this and they indicate that their anxiety rises in relation to continuing with the practice that does not adequately prepare the patient, verbally and nonverbally, for treatment.
(Chapters 3, 8, 15, **16**, 17)

9. Patient Control During Treatment.

Patients respond positively to the practitioner who affords them a sense of control during the treatment. Doctors who communicate caringly and indicate how the patient can feel some control during the treatment process get high marks from patients. This is especially meaningful for those patients who indicate fear or anxiety in relation to procedures.
(Chapters 7, 15, **16**)

10. Painless Injection. *Every* patient wants this

and every patient remembers those offices that increased their anxiety in relation to this. Give a painless injection and the world will beat a path to your doorstep!
(Chapters 5, **16**)

11. Being Up-To-Date: CE-Treatments-

Equipment. Patients describe the ideal office is one that is "up to date." Most powerful in the patient's mind is being current in continuing education and in quality of technology used.
(Chapters 3, 6, 7, **9**, 10, 11 16, 17, 20)

12. Cohesive Team: Sense of Family. This is a

significant factor to most patients. There is a sense of security that comes from familiarity with the team and a sense of caring that comes via that familiarity. Staff continuity is a major subset of this topic; patients like to see the same friendly faces on each visit. This communicates a stability in the office and reflects positively on the practitioner(s).

(Chapters 1, 2, 3, 4, 5, 7, 9, 14, 15, 16, 17, **18**)

13. Rapid Response in Emergencies. This is a *must* for your patients of record. If they can't rely on you in an emergency, particularly when there is pain, then they are likely to leave your practice. Patients speak glowingly about the offices that helped them in time of need and this frequently leads to referrals.

(Chapters 3, 4, 5, 9, **11**, 16, **17**, 20)

14. Communicate Patient Appreciation. An absolute *must* today. Your patients must hear you state your appreciation for them, whether they are new patients or patients of record. If you don't *sincerely* communicate appreciation for the patient, you increase the likelihood of their leaving your practice.

(Chapters 3, 5, 9, 11, **17, 20**)

15. Patients Appreciate Active Listeners. Patients equate active listening with caring. Active listening means being *in the moment*, responding to patients' needs and concerns, and taking seriously their questions. This is rare today and is universally highly valued by patients.

(Chapters 3, 5, 7, **9**, 11, **14, 15**, 16, 17)

16. Explain Fees and Offer Payment Plans. A patient may be very satisfied with your practice, but if there is a serious misunderstanding on fees or insurance, it may be reason enough for them to seek another office. Explain thoroughly and privately what patients need to know about fees, and give a *written* treatment plan to ensure comprehension. Patients appreciate it when the staff helps them understand details of payment plans or features of their insurance coverage. Frequent complaints about high fees may be an indication that the practice is not adequately educating the patient or is not effectively developing value for the treatment and the practice.

(Chapters 3, 5, 8, 9, 11, 17, **19**)

17. TLC Call. Patients consistently state that the practitioner who calls them after a difficult treatment is a very caring caregiver. This is very significant to patients and increases the feelings of mutual appreciation. This can also lead to patient referrals.

(Chapters 5, 7, 9, **11**, 17, 20)

18. Varied and Convenient Hours. Patients say that the caring office has hours that accommodate the range of patient needs. Having some extended hours and some Saturday hours can increase your referrals and increase the likelihood of patients remaining in your practice. Having varied hours communicates an awareness of the patient's time frames.

(Chapters 1, 5, **9**, 11, 17, 20)

19. Be On Time. Patients consider 15 minutes past their time slot as the longest acceptable waiting time. If your office *consistently* keeps patients waiting, you are at risk for patients moving away to other offices.

(Chapters 3, 5, 7, **9**, 11, 17, 20)

20. Appointment Availability. Patients say that if it is the "first time" appointment to a dental practice, they would like to have an appointment within two weeks. If it is an appointment for a patient-of-record, they want the appointment within three weeks, but would find 30 days acceptable. If the office is consistently booked more than 30 days out, this can be discouraging to a patient and may result in their looking elsewhere for an office that can meet their needs more readily.

(Chapters 3, 5, **9**, 11, 17, 20)

21. Accessibility and Safety. The more difficult it is to visit your office, the easier you make it for your patient to find another more accessible practice. Parking, traffic, and safety are all issues of importance to patients. Wheelchair accessibility, both inside and outside of the office, is also crucial and is becoming even more so.

(Chapters 1, 3, **4**, 6, 9, 17, 20)

    22. Loosen Up! This is a message frequently voiced by patients! They state they would feel more at ease in the office if the practitioner were more at ease, not lax, but friendlier and more personable. When the dentist loosens up a bit, it helps the patient to loosen up too! (Chapters 2, 4, 5, 7, 9, 11, **14**, 15, 16, 17, 18)

> *"No technology, no drugs, no power over the patients takes the place of caring."*[1]

CARPE DIEM !

References

[1] Moyers, Bill. *Healing and the Mind*, Doubleday, New York, NY, 1993.

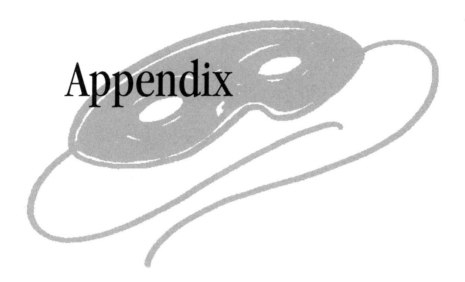

Appendix

WRITTEN SURVEY STATISTICS

PATIENT SURVEY OF 1993-1994, CONDUCTED BY SUZANNE BOSWELL PRESENTATIONS, DALLAS, TX

236 Respondents   Gender: 52% Female, 48% Male
Residence: 70% Texas, 30% Nationwide
Age: 17-24:   2%
        25-35:   12%
        36-50:   48%
        51-65:   36%
        66 and up: 3%

Respondents had received treatment in the following offices within the preceding 10 years:

General dentist: 98.5%
Orthodontist: 7.2%
Periodontist: 5.0%
Endodontist: 3.5%
Other: 1.5%

Respondent employment:

Professional, Executive, Business owner: 18.0%
Management: 31.0%
Sales: 15.5%
Blue collar/manual labor: 12.0%
Clerical/hourly: 8.0%
Students: 4.8%
Retired: 3.2%
No answer: 1.5%
Other: 6.0%

Dentist survey of 1994, conducted by
Suzanne Boswell Presentations, Dallas, TX

197 Respondents   Practice Location: 100% Texas offices

Gender: 32% Female,   68% Male

Number of years in practice: Ranged from 1-45 years.
Average: 14.5 years

Type of practice:

General dentistry: 85.0%

Orthodontics: 7.0%

Periodontics: 2.5%

Pedodontics: 2.0%

Prosthodontics: 0.6%

Endodontics: 0.6%

Other: 2.3%

Number of dentists in the practice:

1:                        68.0%

2-3:   29.5%

4 or more: 1.5%

No answer: 1.0%

*Multiple responses accepted. Percentages do not equal 100%.

**This percentage includes parents of dependent children who were patients in an orthodontic office.

/

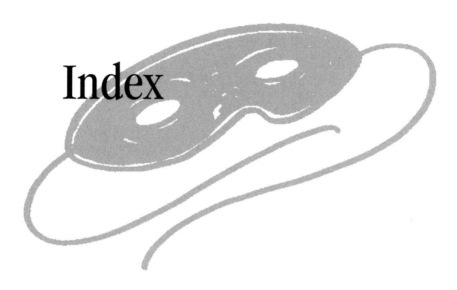

Index

A

Active listening, 187-188

Advertising, 439-445, 469-471: yellow page/magazine, 443-445; specialty items, 469-471

Advice on doctor selection, 124-129

After appointment, 479-492: patient expectations vs. reality, 480-483; potential referrals, 483-486; post-appointment services, 486-489; message to practitioners, 490-491

After hours calls, 201-204

Aging society, 1-13: older patients, 2-3; baby boomers, 3-5; influentials group, 5-6; respect and aging, 6-9; changing values, 9-10; patient survey/focus group comments, 10-11; tips, 11-12

Alternative treatments, 77-91: SEE ALSO Mind-body connect

B

C

D

G

H

High tech/high touch practice, 138-145
Hypnosis and biofeedback, 86-87

I

Immersion (patient), 384-387, 390-395: example, 390-393;
    and behavior modification, 394-395
Impression (management/self-presentation), 111-500: patient
    perceptions, 115-117; patient perspectives, 118-119; new
    patient vs. patient of record, 118-119; obstacles/
    opportunities, 119. SEE ALSO individual chapter topics.
Infection control (patient concerns), 253-254
Influentials group, 5-6
Informed consent, 95-106. SEE ALSO Patient rights.
Internal vs. external marketing, 438-439
Interruption or opportunity (telephone call), 174-175

L

Language in practice, 15-20
Layout/design (office), 158-160: patient likes, 158-159; patient
    dislikes, 159-160
Lighting (office), 220
Little things (patient's viewpoint), 354-355

M

P

T

U

V

W

Y